Veterinary
Endosurgery

VETERINARY ENDOSURGERY

Lynetta J. Freeman, DVM, MS, Dipl ACVS
Research Fellow, Surgical Research and Development
Ethicon Endo-Surgery Inc.
Cincinnati, Ohio

*with 375 illustrations
including 32 color plates*

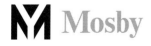

St. Louis Baltimore Boston Carlsbad Chicago Naples New York Philadelphia Portland
London Madrid Mexico City Singapore Sydney Tokyo Toronto Wiesbaden

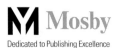

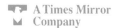

Publisher: John A. Schrefer
Executive Editor: Linda L. Duncan
Senior Developmental Editor: Teri Merchant
Project Manager: Mark Spann
Senior Production Editor: Anne Salmo
Composition Specialist: Julie Janis
Book Design Manager: Judi Lang
Manufacturing Manager: Betty Mueller

A NOTE TO THE READER: The views represented in this book should not be attributed to Ethicon-Endosurgery, Inc., its affiliated companies, or its customers.

Composition by Mosby Electronic Production
Lithography/color film by Top Graphics
Printing/binding by Maple-Vail Book Mfg Group

Mosby, Inc.
11830 Westline Industrial Drive
St. Louis, Missouri 63146

Library of Congress Cataloging in Publication Data
Veterinary endosurgery / [edited by] Lynetta J. Freeman.
     p.   cm.
    Includes bibliographical references and index.
    ISBN 0-8151-3321-9
    1. Veterinary endoscopic surgery.   I. Freeman, Lynetta J.
SF914.2.V48   1998
636.089'705—dc21
                                                 98-25971
                                                     CIP

99 00 01 02 03 / 9 8 7 6 5 4 3 2 1

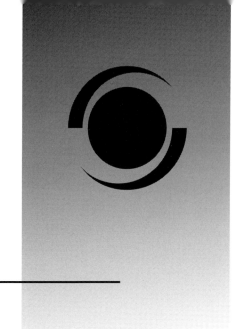

CONTRIBUTORS

James E. Bailey, DVM, MS, Dipl ACVA
Assistant Professor
Department of Large Animal Clinical Sciences
College of Veterinary Medicine
University of Florida
Gainesville, Florida

Robert A. Cook, VMD
Chief Veterinarian and Director
Wildlife Health Sciences
NYZS The Wildlife Conservation Society
Bronx, New York

Lynetta J. Freeman, DVM, MS, Dipl ACVS
Research Fellow, Surgical R&D
Ethicon Endo-Surgery, Inc.
Cincinnati, Ohio

Dean A. Hendrickson, DVM, MS, Dipl ACVS
Assistant Professor
Department of Clinical Sciences
Veterinary Teaching Hospital
Colorado State University
Fort Collins, Colorado

Ronald J. Kolata, DVM, MS, Dipl ACVS
Research Fellow Surgical R&D
Ethicon Endo-Surgery, Inc.
Cincinnati, Ohio

Timothy C. McCarthy, DVM, PhD, Dipl ACVS
Surgical Specialty Clinic
Beaverton, Oregon

Luisito S. Pablo, DVM, MS, Dipl ACVA
Assistant Professor
Department of Large Animal Clinical Sciences
College of Veterinary Medicine
University of Florida
Gainesville, Florida

Laura Potter, DVM, MS
Principal Scientist Surgical R&D
Ethicon Endo-Surgery, Inc.
Cincinnati, Ohio

Ray G. Rudd, DVM, MS, Dipl ACVS
Braelinn Village Animal Hospital
Peachtree City, Georgia

David R. Stoloff, DVM, MS, Dipl ACVS
Research Fellow
Ethicon, Inc.
Somerville, New Jersey

Suzanne E. Thompson, DVM, MS, Dipl ACVS
Principal Scientist Surgical R&D
Ethicon Endo-Surgery, Inc.
Cincinnati, Ohio

Steven Trostle, DVM, MS, Dipl ACVS
Assistant Clinical Professor
Head, Department of Surgical Services
Department of Surgical Science
University of Wisconsin—VMTH
Madison, Wisconsin

To my teachers

FOREWORD

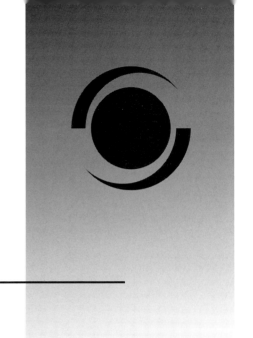

The primary objective of surgery is restoration of structure and function. In all surgery, and especially when working with injured or devitalized tissue, surgeons must make every effort not to inflict additional damage that might interfere with the healing process. As J.H. Bradshaw pointed out 70 years ago, gentleness is the key:[1]

> Now the welfare of the patient is our first consideration, not the welfare of our pockets, or our fame as an operator. In order to best conserve that welfare in our surgical work, we must always keep in mind that every wound . . . is like a sensitive plant. It responds to gentle treatment and resents brutality. It is, moreover, in our own interest to be gentle, for we shall find that we get full compensation for value received: our wounds will heal better, our results will be better, our reputations will be better, and we shall have better satisfaction with ourselves and our work.

The minimally invasive approach of endoscopic surgery, which is still in its infancy, is a major advance in the cause of gentle surgery. This book, written by pioneers in veterinary endoscopic surgery, is a significant contribution to that cause. Detailed descriptions of basic principles and specific procedures, with a generous supply of illustrations, provide guidance and encouragement to inexperienced endoscopic surgeons. Adequate warning is given when a procedure requires well-developed skills, while hints of procedures yet to be perfected keep this rapidly expanding field in responsible perspective.

The authors acknowledge that many of the instruments now in use will eventually become obsolete, but the surgical principles behind them will endure. As the benefits of minimally invasive surgery become more widely known and appreciated, veterinary laparoscopic, thoracoscopic, and arthroscopic surgery are bound to become more widely practiced. I am confident that this book will play an important role in helping that happen.

Ghery D. Pettit, DVM
Pullman, Washington

---

[1]Bradshaw JH: The gentle touch in surgery. *Surg Gyn Obstet* 45:840, 1927.

PREFACE

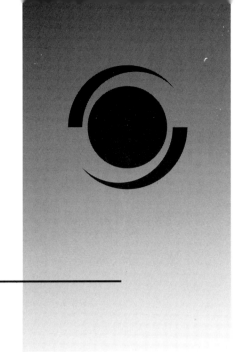

Minimally invasive surgery is a collective term for surgical techniques designed to minimize the extent of an anatomic approach while maintaining precision and efficiency. In humans, minimally invasive techniques began with laparoscopic cholecystectomy in 1988 and grew to nearly 500,000 procedures performed in 1993. General surgeons now consider it possible to use minimally invasive techniques for nearly all conventional open procedures.

Minimally invasive surgery was made possible through an extensive collaboration between physicians and industry in developing the tools and technology that enabled the procedures to be performed safely. Many of the authors of this text have participated in this effort by developing new instrumentation and validating the feasibility of the procedures in preclinical studies in animals. Whenever possible, the authors have indicated the feasibility and advisability of performing these procedures in a veterinary clinical setting. Because many of the techniques have not been applied in a clinical setting, dramatic patient benefits seen in human surgery have not been validated in animals. The authors have chosen to present the data in a concise manner, confident that wise veterinary surgeons, researchers, and clinicians will be able to apply this knowledge to safely and appropriately propagate veterinary minimally invasive surgery.

Most minimally invasive procedures in veterinary medicine are technically feasible and may be accepted as standard practice in the future. Except for arthroscopy, minimally invasive procedures have been performed infrequently in animals. Clinical studies that compare open and minimally invasive approaches are difficult to perform because of the need for special equipment and the technical difficulty of the procedures, making surgeons less willing to attempt them. An experienced operative team must be developed. Just as in human surgery, obtaining the necessary knowledge and skills is challenging. High-quality postgraduate courses to teach the techniques are critical.

Clinicians continue to explore whether procedures can be justified based on economic parameters in human surgery. Except in a few instances, veterinarians lack the benefits of having a third-party payer. To have the proper equipment to quickly and efficiently perform most procedures requires a considerable initial financial investment. The cost-effectiveness of minimally invasive procedures has not been and may not be demonstrated in animals.

Some minimally invasive techniques are unlikely to be performed in a clinical setting in animals in the foreseeable future. Yet, techniques are constantly evolving. Minimally invasive spinal surgery, plastic and reconstructive procedures, and cardiovascular procedures are examples of applications performed in humans that will probably not see wide adoption in veterinary medicine; therefore, we have chosen not to discuss them in this text.

The benefits of minimally invasive approaches are documented in human surgery. Undoubtedly, many of these benefits will apply to animals. This text is intended to aid investigators in identifying the place of minimally invasive surgery in veterinary medicine. Thank you for giving us the opportunity to share our experiences.

Lynetta J. Freeman
March 20, 1998
Cincinnati, Ohio

ACKNOWLEDGMENTS

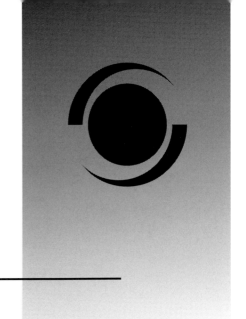

The authors would like to thank Ethicon Endo-Surgery and Ethicon, Inc. for giving us the opportunity to participate in the minimally invasive surgical revolution. These companies forged a vision for the future and promoted the judicious use of animals in conducting the preclinical studies necessary to demonstrate the functionality of products before their release for human clinical work. Recognizing the potential value of these techniques to minimize pain and morbidity in animals, they have allowed us to publish the results of our work.

The medical illustrator, Felecia Paras, deserves special recognition for taking our videotapes and hand-drawn "stick-figures" and creating such wonderful illustrations.

Dr. Ghery D. Pettit applied his knowledge, his pencil, and his sense of humor in revising each chapter to ensure accuracy and consistent style and syntax. Using his experience as a veterinary surgeon, Dr. Pettit challenged us to clarify what procedures are feasible and what procedures are rational.

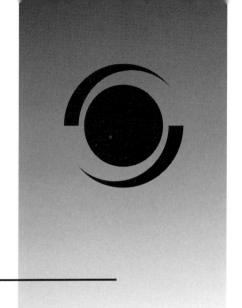

INTRODUCTION

Endoscopic surgery is a minimally invasive surgical approach in which visibility is provided by endoscopes. Endoscopic surgery is also referred to as *laparoscopic, celioscopic,* or *pelviscopic surgery* if procedures involve an approach to the abdomen, and *thoracoscopic, pleuroscopic,* or *video-assisted thoracoscopic surgery (VATS)* if procedures involve an approach to the thorax. The optic device used for viewing the body cavity is referred to as a *laparoscope, thoracoscope, arthroscope,* or *cystoscope,* named for viewing the abdomen, thorax, joints, and bladder, respectively.

Surgical procedures are performed through numerous small-diameter openings. These openings are made with the trocar, which typically includes an obturator and cannula. The obturator is the piercing element that punctures the body to make the opening. Once the puncture is made, the obturator is withdrawn from the cannula. The cannula then provides a small-diameter passageway into and through the body wall to provide access for additional surgical instrumentation to the surgical site.

In laparoscopic surgery, the optical cavity is usually created and maintained by insufflation with carbon dioxide (CO_2). During thoracoscopic surgery, exposure is obtained by low-pressure insufflation of the thorax with CO_2 or by one-lung ventilation. The adverse effects of these maneuvers must be weighed against the advantages of less traumatic exposure of the surgical site. In arthroscopic surgery, effects of the distention media on articular cartilage must be considered.

The fundamental advantage of minimally invasive procedures over open procedures in humans is reduced postoperative morbidity, resulting in less postoperative pain and perioperative morbidity, and shorter hospital stay and convalescence. The benefits of less invasive approaches are now validated in human surgery by procedure adoption rates. Laparoscopic cholecystectomy has been established as the gold standard for the surgical treatment of gallbladder disease. Diagnostic laparoscopy is commonly used to stage for malignancy. Benign diseases of the colon are approached laparoscopically. Laparoscopic appendectomy, antireflux surgery, adhesiolysis, small-bowel resection, hernia repair, splenectomy, lymphadenectomy, and liver biopsy are performed routinely in human surgery.

The physiologic responses that account for the improved clinical outcome have been studied extensively. The open surgical incision is accurate and fast, and exposes the operative site, but, unfortunately, it does so at the expense of tissue trauma. Surgical trauma initiates a stress response, which causes hypermetabolism, increased myocardial oxygen demand, increased pulmonary workload, increased renal workload, impaired bowel motility, and impaired immune function.[1] The biologic response to surgery depends on how severe the injury is relative to the animal's ability to recover.

The hypermetabolic stress response is the dominant physiologic response to injury in humans.[2] The severity and duration of the stress response is related to the severity of tissue injury.[1]

Catabolism begins with the skin incision and lasts 24 to 48 hours for a major abdominal operation. During catabolism, fat is oxidized and protein is broken down to provide energy and amino acid precursors for gluconeogenesis. Anabolism begins at about day 3 and lasts for 4 to 6 weeks after major abdominal operations in humans.[1] During this phase, a positive nitrogen balance is achieved, resulting in weight gain. After nitrogen equilibrium is reached, body fat is again deposited. The degree to which these same processes occur in animals has not been studied extensively.

In human studies comparing open and laparoscopic cholecystectomy procedures, laparoscopy resulted in fewer neuroendocrine and cytokine responses compared with the open approach. By comparing postsurgical serum catecholamine, cortisol, and glucose levels to baseline values, investigators demonstrated that these stress indicators increased less and returned to baseline more quickly after laparoscopic cholecystectomy compared with the open procedure.[3] Indicators of the cytokine response, such as interleukin-6 and C-reactive protein, leukocytosis, and erythrocyte sedimentation rate, were all less with the laparoscopic approach.[4,5] Measures of leukocyte activation and free radical mediators, including malondialdehyde, oxidized glutathione, and myeloperoxidase, were lower in patients undergoing laparoscopic cholecystectomy compared with open cholecystectomy.[6]

Animal studies indicate that cell-mediated immunity is less impaired following laparoscopic surgical techniques compared with open approaches. Pigs that underwent laparoscopic colon resection showed a 20% greater response in tests of delayed-type hypersensitivity than did those that underwent an open colon resection.[7] Tumors grow more slowly in animals undergoing laparoscopy, compared with those undergoing laparotomy.[8]

Human studies suggest that pulmonary complications are minimized with less invasive approaches.[9] Because there is less pain with deep inspiration, there is less chest wall splinting, resulting in better ventilation, larger total lung capacity, and improved oxygen saturation. Pulmonary function returned to baseline 4 to 10 days sooner following laparoscopic, rather than open, procedures.[10]

Gastrointestinal (GI) function returns more rapidly following minimally invasive surgery. Myoelectrical activity and intestinal motility were studied in dogs undergoing open and laparoscopic cholecystectomy.[11-13] GI transit times were compared following open colotomy and laparoscopic or laparoscopic-assisted colectomy.[14-15] These studies demonstrated a more rapid return of GI function with less invasive procedures.

Laparoscopy results in fewer intraabdominal adhesions. Rabbits that underwent laser incision of the uterine horn and peritoneum had no adhesions when laparoscopy was used, but all had adhesions when the same techniques were performed by laparotomy.[16] Studies in rabbits and dogs suggest that there is no difference in adhesions if the peritoneum is removed using either of the two techniques, but fewer wound adhesions are seen with the laparoscopic approach.[17,18] By avoiding retractors, packing, and tissue handling, minimally invasive approaches may reduce injury to the abdominal wall and viscera. A closed approach may reduce tissue dessication and foreign body contamination.

Overall, wound complications are reduced when smaller incisions are used. During the early stages of laparoscopic surgery, hernias at 10-mm trocar sites were occasionally noted when the fascia was not sutured. Large incisional hernias that occurred in up to 20% of morbidly obese humans following open gastric bypass procedures have been virtually eliminated by using minimally invasive approaches.[19]

In veterinary surgery, improvement in postoperative ambulation is evidence of the merits of arthroscopy and thoracoscopic surgical procedures, but these procedures are not yet considered the gold standard. It will take time to determine if minimizing the physiologic responses by minimally invasive surgery results in improved clinical outcomes in animals.

REFERENCES

1. Wilmore DW: Homeostasis: bodily changes in trauma and surgery. In Sabiston DC JR, editor: Textbook of surgery: the biological basis of modern surgical practice, ed 15, Philadelphia, 1996, WB Saunders.
2. O'Riordain M, Ross JA, Fearon KCH: The inflammatory and metabolic response to open surgery and minimally invasive surgery. In Patterson-Brown S, Garden J, editors: Principles and practice of surgical laparoscopy. London, 1994, WB Saunders.
3. Schauer PR, Sirinek KR: The laparoscopic approach reduces the endocrine response to elective cholecystectomy. *Am Surg* 61:106-111, 1995.
4. Roumen RMH et al: Serum interleukin-6 and C-reactive protein responses in patients after laparoscopic or conventional cholecystectomy. *Eur Surg Res* 158:541-544, 1992.
5. Jaberansari MT et al: Inflammatory mediators and surgical trauma regarding laparoscopic access: acute phase response. *Acta Chir Hung* 36:138-140, 1997.
6. Gal I et al: Inflammatory mediators and surgical trauma regarding laparoscopic access: free radical mediated reactions. *Acta Chir Hung* 36:97-99, 1997.
7. Bessler M et al: Is immune function better preserved after laparoscopic versus open colon resection? *Surg Endosc* 8:881-883, 1994.
8. Allendorf JDF et al: Tumor growth after laparotomy or laparoscopy: a preliminary study. *Surg Endosc* 9:49-52, 1995.
9. Karayiannakis AJ et al: Postoperative pulmonary function after laparoscopic and open cholecystectomy. *Br J Anesth* 77:448-452, 1996.
10. Schauer PR et al: Pulmonary function after laparoscopic cholecystectomy. *Surgery* 114:389-397, 1993.
11. Schmieg RE et al: Recovery of gastrointestinal motility after laparoscopic cholecystectomy. *Surg Forum* 44:135, 1993.
12. Ludwig KA et al: Myoelectric motility patterns following open versus laparoscopic cholecystectomy. *J Laparoendosc Surg* 3:461-466, 1993.
13. Schippers E et al: Intestinal motility after laparoscopic vs. conventional cholecystectomy: an animal experiment study and clinical observation. *Langenbecks Arch Chir* 377:14-18, 1992.
14. Hotokezaka M, Combs MJ, Schirmer BD: Recovery of gastrointestinal motility following open versus laparoscopic colon resection in dogs. *Dig Dis Sci* 41:705-710, 1996.
15. Davies W et al: Laparoscopic colectomy shortens postoperative ileus in a canine model. *Surgery* 121:550-555, 1997.
16. Luciano AA et al: A comparative study of postoperative adhesions following laser surgery by laparoscopy versus laparotomy in the rabbit model. *Obstet Gynecol* 74:220-224, 1989.
17. Jorgensen JO, Lalak NJ, Hunt DR: Is laparoscopy associated with a lower rate of postoperative adhesions than laparotomy?: a comparative study in the rabbit. *Aust N Z J Surg* 65:342-344, 1995.
18. Tittel A et al: Laparoscopy versus laparotomy: an animal experiment study comparing adhesion formation in the dog. *Langenbecks Arch Chir* 379:95-98, 1994.
19. Wittgrove AC, Clark GW, Schubert KR: Laparoscopic gastric bypass, roux-en-Y: technique and results in 75 patients with 3-30 months follow-up. *Obesity Surg* 6:500-504, 1996.

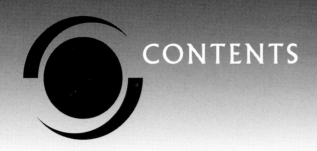

CONTENTS

Veterinary
Endosurgery

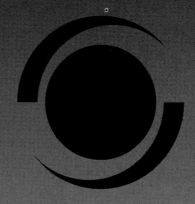

PART ONE

PRINCIPLES OF ENDOSURGERY

CHAPTER 1

OPERATING ROOM SETUP, EQUIPMENT, AND INSTRUMENTATION

Lynetta J. Freeman

Endoscopy means "to look inside." Usually the term is reserved for examining the interior of hollow viscera such as bronchi or the intestinal tract, but it can also be applied to examination of the abdominal cavity (laparoscopy) or the thorax (thoracoscopy). Minimally invasive surgery is a collection of surgical techniques designed to minimize the extent of the anatomic approach while still maintaining precision and efficiency. Endoscopic surgery involves performing a minimally invasive surgical procedure with visualization provided by an endoscope. Laparoscopic and thoracoscopic surgeries entail endoscopic surgical approaches to the abdomen and thorax, respectively.

Team Preparation

Endoscopic surgery requires sophisticated equipment and a smoothly functioning team. Veterinarians who plan to use minimally invasive techniques must be certain that the operating room staff understands the proper use of all the equipment because working as a team improves operating room efficiency and helps avoid complications (Fig. 1-1).

Because the surgeon will be involved in each procedure, support staff must be qualified to identify and solve unexpected system failures. The ideal time for training is before a clinical procedure. Written procedures for setting up, using, and cleaning all equipment should

be developed and followed. Using preoperative checklists minimizes errors (Boxes 1-1 and 1-2).[1] A troubleshooting guide published by the Society of American Gastrointestinal Endoscopic Surgeons (SAGES) is available (Table 1-1).

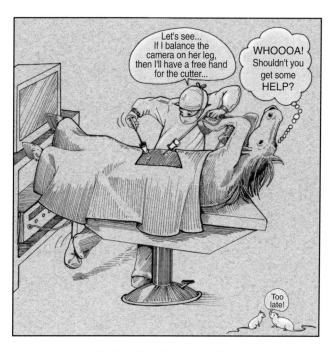

Fig. 1-1　Somebody help him!

BOX 1-1

PREOPERATIVE CHECKLIST FOR LAPAROSCOPIC SURGERY

2 Days Ahead
- Check CO_2 supply
- Ensure equipment availability and compatibility
- Determine the necessary instrumentation
- Prepare instruments for sterilization
- Set up operating room suite, video cart

1-2 days ahead
- Sterilize equipment

Morning of Surgery
- Review operating room checklist

As team members, the nursing staff makes significant contributions in the selection, ordering, and maintenance of instruments and equipment. Having the staff communicate with instrument and equipment representatives enables them to obtain rapid and efficient service and technologic support.

Make the operating room team aware that an unexpected need to convert to an open procedure will require rapid and efficient entry. Teach the team to anticipate a need to control hemorrhage rapidly. This will ensure that suction, electrocautery, and irrigation systems are set up and functioning properly when needed. To enable assistants to pass surgical instruments efficiently, teach them the basic steps of the procedure and the instrumentation required for each step.

Develop "case cards" for each procedure, tailored to the surgeon's preference to ensure that laparoscopic equipment is prepared and available (Box 1-3). A laparoscopic cart, fully stocked with laparoscopic instruments, sutures, backup cables, cords, and tubing, is ideal.

BOX 1-2

OPERATING ROOM CHECKLIST FOR LAPAROSCOPY

Insufflation
- CO_2 tank full and spare available
- CO_2 line attached
- CO_2 coming through insufflator line
- Insufflator pressure gauge responds to kinking tube
  Pressure rises to >15 mm Hg
  CO_2 flow drops to 0 L/min

Laparoscopic Equipment
- Light source operational and spare bulb available
- Light guide cable and light source attached to telescope
- Camera sterilized or sterile sleeve available
- Camera control unit operational and attached to monitor
- Camera attached to telescope and camera control unit
- Camera white-balanced
- Camera focused
- Monitor is operational
- Image on monitor is sharp and has true colors
- VCR operational and case information recorded, videotape loaded

Suction/Irrigation
- Irrigation fluids provided
- Fluid flows through irrigator/aspirator system
- Suction unit connected to suction line of irrigator/aspirator system
- Fluid easily aspirated from basin

Electrosurgical Unit
- Attach grounding pad to patient
- Sterilize cautery cords and attach to instruments
- Place foot pedal next to surgeon
- Inspect electrosurgical instruments to ensure intact insulation
- Select generator power setting

UltraCision Setup
- Connect handpiece to generator
- Attach appropriate adapter to handpiece
- Attach instrument
- Tighten instrument with wrench
- Set generator to level 3
- Place foot pedal next to surgeon's dominant foot

UltraCision Equipment
- UltraCision generator
- UltraCision foot pedal
- 1 handpiece
- 1 LCS device
- 1 LCS adapter
- 1 UltraCision wrench
- 1 5-mm dissection hook (blunt)
- 1 5-mm dissection hook (sharp)
- 1 5-mm ball coagulator

TABLE 1-1

Troubleshooting Guide

PROBLEM	POSSIBLE CAUSE	SOLUTION
No power	Power switch off	Turn power on
	Power cord not plugged in	Plug cord in
	Multioutlet switch is off	Turn on switch
	Circuit breaker tripped	Check circuit box
No picture	No power	See above
	Equipment sequence incomplete	Each unit of equipment must have power to activate the chain; check monitor, camera, light source, and VCR
	Camera placed on dark surface	Turn camera face up
Inadequate light	Light setting manual	Try automatic
	Lightbulb blown	Replace bulb
	Light cable has broken fibers	Replace cable
	Automatic light reflecting off metal	Reposition instruments
	Warm-up cycle not complete	Wait required cycle time
	Scope is too small	Position scope closer to structure
Fogging/haze of picture	Tissue or condensation on scope lens	Quickly touch the scope to tissue, avoiding delay; place the scope in warm water
	Condensation on the camera, eyepiece, or filter	Dismantle the camera; thoroughly dry each lens with 4 × 4
	Out of focus	Focus camera
	Electrocautery plume	Use suction; watch pressure readings
Picture fuzzy	Cracked lens of scope	Manufacturer must repair
Picture grainy	Cable connections loose	Tighten all connections
	Cable lines crossed	Check for correct cable placement
	Cable not grounded	Remove any cables not in use
	Incorrect 75-ohm setting	Refer to operating instructions
Color not acceptable	Camera not "white balanced"	White-balance camera before procedure
	Monitor color controls set incorrectly	Use reset feature on monitor color control
Record button on VCR will not engage	No tape in VCR	Insert tape. Record and play buttons must be depressed simultaneously
Insufflator alarms	CO_2 tubing attached	Tubing crimped. Stopcock turned off
	Trocar insertion taking place	Alarm may temporarily sound during trocar insertion
Exposure compromised because of CO_2 leakage	CO_2 tubing partially occluded	Straighten tubing
	Stopcock partially closed	Fully open valves
	Leakage around trocars	Correct leakage
	Trocars displaced	Reinsert trocar
	CO_2 ports left open on secondary ports	Close stopcock
	Leakage around external gasket	Change reducer cap or trocar
	Leakage through instrument	Use reducer cap or "blocker"
	Using a 5-mm instrument through a 10-mm trocar	Exchange instrumentation

---

BOX-1-3

SAMPLE SURGEON'S PREFERENCE CARD

Laparoscopy Tray—Metals

2 Brown Adson tissue forceps
3 Allis tissue forceps
2 DeBakey tissue forceps
4 Kelly forceps
1 Mayo scissors, curved
1 Metzenbaum scissors, curved
1 Needle holder
1 Saline bowl
2 Senn retractors
1 Suture scissors
Towel clamps
Balfour retractor

Thoracoscopy Tray (add the following instruments):

2 Duvall lung clamps
2 Pennington lung clamps
1 Metzenbaum scissors, long
2 Right-angle forceps, long
1 Finochietto retractor

Access:

- 1 Veress needle
- 1 10-mL syringe
- 2 #10 scalpel blades

Trocars:

- 2 5-mm trocars and stability threads
- 2 10/12 mm trocars and stability threads
- 2 reducer caps
- 1 10/12 mm blunt-tip trocar

Clip Appliers:

- 1 5-mm clip applier
- 1 medium clip applier
- 1 large clip applier

Staplers:

- 35-mm endoscopic linear cutter
- White cartridges
- Blue cartridges

Bipolar Forceps

5-mm Instruments:

- 2 grasping forceps
- 1 dissecting forceps, straight
- 1 dissecting forceps, curved
- 1 curved scissors

10-mm Instruments:

- 3 Babcock forceps
- 1 bowel clamp
- 1 Kelly forceps
- 1 right-angle forceps
- 1 scissors

Other:

- 3 cherry dissectors
- 3 Kittner dissectors
- 1 Endoloop Introducer
- 7 Endoloops
- 1 Suction Irrigation System
- Antifog agent
- Suture
- 2 laparoscopic needle holders
- 1 reusable knot pusher

Operating Room Layout

Carefully plan the position of the surgery table, surgeon, assistant, camera operators, video monitor, anesthesia machine, electrocautery unit, and suction device so the staff can circulate freely about the room. Three basic operating room setups are recognized (Figs. 1-2 to 1-4).

Plan to point the surgical telescope *toward* the video monitor for most of the surgical procedure. Place the monitor at the foot of the table for procedures caudal to the umbilicus or directed toward the diaphragm for procedures in the thoracic cavity (Fig. 1-2). Place the monitor at the head of the table for procedures in the cranial parts of the abdominal and thoracic cavities (Fig. 1-3). If a procedure involves working cranially and caudally, place monitors at both ends of the table. Minimally invasive surgery on animals positioned in lateral recumbency requires positioning the monitor at the animal's back (Fig. 1-4).

Consult with the anesthetist to place the anesthesia equipment in the best location for access and monitoring. Caudal abdominal and thoracic procedures do not usually cause a problem because the video monitor is at the foot of the table. However, positioning both the anesthesia equipment and the video monitor at the animal's head may limit access to the anesthetic equipment or the surgical field.

Position the insufflator at eye level next to the video monitor so the surgeon or assistant can monitor the abdominal pressure. Consider using a cart that stacks the monitor, insufflator, camera, and light source to minimize the crossing of cords, cables, and tubing to the operative field (Fig. 1-5). Ensure that the electrical current supplied to the operating room is capable of simultaneously operating all equipment without blowing a fuse.

To minimize the potential for electrical interference between the electrosurgical unit (ESU) and the video monitor, plug the ESU into a separate electrical outlet from the video cart. Otherwise, activation of the ESU may cause a series of lines to cross the monitor, obscuring vision of the operative site.

Allow the camera operator to stand on the side of the animal that is most comfortable for him or her. If possible, the camera operator should hold the camera with

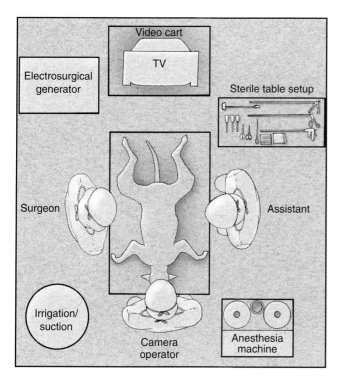

Fig. 1-2   Room setup for caudal abdominal and thoracic procedures.

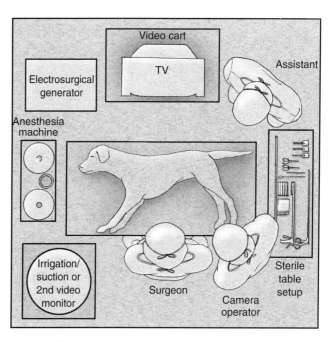

Fig. 1-4   Room setup with animal in lateral recumbency.

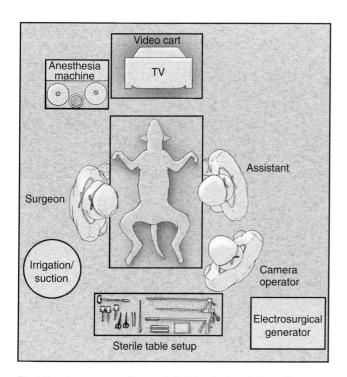

Fig. 1-3   Room setup for cranial abdominal and thoracic procedures.

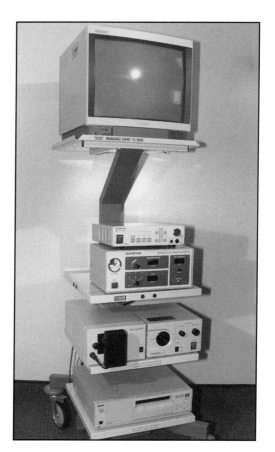

Fig. 1-5   Portable cart for videoendoscopic system.

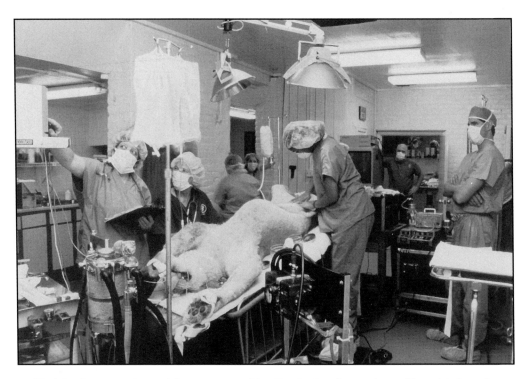

Fig. 1-6   Laparoscopic ovariohysterectomy with a lion in dorsal recumbency. The pelvis is positioned next to the video monitor and elevated approximately 45°. The surgeons stand on surgical lifts.

the dominant hand. The surgeon moves about the table as necessary and should plan to perform most of the procedure with the dominant hand. The assistant should stand opposite the surgeon.

Equipment

SURGERY TABLE

The ideal surgical table can be lowered, raised, and tilted in either direction. Lowering or raising the table to the waist height of the operating team makes the team members more comfortable and improves efficiency and endurance. Provide lifts to improve access to the surgical site. Ideally the surgeon holds his or her arms close to the body with the shoulder in a neutral position and the elbows at 90°.

Be prepared to tilt the end of the table next to the video monitor approximately 60° to improve visualization of the operative site (Fig. 1-6). Conventional veterinary surgery tables require a wider base to keep them from tipping over when heavy animals are positioned on one end of the table and the table is tilted.

VIDEOIMAGING EQUIPMENT
Surgical Telescopes (Endoscope, Laparoscope)

Endoscopes can be flexible or rigid. Flexible endoscopes are usually used for gastrointestinal endoscopy and examination of the respiratory system. Rigid endoscopes

are also called *telescopes.* Telescopes are often named for the anatomic region in which they are used (e.g., laparoscope, thoracoscope, arthroscope).

Rigid endoscopes provide the most light, the largest field of view, and the greatest clarity of vision. Rigid scopes have a central lens chain and fiberoptic bundles that project light into the body cavity (Fig. 1-7). In general, large scopes admit more light, have a larger field of view, and provide greater image resolution. Small scopes can transmit a clear view if they are positioned close to the object being examined. Laparoscopes with an outside diameter of 10 mm are preferred for most operative procedures in larger animals. Scopes that are 5 mm or smaller are ideal for performing diagnostic laparoscopy and thoracoscopy. The 2.7- and 2.2-mm arthroscopes are best for joints. The 1.7-mm endoscopes are best for very small animals (Fig. 1-8).

An operating endoscope is a rigid scope that has a channel for inserting instruments. Operating endoscopes are ideal for limited access techniques using a single puncture. They are ideally suited for obtaining biopsy specimens.

Endoscopes are designed with various viewing angles to improve vision of the operative site. The 0° scope provides the surgeon with a visual field that is in line with the true field (Fig. 1-9, *A*).[2] An angled view obtained with a 30° scope enables one to look over the top of tissue and into recesses and helps keep the scope out of the way of

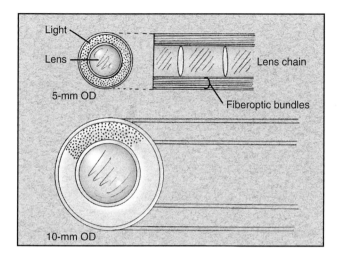

Fig. 1-7 Light is delivered into the abdominal or thoracic cavities by a fiber bundle surrounding the rod lens.

the operative instruments. The angled view is opposite the insertion of the light guide cable (Fig. 1-9, *B*). Thirty and 45° scopes are useful in some abdominal and thoracic procedures to maximize visibility of the operative field. The camera is held stable and the light guide cable is used to rotate the scope to obtain the desired view (Fig. 1-10).

The field of vision refers to the borders of the field of view. By rotating an angled scope 180°, the wider viewing angle produces a larger field of view.[3] Moving a surgical telescope closer to an object magnifies it. As scopes move closer to an object, the camera operator may need to adjust the focus. An experienced camera operator who can maintain the orientation of the surgical field while changing the position of the scope relative to the camera and the light guide cable is a valuable asset to the surgical procedure.

If the telescope image appears slightly out of focus, the problem may be fogging. Fogging can occur at any of three sites: the distal end, the lens chain, or the camera interface. When a cold scope is inserted into a warm cavity, water vapor condenses on the lens, causing the distal end of the scope to become fogged. Prewarming the scope in a water bath at 50° C for 3 minutes is usually effective. Telescope warmers are commercially available. A sterile thermos bottle filled with warm saline keeps several scopes warmed and available for use.

Commercial antifog solutions* can be wiped on the lens to reduce fogging (Fig. 1-11). Placing the scope against tissue for a few seconds is also effective. This method is not ideal for routine use because tissue fluids build up on the lens, resulting in a distorted image and difficulty cleaning the scope. In difficult cases, iodine solution can be wiped on the lens. Although the solution results in temporary color distortion and is difficult to

*FRED Anti-Fog Solution, Dexide, Inc, Fort Worth, Texas. 76181.

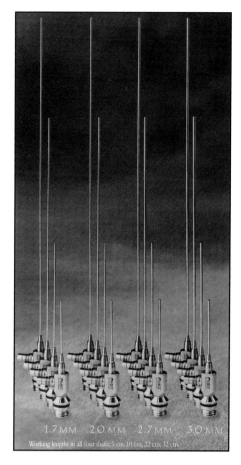

Fig. 1-8 Minilaparoscopy scopes are available in 5-, 10-, 22-, and 32-cm lengths. (Courtesy MIST, Inc, Smithfield, NC.)

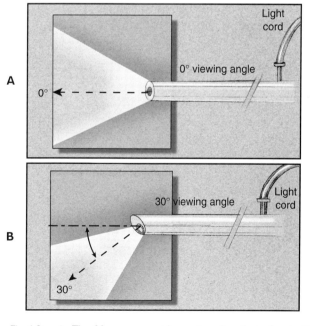

Fig. 1-9 **A,** The 0° scope provides a view directly in front of the scope. **B,** When a 30° laparoscope is used, the camera operator must hold the camera and endoscope so the light cord is "up" if the surgeon wishes to look "down."

remove, it is usually effective. Moving the carbon dioxide (CO_2) attachment to a different port may also help reduce fogging.

Fogging of the lens chain occurs in damaged scopes. If water droplets are seen inside the scope when it is held up to the operating room lights, send it for repair. To reduce fogging at the camera and telescope interface, dry the camera and scope thoroughly during setup. Also, hold the scope so the warmth of the camera operator's hand is not directly over the site of camera attachment.

VIDEOENDOSCOPIC SYSTEMS

A video system consists of a camera, camera control unit, and monitor. The camera is attached to the surgical telescope, and the image is transferred through the control unit to the monitor. Video systems, although expensive, are preferred for minimally invasive surgery because the surgeon, the assistant, and the rest of the operating team are able to view the procedure simultaneously, assist in surgery, and anticipate the surgeon's needs. Further, the telescope and surgical field are less likely to become contaminated with use of a video system. This is very important if it becomes necessary to convert to an open procedure. Video systems are used as an educational tool for clients and students when the procedure is recorded on videotape and reviewed.

Camera

To ensure proper visibility during minimally invasive surgery, a high-quality image is essential (Fig. 1-12). The

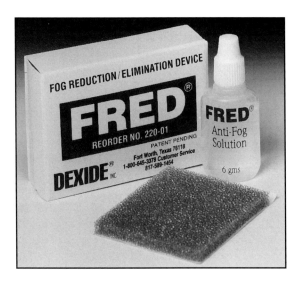

Fig. 1-11   FRED Anti-Fog Solution is supplied with an adhesive-backed sterile sponge. The sponge is saturated with the solution, and the lens is wiped against the sponge. The scope is reinserted. (Courtesy Dexide, Inc, Fort Worth, Texas.)

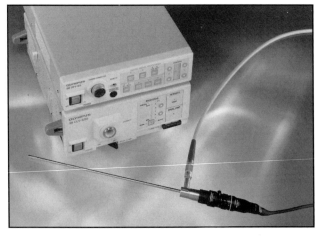

Fig. 1-12   Olympus OTV-S5C Camera Control Unit. The camera has a single chip and features a color bar for video monitor adjustment, automatic white balance, manual color adjustment, brightness adjustment and control, automatic gain control, and image enhancement. (Courtesy Olympus America, Inc, Melville, NY.)

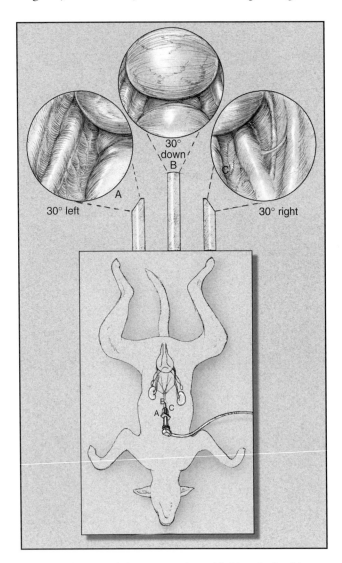

Fig. 1-10   Images of the canine urinary bladder obtained by rotating a 30° scope.

most popular cameras use either one or three chips to convert an image into an electronic signal that can be processed and sent to a video monitor. Single-chip cameras provide 450 lines of resolution. Three-chip cameras use a separate chip for each one of three colors (red, green, blue), provide 600 to 700 lines of resolution, and are seen in the more expensive video camera systems. More lines of resolution provide images of higher quality. Three-chip cameras provide a higher signal-to-noise ratio, which reduces graininess in the picture.

Clarity, or sharpness, of the image is a function of contrast, brightness, color balance, frequency response, and edge enhancement. The human eye relies on contrast rather than color to recognize fine detail.[4] During laparoscopy, bright reflections from shiny or white surfaces, such as the peritoneum, may overload the camera, causing a spilling over into other areas and making the other areas appear white as well. Select a video system with as broad a dynamic range as possible. If the system has poor dynamic range, light-colored objects "white out" and lack detail, whereas objects farther away appear to be dark or lack detail.[5] Most cameras adjust to variations in light intensity during use. An automatic iris measures the available light and adjusts the iris accordingly. Some cameras have a zoom lens or automatic focus capability. Most cameras have a white balance feature that automatically compensates the camera control unit to match the videoscope or camera head used.

Light Source

Older light sources use a tungsten bulb with internal reflectors and are suitable for diagnostic procedures if a video system is not used. Newer high-intensity light sources use mercury, xenon, or halogen bulbs to produce more intense light for videoscopic surgery (Fig. 1-13). If the image is too bright, the surgical field appears "washed out." If the image is too dark, depth perception and fine detail are lost. Newer light sources may have an automatic iris or an automatic light intensity regulator that reduces glare from white images.

The brightness of the image transmitted back to the endoscope depends on the reflective quality of the surface being examined. Pigment and blood-stained tissues absorb light. Brightness also depends on the closeness of the endoscope to the object. Doubling the distance between the endoscope and the tissue being examined increases light dispersion fourfold.[2] Consequently, far more light is required for panoramic views.

Some light sources have a lamp life meter and a built-in spare bulb feature that can be switched easily if a bulb burns out during the procedure. Without that feature, an extra bulb should always be readily available. Teach a staff member how to change the bulb in case it goes out during an operation. Label the light source with the date of the last bulb change to help predict when a bulb change may become necessary.

Light Guide Cable

The delivered light is only as good as the fiberoptic cord transmitting it. If there is poor light, check the integrity of the cord fibers. Broken fibers appear as black "holes" in the light the cable projects onto a white surface (Fig. 1-14). If more than 20% of the surface is blackened,

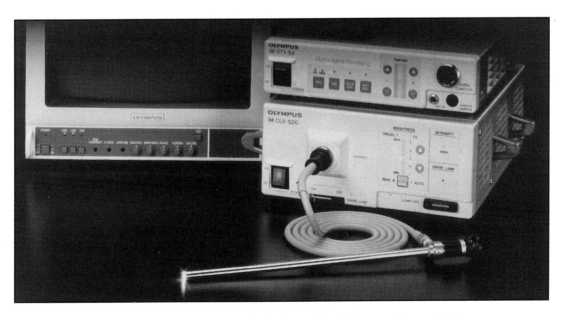

Fig. 1-13   Olympus OES CLV-S20 Xenon Light Source. The light source features brightness control with manual and automatic control, a lamp life meter, and an emergency lamp switch. [Courtesy Olympus America, Inc, Melville, NY.]

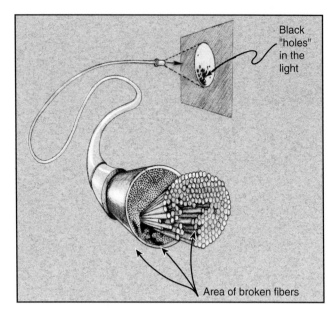

Black "holes" in the light

Area of broken fibers

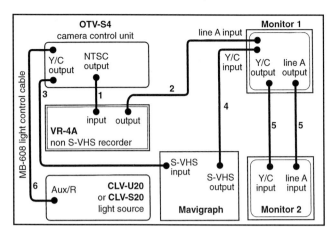

OTV-S4
camera control unit

line A input

Monitor 1

Y/C output   NTSC output

Y/C input   Y/C output   line A output

MB-608 light control cable

3   1   2   4

input   output

VR-4A
non S-VHS recorder

S-VHS input

5   5

S-VHS output

Y/C input   line A input

6   Aux/R   CLV-U20
or CLV-S20
light source

Mavigraph

Monitor 2

Fig. 1-15   Wiring diagram for a single-chip camera. (Courtesy Olympus America, Inc, Melville, NY.)

Fig. 1-14   Broken fibers appear as black dots on the end of the light guide cable. To detect broken fibers, hold the cord up to the surgery light and look at the opposite end, or connect the light cord to the light source and shine the light against a wall.

the cord should be replaced.[6] Before connecting the light guide cable to the laparoscope, make certain that the ends are clean. Adapters are available to allow light guide cables to be compatible with more than one manufacturer's system. Avoid laying the bare cable on surgical drapes because the heat generated can singe or burn the patient. Avoid shining the light into anyone's eyes when the light cord is attached to the scope.

Monitor

Use a monitor with a minimum of 400 lines of resolution if using a single-chip camera and 700 lines of resolution if using a three-chip camera. Two monitors, one facing each surgeon, are ideal for maximum comfort and visibility. Video monitors and all other electronic equipment must be grounded and of medical grade for safety in the operating room. The camera control unit contains a switch to display a color bar on the video monitor. Refer to the monitor's instruction manual to adjust the colors of the color bar.

Recording Devices

Standard videocassette recorders or super VHS recorders allow documentation of the operative procedure. The super VHS systems provide superior image quality; however, the tapes require a super VHS system for optimal image quality during viewing. Videoprinters store and print images as hard copies. Digital recording devices capture images that can later be incorporated into computer graphics presentation media.

Video Cart

A good video cart is sturdy enough to support all of the equipment and has a wide wheel base to make it easy to roll around the surgical suite (see Fig. 1-5). Drawers in the cart are convenient for storing videotapes, cords, and cables. A power strip with electrical surge protection is an excellent feature. A canister for securing the CO_2 tanks is also desirable. Some carts have a side shelf for securing the irrigation and aspiration device. Security measures may include locks for the monitor and for the front and back of the cart. Maintaining a stocked video cart saves valuable setup time. All wiring systems are similar (Fig. 1-15), but each manufacturer's system is specific. Follow the instruction manual for each system.

Insufflator

Electronically controlled insufflators offer the advantage of continuously monitoring the abdominal pressure and maintaining a preset constant pressure (Fig. 1-16). A gas supply gauge indicates the amount of CO_2 in the tank. One can monitor intraabdominal pressure, the CO_2 flow rate, and the total volume of CO_2 instilled. Depending on the manufacturer, the CO_2 flow rate can be regulated as low (1 L/min), medium, or high (6 to 10 L/min), or adjusted from 1 to 15 L/min in 0.1-L increments. The flow rate may be restricted by the insufflation tubing. The CO_2 insufflation tubing has Luer-Lok connectors at each end for attachment to the insufflator and the Veress needle for insufflation or to the stopcock of the trocar during the surgical procedure.

ENERGY SOURCES

Laparoscopic surgical procedures almost always need a means to control hemorrhage. Electrosurgery is preferred by most surgeons (Fig. 1-17), although an ultrasonic cut-

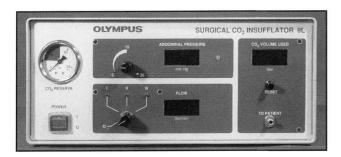

Fig. 1-16 High-flow automatic insufflator. The insufflator features a pressure gauge that reads the CO_2 pressure in the E-tank, three levels of flow control with digital readout of current flow rate, a dial to pre-set the desired intraabdominal pressure, and a digital readout of total liters instilled during the surgical procedure. (Courtesy Olympus America, Inc, Melville, NY.)

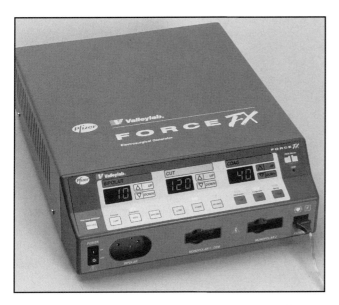

Fig. 1-17 Valleylab Force FX Electrosurgical Generator. The unit features bipolar coagulation; pure and blended monopolar cutting and coagulation; and dessication, fulguration, and spray coagulation capabilities. (Courtesy Valleylab, Inc, Boulder, Colo.)

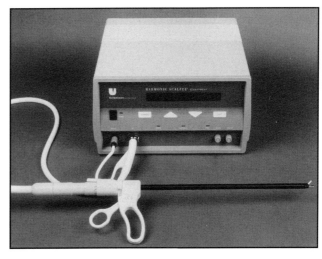

Fig. 1-18 UltraCision Generator and LCS Blade System. The generator sends an electrical signal to the transducer in the handpiece. The transducer converts the electrical energy to mechanical motion. Vibration of the blade at 55,500 cycles per second coagulates blood vessels as tissues are incised. (Courtesy Ethicon Endo-Surgery, Inc, Cincinnati, Ohio.)

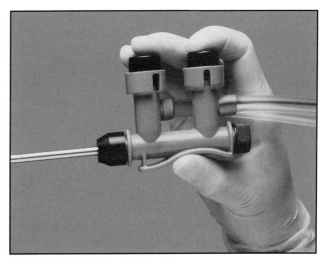

Fig. 1-19 Irrivac-Max Irrigation/Evacuation Device. Two trumpet valves control irrigation and evacuation of fluids through a 10-mm channel. A rear port can be adapted so that 5-mm instruments can be inserted and used simultaneously without leakage. (Courtesy Dexide, Inc, Fort Worth, Texas.)

ting and coagulating unit* is gaining popularity (Fig. 1-18). Laser surgery is used for equine endoscopic applications, but its widespread use awaits further refinement of the technology. Electrosurgical, ultrasonic, and laser equipment are discussed in greater detail in Chapter 4.

IRRIGATION AND ASPIRATION

A clear view of the operative site is imperative. Aspiration/irrigation units remove blood clots and expose bleeding sites to facilitate hemostasis, enable accurate tissue dissection, and minimize postoperative adhesions. Most units combine aspiration and irrigation units into a single device (Fig. 1-19). Various tips are available, including Pool and Yankauer suction tips in 5- and 10-mm sizes. Irrigation is provided by a pressure bag (Fig. 1-20) attached to a plastic bag of lactated Ringer's solution. Irrigation fluids should flow rapidly through

---

*UltraCision, Ethicon Endo-Surgery, Cincinnati, Ohio. 45242.

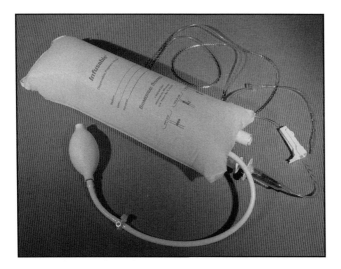

Fig. I-20   Infusable Disposable Pressure Infusor, manufactured by Biomedical Dynamics, Minneapolis, Minn. A 1-L bag of fluids is pressurized by pumping the bulb on the bag. A pressure gauge indicates the pressure. The bag is deflated by opening the stopcock.

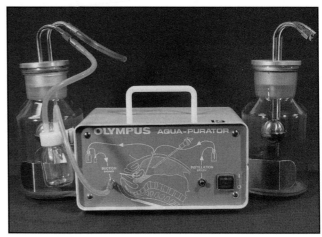

Fig. I-2I   Olympus Aqua-Purator system is a mechanical pump for irrigation and aspiration of fluids during minimally invasive surgery. (Courtesy Olympus America, Inc, Melville, NY.)

the irrigator. Suction can be provided by a portable mechanical suction device (Fig. 1-21) or wall suction. Aspirate fluid from a basin to check the function of the suction apparatus during the operative setup.

LAPAROTOMY PACK

Even with the best operative technique, complications and emergencies occur. Ensure that the animal is properly prepared and draped for open surgery and that a sterile laparotomy pack is available in the room during the surgical procedure.

Procedure Overview

To provide adequate patient support, the operating room team must first understand the surgical sequence of events. The approach and instrumentation differ for laparoscopy and thoracoscopy, and from procedure to procedure. A review of the general sequence of laparoscopy and thoracoscopy will be presented, but the operating room team will want to review procedure-specific instrumentation discussed in later chapters.

For laparoscopy, a Veress needle is used to create a pneumoperitoneum by insufflating the abdomen with CO_2. The insufflation gas lifts the abdominal wall, producing a protective distance between the viscera and abdominal wall and creating a viewing cavity. The needle is removed, and the primary trocar and cannula are then blindly placed through the abdominal wall. The trocar is removed, leaving the outer cannula in place. The animal is then tilted head-down (Trendelenburg position) or head-up (reverse Trendelenburg, or Fowler, position) to

shift abdominal viscera and expose the surgical site. The laparoscope is passed through the primary port, and additional trocars with their outer cannulas are placed under direct vision. The trocar cannulas must be sealed to prevent loss of pneumoperitoneum during the surgical procedure.

For thoracoscopy, a small incision is made in the selected intercostal space and standard curved Kelly forceps are used to bluntly penetrate the thoracic cavity and create a pneumothorax. A rigid cannula is placed bluntly through the intercostal space to protect soft tissues and intercostal nerves. A 30°-angle viewing endoscope is placed through the port and used to visually guide the placement of additional rigid or flexible cannulas. The lung on the side of the proposed procedure must be allowed to collapse for proper visualization. The patient is maintained by one-lung ventilation of the opposite lung. Insufflating the thorax typically is not necessary if the lung is properly collapsed and the trocar cannulas do not require seals.

Instrumentation

INSUFFLATION NEEDLES

Disposable and reusable insufflation needles are available. Disposable needles are always sharp and require less force to penetrate the abdominal fascia. A Veress needle is a type of insufflation needle. To protect abdominal organs from injury by the sharp cutting tip of the needle, Veress needles contain a spring-loaded obturator that advances beyond the sharp tip when the needle enters the abdominal cavity (Fig. 1-22). Most reusable insufflation

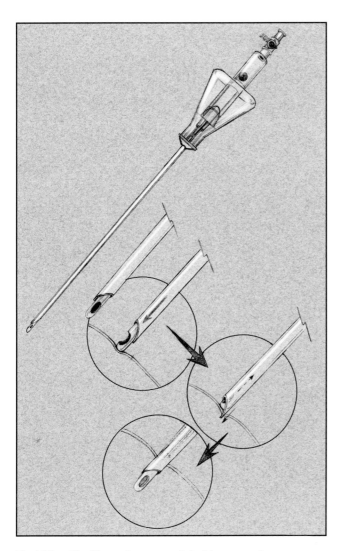

Fig. 1-22 The blunt obturator of the Veress needle retracts as it contacts tissue. When the pressure is released, the obturator springs forward to protect the sharp tip. A red indicator in the needle housing indicates when the needle tip is exposed. The tubing attached to the stopcock provides CO_2 to insufflate the abdomen.

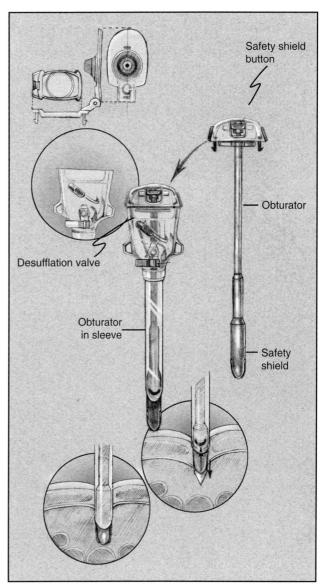

Fig. 1-23 The Endopath TriStar disposable surgical trocar. The obturator has a safety shield that retracts when resistance is met, exposing the cutting tip. When resistance is lost, the safety shield springs forward to protect the internal viscera from the tip of the blade. If the abdominal wall is incompletely penetrated, the safety shield can be reset to allow further penetration.

needles have a stopcock that can open and close the lumen of the needle. The hub of the needle connects to the insufflation tubing.

TROCARS

A trocar is a sharp-pointed instrument (obturator) enclosed in a sleeve (cannula).[7] The obturator usually has a sharp tip to facilitate penetration of fascia, muscle, and peritoneum. The obturator is removed and the cannula remains in place to guide the introduction of instruments. Standard endoscopic trocars have a valve to prevent loss of pneumoperitoneum during insertion and removal of instruments. Most have a stopcock for insufflation of CO_2 (Fig. 1-23).

Reusable trocars are made of stainless steel (Fig. 1-24). The spring-loaded, trumpet-type valve requires disassembly for cleaning. The obturator tip becomes dull with repeated use and requires periodic resharpening.

Disposable trocars have a safety shield, which is a plastic covering over the trocar tip. The cover retracts when the trocar meets resistance and springs forward when the abdominal cavity is penetrated, much like the obturator in a Veress needle (Fig. 1-25).

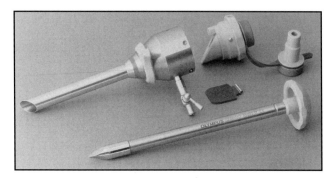

Fig. I-24   Reusable trocar. External gaskets prevent loss of pneumoperitoneum. A trumpet valve inside the cannula is depressed when instruments are inserted and removed. After insertion, the trocar is held steady while the cannula is advanced over the trocar tip to ensure that the cannula will be inside the abdominal cavity. (Courtesy Olympus America Inc, Melville, NY.)

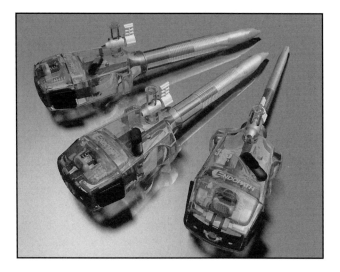

Fig. I-25   Disposable trocars. A 45° flapper valve and an external gasket prevent loss of pneumoperitoneum when instruments are inserted. A desufflator lever controls the flapper valve to allow specimen extraction. Insufflation tubing is attached at the stopcock. The trocar's clear housing allows the surgeon to monitor progress of tissue extraction. (Courtesy Ethicon Endo-Surgery, Inc, Cincinnati, Ohio.)

OPEN PORT PLACEMENT

Open techniques for inserting the first trocar (primary port) were developed to avoid Veress needle and trocar injuries to intraabdominal organs that are a hazard in closed (blind) methods. Open techniques may be slightly more difficult and time consuming, and they require a relatively large incision in obese animals and those with thick abdominal walls. Nevertheless, they are preferred if one suspects adhesions to the abdominal midline. In ruminants, the open technique is used to avoid penetrating

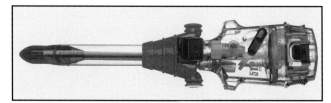

Fig. I-26   A Hasson-type trocar is designed to allow a surgeon to place the primary port in an open manner. The skin, subcutaneous tissue, fascia, and peritoneum are incised. Two size 0 sutures are passed through the edge of the fascia and secured to the tying posts on the olive plug. The amount of the trocar sleeve to be left inside the abdominal cavity is adjusted and secured. The obturator is then removed.

the rumen. The Hasson trocar system is a trocar that facilitates an open technique for primary port placement. The Hasson system consists of a blunt obturator and a cannula with an olive plug with tying posts to secure the sutures placed in the abdominal wall (Fig. 1-26).

THORACIC TROCAR SYSTEM

Thoracoscopic procedures usually do not require a sealed cavity because they rely on collapse of one lung and the curvature of the ribs to establish and maintain an optical cavity. Trocars specifically designed for access to the thorax are available. A rigid cannula for the endoscope port protects the scope from bending when pressure is applied to the ribs. A flexible trocar cannula protects the intercostal artery, vein, nerve, and muscle during repeated insertion of instruments (Fig. 1-27).

CANNULA STABILIZATION

When instruments are inserted and removed, the trocar cannulas slide in and out of the abdomen. If the cannulas are dislodged, there is loss of pneumoperitoneum, collapse of the abdomen, and loss of visibility of the operative site. The procedure is delayed while trocars are reinserted and the pneumoperitoneum is reestablished. To stabilize the cannula in the abdominal wall, manufacturers designed screw threads that fit over the outside of the trocar cannula. Others used a textured surface on the outer cannula wall or incorporated a balloon or other locking device, which is expanded inside the abdominal cavity (Fig. 1-28). Surgeons also use sutures from the skin to the cannula or pads that adhere to the skin and clamp on the outside of the cannula (Fig. 1-29).

REDUCERS

Preventing loss of pneumoperitoneum requires a seal between an instrument that is inserted and the trocar cannula. Usually a gasket is located near the external opening of the trocar cannula. To reduce the size of the external gasket of a large trocar, reducers fit either on top

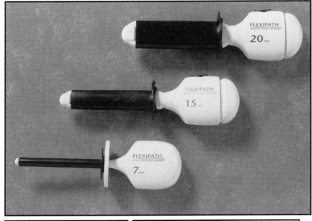

A

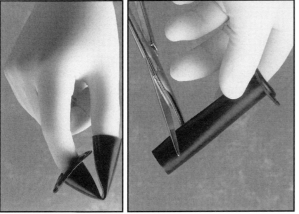

B

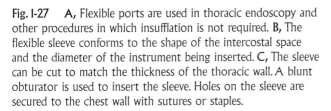

Fig. I-27 **A,** Flexible ports are used in thoracic endoscopy and other procedures in which insufflation is not required. **B,** The flexible sleeve conforms to the shape of the intercostal space and the diameter of the instrument being inserted. **C,** The sleeve can be cut to match the thickness of the thoracic wall. A blunt obturator is used to insert the sleeve. Holes on the sleeve are secured to the chest wall with sutures or staples.

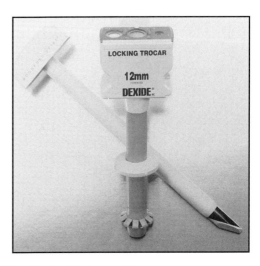

Fig. I-28 The Dexide, Inc., locking trocar has a patented intraabdominal locking device to prevent accidental withdrawal of the trocar. (Courtesy Dexide, Inc, Fort Worth, Texas.)

C

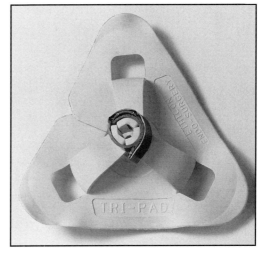

Fig. I-29 External stability pads have a hydrogel adhesive that sticks to the skin surface. The device is placed after the trocar is inserted. A collar secures the trocar in place. (Courtesy Ethicon Endo-Surgery, Inc, Cincinnati, Ohio.)

of the trocar or inside the trocar sleeve. The reducer allows insertion of smaller instruments without loss of pneumoperitoneum. Reducers must be compatible with specific trocars.

LARGE TROCARS

Large trocars (18 to 33 mm) are used to insert large staplers and remove large tissue specimens (Fig. 1-30). In one disposable version, an exchange rod facilitates replacing a smaller trocar with a larger one. The exchange rod ensures that the larger trocar follows the path created by the smaller one.

EXPOSURE, RETRACTION, AND TISSUE HANDLING

Retraction is necessary to improve exposure of the operative site. A retractor may be as simple as a striated stainless steel probe. Some disposable retractors have finger-like projections that extend like a fan to provide a wide retracting surface. One minimally traumatic retractor has a 20-cc air-filled bladder to act as a paddle inside the abdominal cavity (Fig. 1-31).

Plastic and reconstructive surgeons use specially designed scope-holding retractors to elevate the skin and subcutaneous tissue in minimally invasive cosmetic procedures. Cardiothoracic surgeons perform minimally invasive techniques with a scope-holding retractor to harvest the saphenous vein. Veterinarians may find applications for these devices in exploring fistulous tracts (Fig. 1-32).

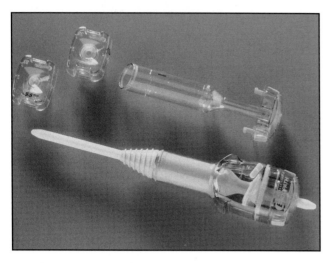

Fig. I-30   Large cannulas are inserted with a threaded conical tip trocar through an existing port site. The instrument is passed over an exchange rod. Reducer caps convert the trocar so 5- and 10-mm instruments can be inserted without loss of pneumoperitoneum. A specimen extractor cannula is available for removing large, potentially infected or malignant tissues.

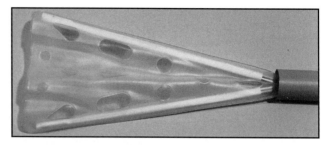

Fig. I-31   Endopath Inflatable Large Organ Retractor. The inflatable paddle provides cushioned retraction of internal organs, notably the liver, lung, colon, stomach, or urinary bladder. (Courtesy Ethicon Endo-Surgery, Inc, Cincinnati, Ohio.)

Grasping forceps, dissecting forceps, and scissors are used for dissection and tissue handling. Reusable and disposable devices are available.

Grasping Forceps

Features of grasping instruments to consider are compatibility with electrocautery, the ratchet mechanism, single- or double-action closure, rotation or articulation, and end-effector configuration (Fig. 1-33).[8] Grasping instruments may be compatible with either monopolar or bipolar electrocautery but usually not both. Insulation along the outside of the shaft prevents arcing to the trocar cannula and adjacent tissues. When using cautery, one should ensure that the protective insulation is intact.

The ratchet mechanism allows a grasper to be fixed on tissue. A ratchet is desirable when tissue must be held securely for a long period. Bar-type ratchets, similar to those in open surgical instruments, are used in many grasping instruments.[9] The instrument is closed to exert constant pressure on the tissue, allowing the operator to relax his or her grip. To open the ratchet, the instrument must be closed slightly to allow the ratchet to clear the fixed position.

The jaw mechanism may be single or double action.[9] In a single-action instrument, only the upper jaw moves. In double-action instruments, both jaws move. Needle holders and microscissors are usually single action. Most surgeons prefer double-action instruments for tissue handling and fine dissection.

Rotation and articulation of the instrument shaft improves access and maneuverability. These features are available in some disposable instruments. Pressing a wheel on the instrument shaft with a finger causes the shaft to rotate. In articulating devices, pushing a knob down the shaft of the instrument causes the tip to angulate up to 90°.

Instrument jaws are called *end effectors* (Fig. 1-34). They are broadly classified as traumatic or atraumatic; however, any instrument is traumatic if used improperly. Atraumatic forceps have fine serrations inside the jaws to hold delicate tissue firmly. The shape of the tip may be blunt, dolphin-nosed, duck-bill, curved, or angled. Bowel clamps and Babcock, Allis, and DeBakey tissue forceps are available as 10-mm instruments (Fig. 1-35). Ring forceps, lung clamps, and Glassman-type forceps are also available. Traumatic grasping forceps have teeth and are used to grasp tissue that is to be removed.

Dissecting Forceps

Curved dissectors, Maryland dissectors, right-angle forceps, and Kelly forceps are useful for isolating and identifying blood vessels. Cherry or peanut dissectors are also useful for blunt dissection.

Scissors

Sharp dissection is performed with a cutting instrument. Scissors, with or without electrocautery, are used the most. Curved Metzenbaum-type scissors are preferred for routine cutting and are available with 5-mm and 10-mm shafts. Hook-type scissors are used for cutting sutures and tubular structures. Straight scissors, including microscissors, are chosen for very fine dissection. Disposable scissors eliminate the need for resharpening.

LIGATION/HEMOSTASIS

Two means of controlling bleeding are ligation with clip appliers and sutures. Reusable single-ligating clip appliers and disposable multiple-clip appliers come in several sizes

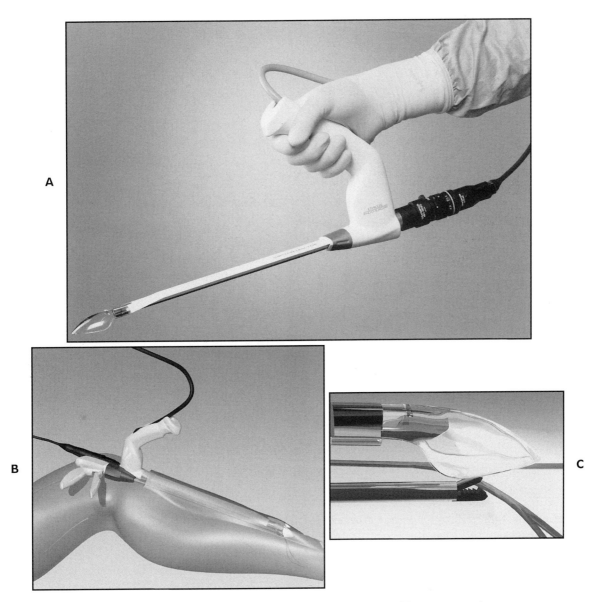

Fig. 1-32   A, An endoscope-holding retractor was developed to enable surgeons to harvest the saphenous vein through small incisions in the leg. A 30°, 5-mm scope is positioned to look "down." The light guide cable is secured in the handle. A direct coupler attaches the video camera to the eyepiece of the telescope, and the image is projected on a video monitor. The spoon-shaped device performs dissection between the skin and saphenous vein. **B,** A 5-mm endoscopic clip applier is inserted along the dissection path adjacent to the telescope. **C,** With visibility provided by the scope, side branches of the saphenous vein are ligated with clips and transected with scissors. Finally, the vein is ligated distally, cut, and removed. (**A** to **C** courtesy Ethicon Endo-Surgery, Inc, Cincinnati, Ohio.)

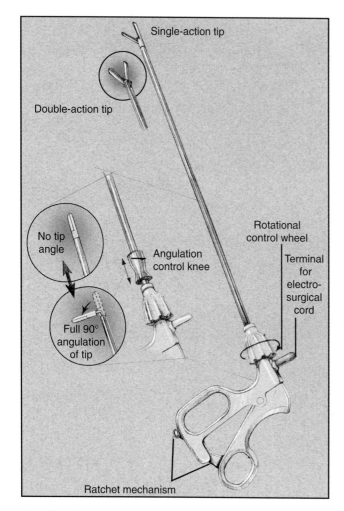

Fig. 1-33   Features of grasping forceps include a ratchet mechanism for closure, a rotation knob, an attachment post for electrocautery, and single- or double-action jaw movement.

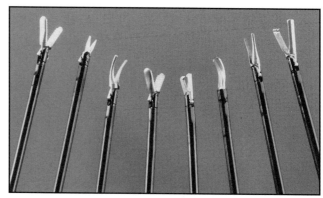

Fig. 1-34   Several jaw configurations are available in 5-mm instruments.

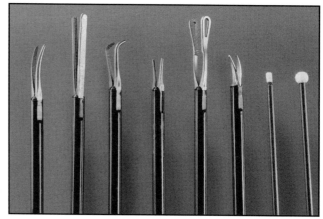

Fig. 1-35   Ten-mm instruments.

(Figs. 1-36 and 1-37). Clip appliers made by different manufacturers may not be compatible with all trocars.

Several suture products are available for ligation, including a pre-tied loop ligature* for pedicles. If the tissue to be ligated is not a free pedicle, extracorporeal or intracorporeal knotting techniques are used.

Generalized oozing or bleeding from solid organs, such as the liver or spleen, can be a problem in some procedures. Local compression, irrigation of the field with lactated Ringer's solution, and application of topical hemostatic agents, such as microfibrillar collagen and thrombin, may be used.

TISSUE APPOSITION AND ANASTOMOSIS
A disposable endoscopic linear stapler is an efficient means of joining tissues (Fig. 1-38). Such devices apply either four or six staggered rows of B-shaped staples and

*Endoloop Pre-tied Loop Ligature, Ethicon, Inc., Somerville, N.J. 08876.

cut between the middle rows. Staple lines are 30 to 60 mm long. Tissue thickness determines cartridge selection. White cartridges, indicated for tissue that is easily compressed to 1.0 mm, are used on vascular tissues, isolated blood vessels, and thin bowel or pulmonary tissue. Blue cartridges, indicated for tissue that is easily compressed to 1.5 mm, are used on bowel and pulmonary tissues. Green cartridges are indicated for 2.0 mm-thick tissue such as stomach, lung, or thicker bowel.

Tissue, such as peritoneum, can also be apposed by using a stapling device developed for fixing mesh to the inguinal floor in hernia repair. Hernia staplers apply box-shaped staples that are similar to skin staples.

Tissue apposition and anastomosis with sutures are accomplished in the same fashion as in open surgery. Laparoscopic needle holders facilitate intracorporeal suturing (Fig. 1-39).

TISSUE REMOVAL
Tissue removal is easier with specialty devices such as disposable specimen bags and morcellators. If the tissue is infected or malignant, one should consider placing it in

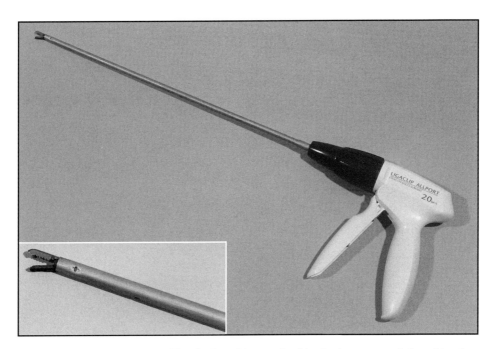

Fig. 1-36 Five-mm clip applier. The clip (*inset*) is contained in the instrument shaft and is advanced after the jaws of the applier are closed on tissue.

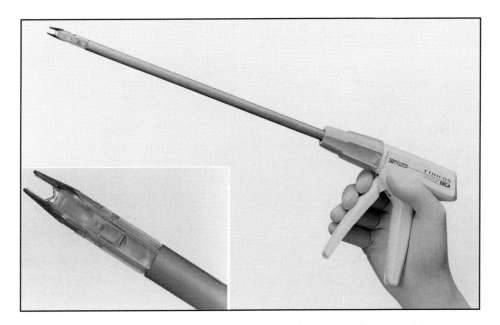

Fig. 1-37 Ten-mm clip applier. A magnified view of the clip is shown in the inset.

a bag while it is still in the body to prevent contamination of the trocar site (Fig. 1-40). Morcellators cut the tissue into pieces small enough for extraction through a 10-mm port. Some morcellators simultaneously aspirate the tissue fragments as they are morcellated.

CLOSURE

The final step in a laparoscopic procedure is to remove the laparoscopic cannulas. Several devices are available for closure of the trocar sites. Alternatively, trocar sites are closed with conventional sutures, as in open surgery. The J-needle facilitates closures of port sites.

Cleaning and Sterilizing Instruments and Equipment

The most effective way to clean instruments after use is to rinse them in cold water and wash them thoroughly

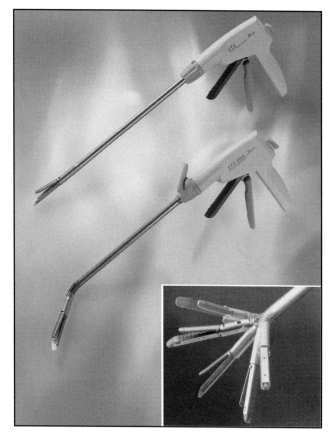

Fig. I-38 Endopath ETS Endoscopic Transecting Stapler. The device applies six staggered rows of staples (*inset*) and cuts between the middle rows. An articulation knob on the instrument deflects the tip 45° in two directions. (Courtesy Ethicon Endo-Surgery, Inc, Cincinnati, Ohio.)

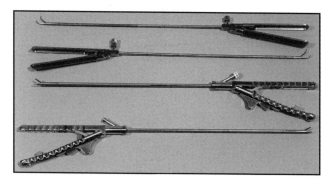

Fig. I-39 Laparoscopic needle holders. *Top to bottom:* Storz reusable needle holders, Storz assist device, and Ethicon reusable needle holders.

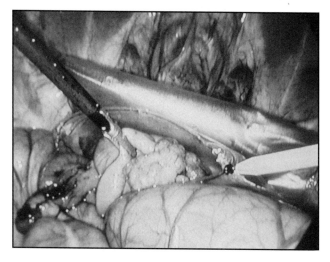

Fig. I-40 Placement of a uterus into a disposable specimen retrieval bag. The neck of the bag is closed and brought to the abdominal wall for extraction.

with soap and a brush. Disassemble and clean reusable instruments. Handle sharp instruments, such as Veress needles, trocars, and scissors, carefully to prevent injury. Treat disposable products as medical waste.

Use steam, gas, or liquid chemical sterilants to sterilize items entering the abdominal or thoracic cavities or the operative field.[9,10] Process metal instruments in the same manner as those used in open surgery, using a steam autoclave. For plastic items, ethylene oxide is usually used. Be sure to follow the manufacturer's recommendations for cycle and aeration times.

Instruments must be cleaned thoroughly before they are immersed in chemical sterilants. One common practice is to soak instruments for 30 minutes in a 2% glutaraldehyde-based solution. Follow the manufacturer's recommendations for use. Remember to replace the solution every 28 days. Rinse instruments thoroughly with sterile saline before use. Use aseptic technique when removing, rinsing, and transferring instruments to the operative field. Provide adequate ventilation, because chemical vapors may irritate mucous membranes.

Surgical telescopes and light guide cables should be sterilized with ethylene oxide at 50° to 60° C for 2 to 3 hours or soaked in a chemical germicide. Steam autoclaving damages the optics. Cameras can be sterilized with ethylene oxide, soaked in a chemical germicide, or used in a sterile plastic sleeve to avoid contamination of the operative field. For the fastest turnover between cases and to prolong the life of the camera, a plastic sleeve is preferred.

Two new processes are available for sterilizing laparoscopic equipment. One unit uses a peracetic acid germicide and runs a rinse cycle after the chemical sterilization* (Fig. 1-41). Another combines radio waves with hydrogen peroxide to create a gas plasma.† Free radicals

---

*Steris, Steris Corp., Menton, Ohio 44060.
†Sterrad, Johnson & Johnson Medical, Inc. Arlington, Texas 76014.

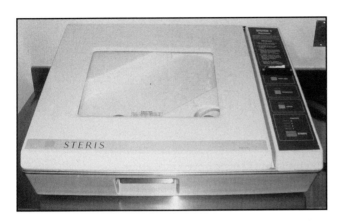

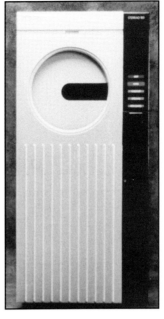

Fig. 1-41   The Steris system for sterilizing endoscopic equipment uses a peracetic acid germicide and runs a rinse cycle after the chemical sterilization. The instruments must be used immediately after sterilization.

Fig. 1-42   The Sterrad system for sterilizing endoscopic equipment combines radio waves with hydrogen peroxide to create a gas plasma that disrupts cell membranes. The instruments can be processed in special packs and stored. No aeration is required. (Courtesy Johnson & Johnson Advanced Sterilization, Irvine, Calif.)

in the plasma cloud interact with cell membranes, enzymes, and nucleic acids to disrupt the life function of microorganisms (Fig. 1-42). The process requires approximately 1 hour, and no aeration is required. The system is compatible with most materials except liquids and fabrics.[11]

Low infection rates have been reported in human laparoscopy, probably because of short operative times and minimal tissue injury. Some veterinarians have attempted to reuse disposable instruments to reduce costs, but disposable instruments are designed for a single use. Proper cleaning between patients cannot be ensured. Preventing equipment-related infections requires meticulous care in preparing for surgery.

REFERENCES

1. Clayman RV, Winfield HN: Room set-up and patient positioning. In Soper NJ et al, editors: Essentials of laparoscopy. St. Louis, 1994, Quality Medical Publishing.
2. Buyalos RP: Principles of endoscopic optics and lighting. In Azziz R, Murphy AA, editors: Practical manual of operative laparoscopy and hysteroscopy. New York, 1992, Springer-Verlag.
3. Hill DL: The basics of laparoscopy. In Graber JN et al, editors: Laparoscopic abdominal surgery. New York, 1993, Health Professions Division, McGraw Hill.
4. Cartmill J, Aamodt D: Video systems in laparoscopy. In Graber JN et al, editors: Laparoscopic abdominal surgery. New York, 1993, Health Professions Division, McGraw Hill.
5. Sanfilippo JS, Indman PD: Photo documentation in laparoscopic surgery. In Vitale GC, Sanfilippo JS, Perissat J, editors: Laparoscopic surgery: an atlas for general surgeons. Philadelphia, 1995, Lippincott.
6. Talamini MA, Gadacz TR: Laparoscopic equipment and instrumentation. In Zucker KA, editor: Surgical laparoscopy. St. Louis, 1991, Quality Medical Publishing.
7. Dorland's illustrated medical dictionary, ed 27. Philadelphia, 1988, WB Saunders.
8. Goldstein DS et al: Laparoscopic equipment. In Soper NJ et al, editors: Essentials of laparoscopy. St. Louis, 1994, Quality Medical Publishing.
9. Duppler DW: Laparoscopic instrumentation, videoimaging, and equipment disinfection and sterilization. *Surg Clin North Am* 72:1021-1031, 1992.
10. Ad Hoc Committee on Infection Control in the Handling of Endoscopic Equipment (Association for Practitioners in Infection Control): Guidelines for preparation of laparoscopic instrumentation. *AORN J* 32:65-76, 1980.
11. Sterrad System of Dry Sterilization. Instruction manual.

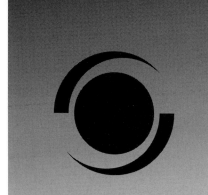

CHAPTER 2

ANESTHETIC AND PHYSIOLOGIC CONSIDERATIONS FOR VETERINARY ENDOSURGERY

James E. Bailey, Luisito S. Pablo

Minimally invasive surgery has been applauded by anesthesiologists for reducing postoperative pain and respiratory difficulties. Smaller entry wounds and limited tissue trauma reduce adhesion formation and a need for narcotic analgesics, and promote earlier ambulation and return to eating and self-sufficiency.[1-10]

To support an animal adequately, anesthetists must understand the principles of endoscopic surgery and the sequence of events for the specific procedure to be performed. The approach and anesthetic considerations differ for laparoscopy and thoracoscopy, and from procedure to procedure. Anesthetists must be familiar with the cardiopulmonary changes associated with increased intraabdominal pressure and elevating or lowering an animal's head. The physiologic changes associated with these maneuvers can be significant and will affect therapeutic choices. Although the anesthetist is not directly involved in the surgery, observing the procedure on a video monitor enables him or her to recognize and take appropriate action against complications such as hemorrhage or pneumothorax.

Physiologic Considerations in Laparoscopy

INSUFFLATION

Abdominal insufflation with gas, also called *pneumoperitoneum*, is used in laparoscopic procedures to produce the requisite viewing space, but with adverse cardiopulmonary effects. The effects vary with the gas used, the presence or absence of mechanical ventilation, and the pressure and duration of insufflation. Insufflation should be applied cautiously in cardiopulmonary-compromised patients.

Pulmonary Effects

As the intraabdominal pressure (IAP) rises, pressure on the diaphragm alters pulmonary mechanics (Table 2-1). Elevated IAP causes bulging of the diaphragm, increased intrathoracic pressure, and reduced lung volumes.[11,12] Mechanical ventilation requires increased inspiratory pressure to deliver a fixed tidal volume, and dynamic pulmonary compliance decreases.[13-15] Deadspace ventilation is not increased.[16] Tidal volume and minute ventilation decrease without changes in the respiratory rate in spontaneously ventilating animals.[17] Overall, the thorax, diaphragm, and abdomen interact to minimize the respiratory embarrassment caused by a finite degree of abdominal distention.[18]

Blood Gas Changes

Changes in blood gas values have been observed with increases in abdominal pressure. These changes depend on the insufflation gas used and whether the animal is mechanically ventilated.

$PaCO_2$ A significant rise in arterial partial pressure of carbon dioxide ($PaCO_2$) is expected when the insufflation gas is carbon dioxide (CO_2), regardless of the ventilation mode. This rise is caused by transperitoneal absorption of CO_2. Normal and hypovolemic anesthetized pigs paralyzed with pancuronium and mechanically ventilated with 100% oxygen (O_2) to control $PaCO_2$ were insufflated with CO_2 to an IAP of 15 mm Hg. The $PaCO_2$ level rose significantly after insufflation. However, no change occurred in $PaCO_2$ when the insufflation gas was helium.[16,19] In dorsally recumbent, anesthetized dogs mechanically ventilated with 100% O_2 to stabilize $PaCO_2$ before insufflation, the $PaCO_2$ rose after insufflation with CO_2 gas to increase IAP to 20 mm Hg.

The $PaCO_2$ did not rise when nitrous oxide (N_2O) was the insufflation gas.[20] However, spontaneously ventilating anesthetized dogs insufflated to more than 20 mm Hg IAP with N_2O showed a significant rise in $PaCO_2$.[17]

It has been demonstrated that transperitoneal CO_2 absorption depends on the peritoneal surface area exposed and the length of exposure.[17,20-23] Subcutaneous or retroperitoneal CO_2 appears to be more readily absorbed than intraperitoneal CO_2. Absorption of such extraperitoneal CO_2 increases as the gas dissects tissues, further increasing the exposed surface area.[24,25]

PaO_2 A fall in arterial partial pressure of oxygen (PaO_2) is expected with CO_2 insufflation to an IAP of 10 to 15 mm Hg. If animals are mechanically ventilated with high oxygen concentrations, the decrease may have minimal clinical implications. Dorsally recumbent, anesthetized pigs that were insufflated with helium to an IAP of 15 mm Hg showed no significant changes in PaO_2.[22] Laterally recumbent, anesthetized dogs insufflated with CO_2 or N_2O to IAPs above 10 mm Hg had progressive decreases in PaO_2.[17,26] In another study in dogs, the PaO_2 decreased significantly when the IAP reached 40 mm Hg with CO_2 insufflation, but not with N_2O.[20] However, the PaO_2 declined significantly to a mean of 74 mm Hg in dorsally recumbent, anesthetized dogs insufflated to IAPs >35 mm Hg and ventilated with room air.[11,13] This level of hypoxemia requires monitoring and administration of supplemental oxygen. The decrease in PaO_2 probably results from an increased right-to-left intrapulmonary shunt caused by mechanical compression and atelectasis.[27]

Cardiovascular Effects

Cardiac Output

Although early studies indicated no undue strain on the cardiovascular system,[28] increasing the IAP alters cardiovascular mechanics significantly (Table 2-2). Increasing

TABLE 2-1

Physiologic Effects of Elevated Intraabdominal Pressure on Pulmonary Function

PARAMETER	EFFECT	DISTENTION MEDIA	SPECIES	REFERENCES
Peak inspiratory pressure	Increased	Air	Canine	13
Intrathoracic pressure	Increased	Tyrode's solution	Canine	11
$PaCO_2$	Increased	N_2O, CO_2	Canine, porcine	16,17,19,20,39,145
PaO_2	Decreased	CO_2, N_2O air	Porcine, canine	11,13,17,20,26,145
Pulmonary compliance	Decreased	CO_2	Human	14,15
Tidal volume	Decreased	N_2O	Canine	17
Minute ventilation	Decreased	N_2O	Canine	17

Insufflated abdomen

TABLE 2-2

Physiologic Effects of Elevated Intraabdominal Pressure on Cardiovascular Function

PARAMETER	EFFECT	DISTENTION MEDIA	SPECIES	REFERENCES
Heart rate	Increased	N_2O, N_2, CO_2	Canine, porcine	20,30,39
Mean arterial blood pressure	Increased	N_2O, saline, CO_2	Canine, porcine	20,29,33,39
Pulmonary arterial pressure	Increased	Helium, CO_2	Porcine, canine	19,22,29,39,133
Pulmonary vascular resistance	Increased	Helium, CO_2	Porcine, canine	19,29,39,133
Systemic vascular resistance	Increased	N_2O, saline, CO_2, helium	Porcine, canine	20,22,23,33-35
Venous return	Decreased	CO_2, N_2O, N_2	Canine	20,30
Cardiac output	Decreased	CO_2, helium, N_2O, air, N_2, argon, Tyrode's solution, saline, air bag	Canine, porcine, human	11,13,19,20,22,23,29-36,159,160
Hepatic arterial and portal venous blood flow	Decreased	Lactated Ringer's solution, CO_2, hydroxyethyl starch colloid	Porcine, canine	23,38,41
Abdominal visceral blood flow	Decreased	Air bag, CO_2, helium, Tyrode's solution	Porcine, canine	11,22,23,34
Renal arterial blood flow and glomerular filtration	Decreased	Air bag, Tyrode's solution	Canine	11,34,35

the IAP to more than 15 mm Hg reduces cardiac output. This was shown in several studies in pigs and dogs and occurs when CO_2, helium, N_2O, argon, or N_2 is used as the insufflation gas.* The reduction in cardiac output is exacerbated by adding 1.0 MAC† halothane, or by hypovolemia from hemorrhage, or both.[30,31] Increasing IAP by external compression or fluid instillation into the abdomen confirmed this reduction in cardiac output.[11,33-38]

Increasing the IAP in dorsally recumbent, anesthetized, mechanically ventilated pigs and dogs led to increased heart rates in some studies, but not in others.‡ Reduced venous return was indicated by decreased inferior vena cava blood flow and decreased transmural right atrial pressure (atrial pressure minus pleural pressure) in mechanically ventilated dogs insufflated with CO_2, N_2O, or N_2.[20,30] Mean arterial blood pressure was unchanged in some studies involving similarly treated pigs and dogs but increased in others.§ Pulmonary arterial blood pressure, pulmonary vascular resistance, and systemic vascular resistance were significantly elevated with increases in IAP.¶ Although a decrease in venous return (preload) contributes to the reduced cardiac output, a constant mean arterial blood pressure in the face of increased systemic vascular resistance suggests that increased afterload plays a significant, if not primary, role in the low cardiac output state.[40]

Tissue Perfusion

An IAP >15 mm Hg may lead to reduced abdominal organ perfusion and oliguria. Elevated IAPs are associated with decreased hepatic blood flow, decreased visceral perfusion, and oliguria. Pigs with an IAP >10 mm Hg had significant reductions in hepatic artery and microvascular blood flow.[38] Decreased portal venous blood flow, but not hepatic arterial flow, was recorded in dogs with an IAP of 16 to 20 mm Hg.[23,41] Celiac, mesenteric, and intestinal mucosal arterial blood flow and perfusion of the rectus sheath decreased significantly with an IAP >16 to 20 mm Hg in pigs and dogs.∥ Ileal submucosal tissue oxygen in pigs fell with IAPs >15 mm Hg.[22] Decreased renal arterial blood flow and glomerular filtration, and increased renal vascular resistance occurred in dogs when the IAP was 20 to 40 mm Hg.[11,34,35] Oliguria was the most consistent sign of elevated IAP, occurring in dogs and pigs at 15 to 20 mm Hg.[22,43] Anuria developed in dogs with IAPs >40 mm Hg.[35]

---

*References 13, 19, 20, 22, 23, 29-32.
†MAC, Minimum alveolar concentration of a gas anesthetic that prevents movement in 50% of animals upon application of a noxious stimulus. It represents the potency of an inhalation agent. Surgical planes of anesthesia in humans and animals are achieved at 1.2 to 1.5 times MAC.
‡References 11, 19, 20, 23, 29, 30, 33, 39.
§References 20, 22, 23, 29-31, 33, 37, 39.
¶References 19, 20, 22, 29, 33-35, 39.
∥References 11, 23, 34, 37, 42.

POSTURE

During laparoscopic procedures, the surgical table is tilted to allow better exposure of the area of interest. Head-down tilt of a dorsally recumbent animal, also called *Trendelenburg position*, encourages abdominal organs to slide craniad and exposes a caudal operative site. Head-up tilt of dorsally recumbent animals, also called *reverse Trendelenburg*, or *Fowler, position*, encourages abdominal organs to slide caudad, exposing a cranial operative site. Even without insufflation, anesthetizing an animal and placing it in dorsal recumbency has physiologic consequences that are exacerbated by tilting.[44-47] All inhalation anesthetic agents alter the baroreflex or the pressor reflex, or both, leading to depressed reflex control of circulation in response to tilting.[64-72] Tilt posture should be applied with caution when animals with cardiovascular impairment are anesthetized with inhalation anesthetics.

Head-Down Tilt
Pulmonary Effects

Head-down tilt causes a craniad shift in abdominal contents, which places pressure on the diaphragm, altering pulmonary mechanics (Table 2-3). Compromise of

TABLE 2-3		
Summary of Human Studies Evaluating the Physiologic Effects of Head-Down Posture		
PARAMETER	EFFECT	REFERENCES
Pulmonary compliance	Decreased	51
Tidal volume	Decreased	49,50
Minute ventilation	Decreased	52
Vital capacity	Decreased	48
Pulmonary shunt fraction	Increased	27
Mechanical impedance	Increased	54
Mean arterial blood pressure	Increased	56,161
Pulmonary arterial pressure	Increased	27,161
Cerebral venous, spinal fluid pressure and vascular resistance	Increased	61
Stroke volume	Decreased	56
Index of cardiac contratility	Decreased	56
Cardiac output	Decreased	57

Head-down
Trendelenburg 30°

pulmonary function caused by head-down tilt is greatest in anesthetized, spontaneously ventilating animals. During anesthesia, higher inspiratory pressures will be necessary for adequate lung expansion when positive pressure ventilation is applied. Decreased tidal volume, vital capacity, and pulmonary compliance occurred in healthy human volunteers during head-down tilt.[48-51] Minute volume of ventilation was reduced in healthy humans anesthetized with halothane at 30° head-down tilt, but it was not affected in humans under light epidural anesthesia.[52,53] Pulmonary shunt fraction was increased in humans with coronary artery disease who were "anesthetized" with fentanyl, paralyzed, and placed in 20° head-down tilt.[27] In humans anesthetized with nitrous oxide and isoflurane, increased lung mechanical impedance was attributed to decreased lung volumes in head-down tilt.[54]

Cardiovascular Effects

Head-down tilt also causes significant changes in cardiovascular mechanics (see Table 2-3). This position was advocated for treatment of shock during World War I, and it has been widely used to treat hypotension.[55] However, there is no consistently documented clinical benefit from this maneuver. Baroreceptor reflexes are responsible for the cardiovascular response to head-down tilt: generalized vasodilation and reductions in heart rate, strength of contraction, stroke volume, cardiac output, arterial blood pressure, and perfusion.[56,57] Baroreceptor reflexes triggered this cardiovascular response in morphine/pentobarbital-anesthetized dogs with intact or denervated baroreceptors, and in dogs induced to hypovolemic shock by hemorrhage, when they were moved to 30° head-down tilt.[58,59] The baroreflex sensitivity to hypertension of several species has been ranked as follows: dog > pig > human > calf > horse.[60] Cerebral venous pressure, cerebral spinal fluid pressure, and cerebral vascular resistance are increased in 20° head-down tilt, leading to decreased cerebral blood flow.[61] The anesthesiologist should be prepared for the potentially adverse effects of head-down tilt in hypovolemic and cerebral hypertensive animals.

Head-Up Tilt

Pulmonary Effects

The caudal shift in abdominal contents during head-up tilt relieves pressure on the diaphragm but compromises cardiopulmonary mechanics somewhat (Table 2-4). Only limited impairment of pulmonary mechanics is apparent.[48,52,54]

Cardiovascular Effects

Baroreceptor and pressor reflexes trigger reflex vasoconstriction and increase the heart rate, strength of contraction, and arterial blood pressure. This was evident in morphine/pentobarbital-anesthetized dogs with intact and denervated baroreceptors when moved to 30° head-up tilt.[58] The baroreflex sensitivity to hypotension has been ranked as follows: dog > pig ≅ horse ≅ human > calf.[60] Tilting healthy humans 20° head-up resulted in a fall in carotid arterial blood pressure with a compensatory fall in cerebrovascular resistance that maintained cerebral blood flow.[61] Cardiac output decreased and heart rate and blood pressure increased when healthy humans were passively tilted upright from dorsal recumbency (orthostatic stress).[62,63] The reduction in cardiac output was attributed to reduced venous return. Increased heart rate and blood pressure were consequences of reflex circulatory adjustments.

Standing

Laparoscopic techniques have often been performed in large animals in standing position under sedation.[73-85] Cardiorespiratory depression depends more on the drugs used for sedation and the application of insufflation gas than on position.[46,47] However, lowering of the head from profound sedation activates the baroreceptor reflexes, causing decreased blood pressure and a slower heart rate.[60,86] Using a standard head position is advised when monitoring sedated, standing endosurgical patients.

EFFECT OF COMBINING POSTURE WITH INSUFFLATION

Clinically, anesthesia, posture, and abdominal distention have a combined effect on cardiopulmonary function.

TABLE 2-4

Summary of Human Studies Evaluating the Physiologic Effects of Head-Up Posture

PARAMETER	EFFECT	REFERENCES
Minute ventilation	Decreased	52
Vital capacity	Decreased	48
Heart rate	Increased	62,63
Mean arterial blood pressure	Increased	62,63
Cerebral vascular resistance	Decreased	61
Cardiac output	Decreased	62,63,71,72

Head-up
Reverse Trendelenburg,
or Fowler, 30°

TABLE 2-5

Summary of the Physiologic Effects of Elevated Intraabdominal Pressures and Head-Down Tilt

PARAMETER	EFFECT	REFERENCES
Impedance of lung and chest wall	Increased	87
Peak inspiratory pressure	Increased	91
Deadspace ventilation	Increased	89,92
$PaCO_2$	Increased	90,92-100
PaO_2	Decreased	92-94
Pulmonary compliance	Decreased	14,15
Functional residual capacity	Decreased	88
Vital capacity	Decreased	89
Mean arterial blood pressure	Increased	91,92,98,99,103,105
Left ventricular pressure, dp/dt and end-systolic wall stress	Increased	91,108
Systemic vascular resistance	Increased	99,107
Intracranial pressure	Increased	111
Cardiac output	Decreased	105-107,109,110

Head-down, Trendelenburg 30° insufflated

Insufflated abdomen

Head-Down Tilt with Gas Insufflation
Pulmonary Effects

It might be predicted from the previous discussion that head-down tilt with gas insufflation would have significant pulmonary consequences (Table 2-5). In fact, lung and chest wall impedance were increased; pulmonary compliance, functional residual capacity, and vital capacity were reduced; and demonstrable diaphragmatic elevation was evident in humans undergoing laparoscopy.[14,15,87-90] Mechanical ventilation required elevated peak airway pressures, and there was increased deadspace ventilation in humans and pregnant sheep.[89,91,92] Pulmonary ventilation-perfusion abnormalities led to alterations in blood gas values. The PaO_2 was decreased in mechanically ventilated humans, horses, and pregnant sheep.[92-94] Spontaneously ventilating humans and mechanically ventilated humans, horses, and pregnant sheep became hypercapnic.[90,92-100] The hypercapnia in mechanically ventilated patients occurred with CO_2 but not N_2O abdominal insufflation.[101,102] It was necessary to increase mechanical minute ventilation 20% to 30% to return patients to eucapnia.*

Cardiovascular Effects

Head-down tilt with gas insufflation has been shown to have significant cardiovascular consequences (see Table 2-5). Although heart rate generally remained constant, it was increased in some human studies and decreased in another.[98,105,106] Mean arterial blood pressure was increased in humans and fetal sheep.† Total peripheral resistance, as well as left ventricular pressure and end-systolic wall stress, were increased in humans and pigs.[91,99,107,108] Cardiac output decreased in humans and dogs.[105-107,109,110] A significant increase in intracranial pressure independent of $PaCO_2$ was detected in pigs.[111]

Head-Up Tilt with Gas Insufflation
Pulmonary Effects

It might be supposed that many of the pulmonary effects of gas insufflation would be alleviated by a head-up posture. Indeed, one investigator noted negligible hemodynamic or respiratory changes with pneumoperitoneum in head-up tilt.[97] However, despite surprisingly scant information on gas exchange and carbon dioxide homeostasis during head-up tilt with gas insufflation, there are significant pulmonary consequences (Table 2-6). Compliances of the chest wall and lung, total lung capacity, and functional residual capacity were reduced in human studies.[14,112-116] Lung and chest wall impedance, all regional pleural pressures, and respiratory resistance were increased.[87,112,113] Insufflation of CO_2 gas caused elevation of $PaCO_2$ in humans.[113,116-118] Increases in minute ventilation and peak airway pressure were required to control insufflation-induced hypercapnia.‡

Cardiovascular Effects

Cardiovascular consequences of head-up tilt with gas insufflation were also significant (see Table 2-6). Cardiac output decreased significantly in humans in head-up tilt with abdominal distention.[71,116,121-125] Heart rate, mean arterial blood pressure, pulmonary arterial blood pressure, systemic vascular resistance, and pulmonary vascular resistance were all increased.§ Oliguria occurred in humans with heart disease.[128]

CONCLUSION

The anticipated effects of posture and gas insufflation are summarized in Table 2-7. Most of the physiologic changes are caused by the increased IAP, specifically by CO_2 gas insufflation. It appears that the *Rule of the 15's* (15 mm Hg IAP; 15° tilt up or down) when applying

---

*References 89, 95, 96, 103, 104.
†References 91, 92, 98, 99, 103, 105.
‡References 71, 115, 116, 119, 120.
§References 71, 103, 116, 120-122, 124-127.

TABLE 2-6

Summary of the Physiologic Effects of Elevated Intraabdominal Pressures and Head-Up Tilt

PARAMETER	EFFECT	REFERENCES
Impedance of lung and chest wall	Increased	87
Pleural pressure	Increased	112
Respiratory resistance	Increased	113
$PaCO_2$	Increased	113,116-118
Mechanical minute ventilation	Increased	119,120
Peak inspiratory pressure	Increased	71,115,116,119
Compliance of lung and chest wall	Decreased	14,112-116
Total lung capacity	Decreased	112
Functional residual capacity	Decreased	112,113
Heart rate	Increased	121,124
Mean arterial blood pressure	Increased	71,103,116,120-122, 125-127
Pulmonary arterial blood pressure	Increased	116,124
Pulmonary vascular resistance	Increased	71
Systemic vascular resistance	Increased	71,116,124,125
Cardiac output	Decreased	71,116,121-125

Head-up, Reverse Trendelenburg, or Fowler, 30° insufflated

Insufflated abdomen

TABLE 2-7

Summary of Physiologic Effects of Tilting and Gas Insufflation

	PARAMETER	EFFECT
PULMONARY FUNCTION	Compliance	Decreased
	Functional residual capacity	Decreased
	Vital capacity	Decreased
	Intrathoracic pressure	Increased
	Peak inspiratory pressure	Increased
	Deadspace ventilation	Increased
	$PaCO_2$	Increased
	PaO_2	Decreased
CARDIOVASCULAR FUNCTION	Heart rate	Variable
	Mean arterial blood pressure	Increased
	Systemic vascular resistance	Increased
	Intracranial pressure	Increased
	Cardiac output	Decreased

CO_2 insufflation is an acceptable rule of thumb. Exceeding these limits leads to profound changes in physiologic performance during laparoscopic procedures.

Physiologic Considerations in Thoracoscopy

GAS INSUFFLATION FOR THORACOSCOPY

Insufflating the thorax minimally enhances the optical cavity, and pressures of as little as 5 mm Hg cause a significant reduction in cardiac output and mean arterial blood pressure in pentobarbital/isoflurane-anesthetized pigs.[129] An abnormal lung may require thoracic insufflation for adequate visualization; however, it must be applied with extreme caution. If the technique is used, it should only be applied for a short time, such as the time required to obtain a pleural biopsy. More invasive monitoring, including pulmonary arterial catheterization, is advised. Importantly, most modern insufflators are automated to self-adjust to changes in insufflation pressure. Accidental use of automatic settings in thoracic insufflation could lead to sustained, dangerous insufflation pressures.

Alternatively, limited insufflation of gas can be used to create a viewing space (pneumothorax) and discontinued. Pulmonary and hemodynamic effects of transient insufflation of the thorax with nitrous oxide were examined during thoracic lung biopsy procedures of dogs.* The thorax was insufflated to create pneumothorax and was maintained through the use of valved trocar cannulas. Insufflation pressures were not recorded but were presumed minimal. Ventilation was maintained with standard endotracheal intubation, a fixed tidal volume, and two-lung ventilation. The PaO_2 and total peripheral vascular resistance decreased during the procedure. The end-tidal CO_2 ($ETCO_2$), $PaCO_2$, clinical shunt fraction, systemic mean arterial blood pressure, heart rate, and cardiac output increased. Observed parameters were consistent with hypoventilation and hypercapnia. However, the clinical implications of these changes were considered minimal and acceptable in these normal, healthy patients breathing 100% oxygen.

ONE-LUNG VENTILATION

With the animal in lateral recumbency and using the mediastinum as a point of reference, the term *superior* will be applied to the superior, operative, nondependent, nonventilated lung, and the term *inferior* will be applied to the lower, nonoperative, dependent, ventilated lung (Fig. 2-1). One-lung ventilation, with collapse

---

*Faunt KK et al: Cardiopulmonary effects of two-lung ventilation and diagnostic thoracoscopy in the dog. *AJVR* 1998 (in press).

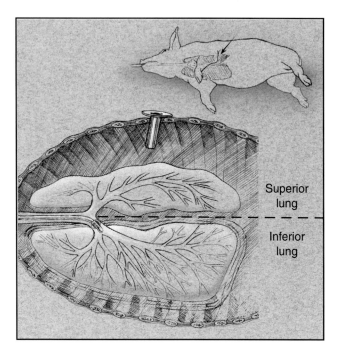

Fig. 2-1 One-lung ventilation. The animal is positioned in lateral recumbency. The mediastinum is used as a reference point for determining superior and inferior. The superior lung is not ventilated and becomes atelectatic to allow more working space inside the thorax. The inferior lung is ventilated.

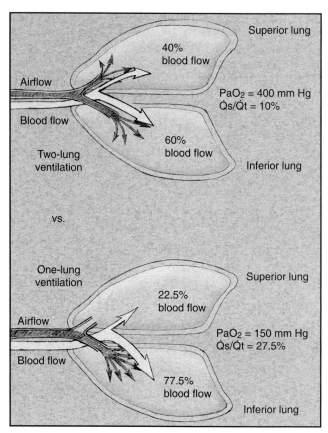

Fig. 2-2 Blood flow and oxygenation during one-lung and two-lung ventilation.

of the superior, operative lung and ventilation of the inferior, nonoperative lung, is mandatory for optimal, safe thoracoscopy. The physiologic consequences of one-lung ventilation have been reviewed.[130]

Ventilation-to-Perfusion Mismatching

One-lung ventilation leads to significant ventilation-to-perfusion mismatching that requires intensive support from the anesthetist. General anesthesia depresses central control mechanisms of respiration and leads to a reduction in lung volumes. Placing the anesthetized animal in lateral recumbency leads to ventilation-to-perfusion mismatching, with most of the tidal volume distributed to the superior lung. Approximately 40% of the cardiac output perfuses the superior lung, and 60% perfuses the inferior lung (Fig. 2-2). Lung volumes and ventilation-to-perfusion matching continue to decrease in the inferior lung as abdominal organs force the diaphragm forward, mediastinal structures compress from above, and restrictive positioning and roll pads compress the thorax. When mechanical ventilation is initiated and the first thoracic trocar is inserted, an open chest situation is created. Selective ventilation of the inferior lung allows the superior, operative lung to collapse (selective atelectasis), and the tidal volume is delivered only to the inferior, nonoperative lung.

Hypoxic Pulmonary Vasoconstriction

Before selective, one-lung ventilation is initiated, 40% of the cardiac output perfuses the superior lung while 60% perfuses the inferior lung (see Fig. 2-2). If the superior lung still received 40% of the blood flow after ventilation to it was discontinued, 40% of the cardiac output would not be involved in gas exchange. A right-to-left transpulmonary shunt would occur through the nonventilated lung. However, active vasoconstrictive mechanisms in the nonventilated lung reduce the blood flow and act to minimize this shunt. The most significant reduction in superior lung blood flow is due to increased pulmonary vascular resistance caused by constriction of the pulmonary vasculature of this atelectatic, hypoxic lung. This hypoxic pulmonary vasoconstriction (HPV) diverts blood flow away from the atelectatic lung and toward the ventilated lung, thus minimizing shunt. Even so, blood flow through the nonventilated superior lung remains 20% to 25% of the cardiac output (see Fig. 2-2). Passive mechanisms also contribute to increasing blood flow to the inferior lung, minimizing the shunt. Gravity creates a vertical gradient for blood flow, making blood flow to the superior lung less than to the inferior lung. Surgical compression and retraction, as well as pulmonary vascular ligation, also act mechanically to restrict blood flow to the superior lung.

Even though the inferior lung receives most of the cardiac output because of passive mechanical and active vasoconstrictive mechanisms, hypoxic compartments can develop in the inferior lung because of anesthesia, lateral posture, and mechanical compression. Obstructive secretions and fluid transudation contribute by causing airway closure. Oxygen is absorbed rapidly in regions with a low ventilation-to-perfusion ratio, producing absorption atelectasis. Hypoxic regions that develop in the inferior lung trigger focal HPV and increase vascular resistance, causing increased blood flow back to the nonventilated, superior lung.

Inhalation anesthetic agents inhibit HPV, but injectable anesthetics do not. With 1.0 MAC equivalent of isoflurane the HPV response is depressed 20%, increasing blood flow to the nonventilated, superior lung from 20% of the cardiac output to 24%. However, animal studies indicate that PaO_2 does not decrease any more with inhalation anesthetic agents than with injectable agents, suggesting that the effect of gas anesthetics on HPV is not extreme and may not be of clinical concern. The beneficial effects of inhalation anesthetics outweigh the minor effect on HPV.

Anesthetic Considerations

PREOPERATIVE EXAMINATION AND PATIENT SELECTION

Laparoscopy and thoracoscopy have important physiologic effects on the cardiovascular and respiratory systems. Physiologically normal animals usually compensate for the cardiopulmonary embarrassment satisfactorily. However, animals with cardiovascular, respiratory, or other concurrent disease may not be able to compensate. The purposes of a preoperative examination are to evaluate the animal's condition, identify coexisting disease, and optimize the cardiopulmonary and metabolic status before anesthesia. Coexisting diseases, such as diabetes and hyperthyroidism, should be regulated before any elective surgical procedure. As with open surgery, animals with systemic disease should have a more extensive examination of cardiopulmonary function before undergoing minimally invasive surgery. Based on the animal's physical status and surgical risk, the preoperative workup may include laboratory tests, chest radiographs, and an electrocardiogram.

ANESTHETIC TECHNIQUE
Premedication

The purpose of premedication is to provide sedation, analgesia, and amnesia while reducing secretions, anxiety,

and nausea and vomiting. Premedicants also smooth induction and reduce anesthetic requirements. Premedicants for endosurgery are not specifically different from those for open procedures. However, some considerations may affect the selection of a specific premedicant. Short-acting or reversible agents would be advised for an outpatient procedure. Anticholinergic agents are useful in thoracoscopy to reduce respiratory secretions, and prevent vasovagal reflex from visceral manipulation during laparoscopy. Administration of phenothiazines, such as acepromazine, may minimize nausea and vomiting, but some patients may not compensate well for the vasodilation they cause. Phenothiazines and barbiturates also will promote splenic engorgement, which might obscure the surgical field of view. Although morphine enhances postural hypotension and may interfere with bile duct surgery by causing spasm of the sphincter of Oddi, the use of narcotics is usually appropriate.[131] Alpha-2 adrenergic agonists, such as xylazine and medetomidine, are usually inappropriate because they significantly reduce cardiac output and increase pulmonary and systemic vascular resistance. These same complications are anticipated with gas insufflation and postural changes and might well be exacerbated with use of alpha-2 agonists. Nevertheless, alpha-2 agonists are useful in providing the profound sedation necessary for standing procedures in large animals.

Preemptive and Preventive Analgesia

Postoperative pain can be minimized by analgesics if they are given before surgical manipulation. *Preemptive analgesia* means minimizing postoperative pain by preventing exorbitant nociceptive signal transmission to the central nervous system, thereby preventing establishment of central sensitization. The term *preemptive analgesia* may be misleading because simply providing nociceptive blockade before stimulation does not ensure complete blockade, nor is it enough to prevent sensitization.[132] Postoperative pain is treated best by pre-, intra- and postoperative analgesic agents. Peripheral nociceptors, sensory nerve inflow, and central nervous system structures must all be addressed. Analgesia can be provided by nonsteroidal antiinflammatory agents, local anesthetics, alpha-2 adrenergic agonists, and opioids that are administered orally, locally, epidurally, intrathecally, and parenterally, alone or in combination. Central sensitization is related to inflammation from surgical manipulation. Minimally invasive surgical techniques minimize surgical manipulation, inflammation, and postoperative pain. Taken together, these maneuvers are better described as *preventive analgesia*.[132]

Anesthetic Maintenance

Minimally invasive surgical procedures differ from conventional surgery or diagnostic laparoscopy in that gas insufflation, tilted posture, and electrosurgery are usually used. Relaxation and a quiet operative field are important in endosurgery. Respiratory embarrassment and a potential for aspiration of gastric contents mandate use of general anesthesia and endotracheal intubation in small animals.

Selection of Inhalation Agent

General anesthesia provides muscle relaxation, analgesia, and amnesia; allows controlled ventilation; and minimizes operative field movement. Inhalation anesthetics are most often used to maintain general anesthesia. As for any surgery, the choice of inhalation anesthetic depends on the animal's condition and coexisting disease states, with a few additions.

NITROUS OXIDE Nitrous oxide (N_2O) is not recommended for several reasons. The cardiovascular effects of N_2O are not as nominal as often implied. N_2O does little to reduce the MAC of inhalation anesthetics in animals, even if the inspired percentage is high. The high percentage of N_2O needed to be effective leads to low inspired oxygen concentrations. It diffuses into hollow viscera, distending the intestine and interfering with the laparoscopic field of vision.

ISOFLURANE AND HALOTHANE Isoflurane is preferred over halothane because equipotent concentrations of isoflurane have less effect on autoregulation of cerebral blood flow, arrhythmogenicity, and cardiac contractility. All inhalation anesthetic agents lead to increased cerebral blood flow. This may be important when elevations in intracranial pressure are of concern, particularly in head-down tilt posture. Cerebral vasculature responds to changes in $PaCO_2$, or the pH change associated with changes in $PaCO_2$, by altering cerebral vascular tone and cerebral blood flow. This autoregulation of cerebral blood flow is altered by halothane but minimally by isoflurane. Therefore, cerebral blood flow may be reduced by reducing $PaCO_2$ during isoflurane, but not halothane, anesthesia. However, cerebral blood flow may be reduced by lowering $PaCO_2$ through hyperventilation immediately before exposure to halothane.

Hypercapnia associated with laparoscopy and thoracoscopy leads to elevated intracranial pressures and catecholamine levels. Halothane enhances myocardial sensitivity to the arrhythmic effect of catecholamines more than isoflurane does. Thus, arrhythmias may be more common with halothane anesthesia.

Two of the principal effects of tilted posture and gas insufflation are reduced cardiac output and increased systemic vascular resistance. Halothane depresses myocardial contractility more than isoflurane, whereas isoflurane tends to cause more vasodilation than halothane. In this way, isoflurane may minimize the cardiovascular effects of posture and insufflation, whereas halothane may exacerbate them.

Local and Regional Anesthesia

Local and regional anesthesia require the animal's cooperation and the anesthetist's patience for a successful outcome. Large animals in standing position under profound sedation have responded favorably to local and regional anesthetics for a limited number of minimally invasive procedures. However, organ manipulation causes pain, spontaneous ventilation is difficult with gas insufflation, and there is poor muscle relaxation.

EPIDURAL ANESTHESIA Epidural anesthesia and analgesia are attractive for intraoperative and postoperative management of pain because they are effective and they minimally depress the physiologic response to stressors such as elevated $PaCO_2$. For example, a single injection of 1 mL/5 kg (20 mL maximum) of 2% lidocaine or 0.5% bupivacaine into the lumbosacral epidural space produces anesthesia caudal to the diaphragm in dogs. However, there is at least partial motor block of the intercostal musculature with associated respiratory depression. More cranial spread depresses respiration further, making epidural anesthesia less than ideal for thoracoscopy.

Unlike single-injection epidural analgesia, selective and continuous epidural analgesia require epidural catheter placement, which introduces more difficulties. There is risk of infection and of causing damage to nervous tissues, as well as problems maintaining the catheters in place. Large animals undergoing standing laparoscopy could have segmental epidural anesthesia or analgesia, but they would remain at risk of posterior paresis, which could cause them to become unstable or drop into recumbency. Paralumbar anesthesia is an alternative for standing procedure in large animals.

INTERCOSTAL NERVE BLOCK Intraoperative and postoperative anesthetic and analgesic techniques for thoracoscopy include, but are not limited to, intercostal nerve block and intrapleural infusion. The ease of application makes these techniques very attractive. Because of overlapping innervation, it is necessary to block at least three consecutive intercostal nerves. It is best to block the intercostal nerve in the space occupied by the cannula, plus two intercostal nerves cranial and two intercostal nerves caudal to the site. In dogs, 0.5 to 1.0 mL of 0.5% bupivacaine (2 mg/kg maximum dose) is injected just caudal to the rib and dorsally near the intervertebral foramen.

INTRAPLEURAL BLOCK Intrapleural block involves simple infusion and diffusion. In dogs, air and fluid are aspirated through a chest tube placed before recovery. Bupivacaine, 1.5 mg/kg of 0.5% solution, is injected into the pleural space through the chest tube, followed immediately by 3 to 5 mL of sterile saline flush. The animal is positioned with the treated side inferior for approximately 20 minutes. Gravity causes the local anesthetic to pool and diffuse into the entry wound site. Pain should be relieved for 3 to 5 hours.

Neuromuscular Blocking Agents

A firm abdominal wall is desirable during insertion of trocars. However, use of neuromuscular blocking agents after cannula placement helps maximize abdominal distention while minimizing intraabdominal pressure. Neuromuscular blocking agents should not be used unless a stable plane of anesthesia and properly controlled ventilation have been established.

Airway Management

Intubation

Endotracheal intubation helps protect against aspiration of gastric contents and allows controlled ventilation to prevent hypercapnia and hypoxia. Intubation techniques and endotracheal tube choices are the same as for standard procedures. If lasers are used, a laser-protected endotracheal tube may be necessary. One-lung ventilation techniques require specialized endotracheal tubes. Changing posture may lead to endotracheal tube migration and endobronchial intubation if the tube is not properly secured.

Ventilation

Management of ventilation in endosurgical patients under general anesthesia is accomplished best by intermittent positive pressure ventilation. In practice, ventilation is increased to compensate for increasing $PaCO_2$.[26,133] Minute ventilation and inspiratory pressure are increased to overcome CO_2 absorption and the pulmonary effects of elevated IAP.[13,119,133] Overall minute ventilation must be increased 20% to 30% to maintain eucapnia.[104]

POSITIVE END-EXPIRATORY PRESSURE Positive end-expiratory pressure (PEEP) prevents airway pressure from returning to zero, keeps small airways splinted open, and prevents atelectasis. Unfortunately, PEEP also compromises venous return, pulmonary vascular resistance, and cardiac output. PEEP has been used in an attempt to improve gas exchange during laparoscopy.[134,135] Although ventilation improved somewhat, PEEP as low as 5 cm H_2O, in association with elevated IAPs, exacerbated the adverse cardiovascular effects of PEEP alone.[29] Positive end-expiratory pressure should be used with caution during laparoscopy.

ABSORPTION ATELECTASIS As small airways connecting to alveoli are underventilated or obstructed, oxygen within the alveoli is absorbed and the alveoli collapse. This is called *absorption atelectasis*. Normally, the nitrogen of room air splints the alveoli open as oxygen is absorbed. Increasing the inspired and alveolar oxygen concentrations and nitrogen washout in this situation promotes absorption atelectasis. Decreasing the inspired oxygen concentration to 50% may help minimize absorption atelectasis. In clinical situations, the beneficial effects of using high inspired O_2 concentrations usually outweigh the potential for causing limited absorption at-

electasis. When ventilation is difficult or PaO_2 values are low, reducing the IAP to the lowest pressure possible without interfering with the surgeon's field of view should be tried first. Neuromuscular blocking agents can be applied to maximize abdominal wall relaxation and distention while minimizing intraabdominal pressure.

PERMISSIVE HYPERCAPNIA The respiratory embarrassment and CO_2 absorption associated with laparoscopy and thoracoscopy are usually managed by maintaining a $PaCO_2$ of 40 mm Hg and a pH of 7.40 (as measured at 37° C). To accomplish this, increased inspiratory pressure, rate, or tidal volume may be necessary. If an animal has lung disease, ventilation with conventional tidal volumes may cause alveolar overdistention and lung injury. If mechanical inspiratory pressures or tidal volumes are intentionally limited to diminish possible alveolar overdistention, hypercapnia may develop. Permissive hypercapnia involves accepting hypercapnia and associated acidemia to avoid the potentially negative effects of mechanical ventilation.[136] Application of permissive hypercapnia is common in equine anesthesia, and its potentially beneficial cardiovascular effects have been described.[137]

EFFECTS OF HYPERCAPNIA Before using permissive hypercapnia, its effects must be understood (Box 2-1). High blood levels and alveolar concentrations of CO_2 can

---

BOX 2-1

EFFECTS OF HYPERCAPNIA

Cardiovascular Effects

↑Cardiac output
↓Peripheral vascular resistance
↑Blood pressure
↓Contractility
Cardiac arrhythmias

Pulmonary Effects

Hypoxemia

Other Physiologic Effects

Oxyhemoglobin dissociation curve shifts to the right, promoting downloading of oxygen from Hb
Tissue acidosis—↓intracellular pH
- Alteration of transmembrane electrolyte transport
- Alteration of glucose utilization
- Alteration of amino acid structure-function relationship
- SANS stimulation
- Release of epinephrine, norepinephrine
- ↑Cerebral blood flow
- ↑Intracranial pressure

contribute to hypoxemia. The alveolar gas equation, $PAO_2 = (PB - PH_2O)F_IO_2 - PaCO_2/R$, in which PAO_2 is the alveolar partial pressure of oxygen, PB is the barometric pressure, PH_2O is the vapor pressure of water, F_IO_2 is the fractional inspired oxygen concentration, $PaCO_2$ is the arterial partial pressure of carbon dioxide, and R is the respiratory quotient ($\dot{V}CO_2/\dot{V}O_2 \cong 0.8$), demonstrates this effect. Hypoxemia may be remedied by administering supplemental oxygen.

Hypercapnia may cause tissue acidosis, resulting in decreased intracellular pH and altered transmembrane electrolyte transport, glucose utilization, and structure-function relationships of amino acids. Neurologic sequelae of hypercapnia include sympathetic nervous stimulation with release of epinephrine and norepinephrine, significant increases in cerebral blood flow, and elevation of intracranial pressures. Hypercapnia also leads to increased cardiac output, decreased peripheral vascular resistance, and increased arterial blood pressure. As pH falls, left ventricular contractility is decreased in dogs, but cardiac output is still increased.[138] Decreasing pH also causes a shift in the oxyhemoglobin dissociation curve to the right, promoting release of oxygen from hemoglobin. Cardiac arrhythmias are reported with $PaCO_2$ levels above 80 mm Hg, but this observation may vary with species.[136,139,140] Type I hearts (dog, cat, human) tend to be more arrhythmic than type II hearts (horse, cow, pig).

Maintaining eucapnia is more important during one-lung ventilation. Hypocapnia may directly inhibit HPV of the nonventilated lung. Hypercapnia may increase pulmonary vascular resistance of the ventilated lung. Both lead to increased shunt.

GUIDELINES FOR USING PERMISSIVE HYPERCAPNIA If permissive hypercapnia is used, the $PaCO_2$ should be maintained below 80 mm Hg, the pH above 7.2, and the PaO_2 well above 60 mm Hg. A blood gas analyzer is mandatory for prompt, accurate decision-making. Neuromuscular blockade may be required to control excessive spontaneous respiratory movements.

One-Lung Ventilation Techniques

Three techniques are used to establish one-lung ventilation: bronchial blockade, endobronchial intubation, and double-lumen endotracheal tube application (Fig. 2-3).

BRONCHIAL BLOCKADE One of the first one-lung ventilation techniques involved simple bronchial blockade with gauze packing. Today, Fogarty occlusion catheters, Foley balloon-tipped catheters, and Swan-Ganz catheters are used to occlude the mainstem bronchus of the nonventilated, superior lung (Fig. 2-4). The balloon-tipped catheter is inserted into the bifurcation of the trachea, and a single-lumen endotracheal tube is passed beside it. A fiberoptic bronchoscope is passed through the lumen of the endotracheal tube to guide the balloon-tipped catheter into the mainstem bronchus of

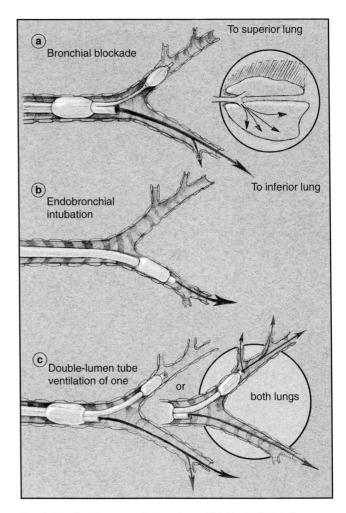

Fig. 2-3 One-lung ventilation. Bronchial blockade (a). A bronchial blocker prevents ventilation of the superior operative lung. The tip of an endotracheal tube remains in the trachea, and the inferior lung is ventilated. Endobronchial intubation (b). An endobronchial tube is placed in the mainstem bronchus of the inferior lung. The inferior lung is ventilated, and the superior lung is allowed to collapse. Double-lumen endotracheal tube (c). The double-lumen tube allows ventilation of both lungs or selective ventilation of either lung.

the superior lung. The endotracheal tube cuff can then be inflated. The bronchial blocker is not inflated until the superior lung has been allowed to collapse. The lumen of the bronchial blocker is used for aspiration and continuous positive airway pressure (CPAP). The Univent* endotracheal tube, which has a built-in, movable, bronchial blocking balloon-tipped catheter, has been used successfully in dogs (Fig. 2-5).[141] Bronchial blockers can be placed easily and swiftly, but they can become dislodged intraoperatively, possibly obstructing ventilation of either or both lungs. Frequent broncho-

*Univent, Fuji Systems Corp, 1-11-1 Ebisu, Shibuya-ku Tokyo 150, Japan.

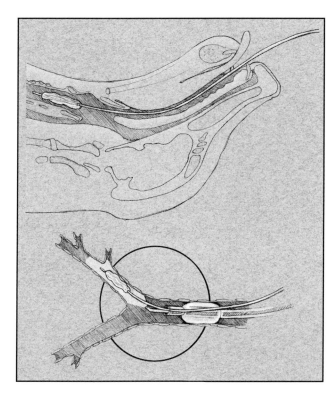

Fig. 2-4 Use of a bronchial blocker for one-lung ventilation. A balloon-tipped catheter is inserted to the bifurcation of the trachea. A single-lumen endotracheal tube is passed beside the catheter. A fiberoptic bronchoscope is passed through the lumen of the endotracheal tube to guide the balloon-tipped catheter into the mainstem bronchus of the superior lung. The endotracheal tube cuff is inflated. The bronchial blocker is inflated after the superior lung has been allowed to collapse.

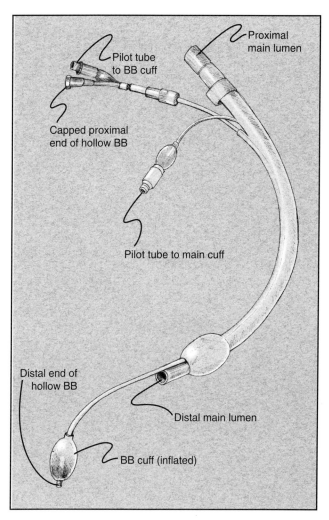

Fig. 2-5 Univent Bronchial Blocker. The bronchial blocker (BB) is an integral part of the endotracheal tube.

scopic monitoring of the balloon blocker position is recommended.

ENDOBRONCHIAL INTUBATION Endobronchial intubation is performed by using an endotracheal tube with a diameter smaller than the bronchus to be intubated (Fig. 2-6). The endotracheal tube is passed into the mainstem bronchus of the ventilated, inferior lung by using a bronchoscope as a guide. Careful placement and rotation to position the end-hole and the side-hole (Murphy eye) of the endobronchial tube prevent occlusion of early branching lobar bronchioles. Inaccurately positioning the bronchial cuff can lead to inadequate ventilation and accidental displacement of the tube. Endobronchial intubation does not provide a means for aspiration or intermittent ventilation of the nonventilated, superior lung. In some species, the right cranial lung lobe may not be ventilated when the right mainstem bronchus is selectively intubated. Infrequently, the tip of the endotracheal tube cannot be guided over the bronchoscope into the desired bronchus. This is usually caused by a mediastinal shift associated with atelectasis of the inferior lung after pro-

longed lateral recumbency, or by a disease process. If the endotracheal tube diameter is appropriate, successful selective intubation is almost always achieved with the animal in dorsal recumbency.

DOUBLE-LUMEN TUBES Double-lumen tubes provide a simple means of controlling ventilation of either lung (see Fig. 2-3, c). The tubes are designed specifically for placement in either right or left human mainstem bronchi. This specific design does not necessarily work in animals. A right- or left-oriented double-lumen endotracheal tube is passed the length of the trachea and rotated to seat in the appropriate mainstem bronchus. Blind placement of the double-lumen endotracheal tube is inaccurate even in humans,[142] so a fiberoptic bronchoscope is passed through the lumen of the endotracheal tube to guide final positioning (Fig. 2-7). Double-lumen tubes allow ventilation, aspiration, and insufflation of either lung, but they offer greater resistance because of their smaller lumen diameter.

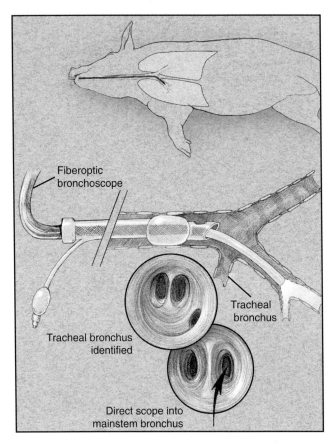

Fig. 2-6 Endobronchial intubation. The single-lumen tube is passed and guided into position with a fiberoptic broncho-scope. The tracheal bronchus assists in identifying the right mainstem bronchus in pigs and oxen.

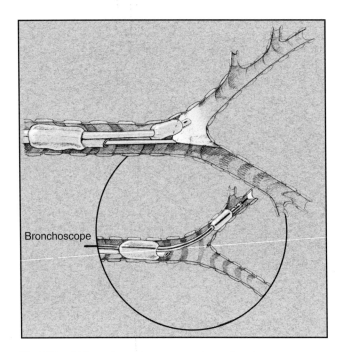

Fig. 2-7 Using a bronchoscope to determine the correct po-sition of a double-lumen tube.

POTENTIAL COMPLICATIONS No matter which tech-nique is chosen for one-lung ventilation, overinflation of the sealing balloon or cuff can cause several problems (Fig. 2-8). Overinflation can cause the tube or catheter to be dislodged from its position. When dislodged, ven-tilation may not be possible and the cuff or balloon may partially or completely obstruct airflow to one or both lungs. Overinflation of the cuff or balloon may displace the tracheal carina to the contralateral side and obstruct airflow, which can lead to inadequate ventilation or in-appropriate collapse of the contralateral lung. Overin-flation can lead to obstruction of cranial lobar bronchi-oles branching from the mainstem bronchus, causing in-adequate ventilation. Overinflation of the endobronchial

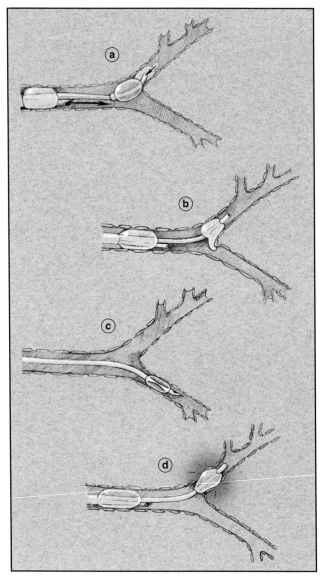

Fig. 2-8 Difficulties with cuff overinflation. The tube backs out of the mainstem bronchus (*a*). The carina deviates or the cuff herniates over the tracheal carina (*b*). The endobronchial tube collapses (*c*). Trachea or mainstem bronchus ruptures (*d*).

tube cuff may also lead to collapse of the tube lumen, particularly when thin-walled or silicone tubes are used. Further overinflation can lead to bronchial or tracheal rupture. With endobronchial intubation, passing the tube too far causes inadequate ventilation of the intubated lung (Fig. 2-9).

TECHNIQUE The choice of method for inducing one-lung ventilation may vary with the species. Pigs and oxen have a tracheal bronchus on the right side that branches well ahead of the mainstem bronchi and supplies ventilation to the right cranial lung lobe (Fig. 2-10). If the right lung is the operative site, endobronchial intubation of the left mainstem bronchus may be the simplest way to establish one-lung ventilation. If the left lung is the operative site, a bronchial blocker placed in the left mainstem bronchus with an endotracheal tube stopping proximal to the tracheal bronchus may provide simpler airway control and more effective ventilation to the right lung. Lobar bronchioles branch early in smaller species. Any cuff or balloon placed in the mainstem bronchus is likely to occlude some of these bronchi despite careful placement. Accidental occlusion of lobar bronchioles or passing the endobronchial tube deep into the airway prevents ventilation of the cranial lung region.

Ensuring proper collapse of the superior lung is the responsibility of the anesthetist (Fig. 2-11). After the surgeon penetrates the parietal pleura, breaking the surface tension and abolishing the negative intrathoracic pressure, the lung will begin to collapse because of its elastic nature. This is not an instantaneous process, so patience is advised. However, delayed collapse may occur for a number of reasons. If adhesions to the thoracic wall prevent collapse, adhesiolysis will be necessary to free the lung. Parenchymal disease of the lung may prevent regional or general lung collapse, possibly requiring conversion to a thoracotomy. Improper collapse of the superior lung can occur with obstruction of gas outflow. With endobronchial intubation, the tube could be incorrectly located, or the cuff overinflated or displaced, obstructing gas escape from the superior lung. Halting ventilation

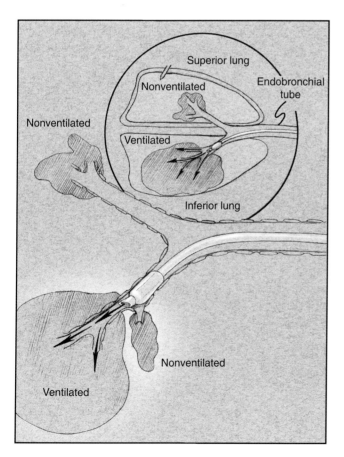

Fig. 2-9   The endobronchial tube may be passed too far, causing inadequate ventilation of the inferior lung.

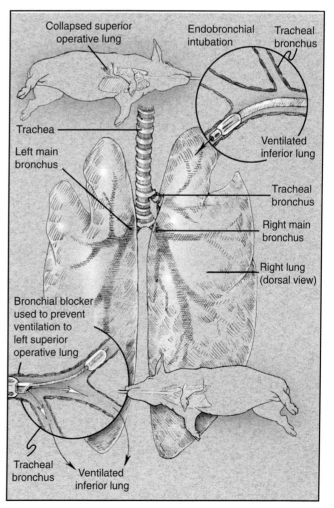

Fig. 2-10   The tracheal bronchus identifies the right lung and is a landmark for endobronchial intubation guided by a fiberoptic bronchoscope. See text for further description.

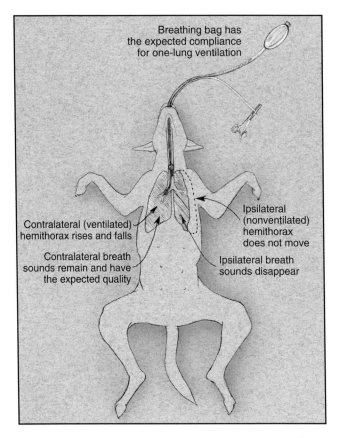

Fig. 2-11 Subjective visual and auditory cues of proper selective intubation.

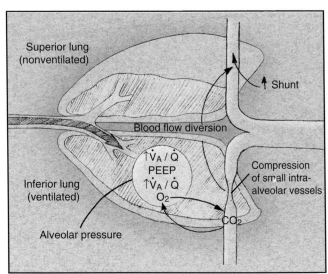

Fig. 2-12 PEEP in the inferior lung increases the vascular resistance and increases the shunt during one-lung ventilation.

and deflating any cuffs or balloons for 30 seconds may assist collapse of the superior lung. Proper replacement must be confirmed by fiberoptic bronchoscopy. Excessive positive pressure ventilation or PEEP of the inferior lung may prevent collapse of the superior lung when using double-lumen tubes. Premature or excessive application of CPAP to the superior lung also prevents proper collapse.

MANAGEMENT One-lung ventilation begins with administration of high concentrations of O_2. Administration of 100% O_2 prevents hypoxic pulmonary vasoconstriction (HPV) in the ventilated, inferior lung, and special ventilation techniques help prevent excessive ventilation-to-perfusion mismatching. The ventilated, inferior lung will be responsible for all gas exchange and will need to carry the normal tidal volume of 10 mL/kg alone. If inspiratory pressure exceeds normal ranges (15 cm H_2O), increased pulmonary vascular resistance will develop and blood flow will increase to the nonventilated, superior lung. High tidal volumes and intermittent hyperventilation are not beneficial. Instead, to maintain eucapnia the respiratory rate must be increased by approximately 20%. Hypocapnia should be avoided because it leads to increased pulmonary vascular resis-

tance in the inferior lung and inhibits HPV in the superior lung.

Ventilation techniques may involve the use of PEEP, CPAP, or both (Fig. 2-12). PEEP is applied to the ventilated, inferior lung to minimize atelectasis. Pressures higher than 5 cm H_2O will increase pulmonary vascular resistance in the inferior lung and increase blood flow through the nonventilated, superior lung.

CPAP is applied to the superior lung by administering 100% O_2 at 5 to 10 cm H_2O. This permits oxygen up-take in the superior lung without preventing hypoxic pulmonary vasoconstriction, but high levels of CPAP obstruct the surgeon's thoracoscopic view. PEEP can be combined with CPAP (Fig. 2-13). PEEP limits atelectasis in the inferior lung. Blood diverted to the superior, nonventilated lung is oxygenated by CPAP. However, this may be technically difficult without specialized equipment.

VIGILANCE MONITORING
Guidelines for routine vigilance monitoring during anesthesia are available from the American College of Veterinary Anesthesiologists (ACVA).[143,144] The anesthetist should also be attentive to the degree of tilt, the IAP, and blood gas levels.

Rule of the 15's
Posture and gas insufflation affect the physiologic status of endosurgical patients. Most of the physiologic effect is due to CO_2 gas insufflation, with associated increases in IAP and CO_2 absorption. Applying the Rule of the 15's (15 mm Hg IAP; 15° tilt up or down) when insufflating the abdomen with CO_2 should be within safe limits for normal animals. Exceeding these limits may lead

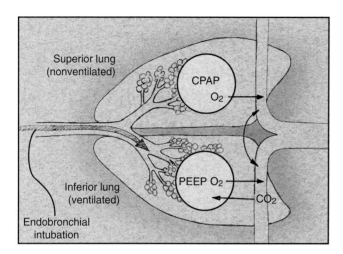

Fig. 2-13 When PEEP is combined with CPAP, blood flow diverted from the lung receiving PEEP is oxygenated in the lung receiving CPAP, and the amount of blood unavailable for gas exchange (left-to-right shunt) is reduced.

to profound changes in physiologic status during endosurgical procedures. Increased abdominal pressure and tilting are increased risks for animals with cardiopulmonary abnormalities.

Ventilation and Gas Exchange Monitoring

Obtaining blood gas values to monitor $PaCO_2$ and PaO_2 is highly recommended, especially during one-lung ventilation. The PaO_2 will provide information on gas exchange and the degree of shunting. Typically, PaO_2 is not decreased to levels of clinical concern when high inspired oxygen concentrations are used in laparoscopy. Nevertheless, hypoventilation, ventilation-to-perfusion mismatching, increased shunt, and elevated $PaCO_2$ may affect oxygenation. Pulse oximetry can be used to provide indirect, moment-to-moment indications of hemoglobin saturation with oxygen. The absorption of CO_2 and adequacy of ventilation must be monitored by measuring $PaCO_2$. Investigators have attempted to use end-tidal carbon dioxide ($ETCO_2$) measurements during CO_2 insufflation to estimate the blood $PaCO_2$. However, the $PaCO_2$-$ETCO_2$ gradient was increased and did not indicate the severity of hypercapnia.* Parameters of ventilation, such as tidal volume, peak inspiratory pressure, and minute volume, should also be monitored.

Blood Pressure Monitoring

Arterial blood pressure may not correlate well with cardiac output or oxygen delivery because the combination of posture changes and gas insufflation result in increased systemic vascular resistance and reduced cardiac output. Central venous pressures will not be accurate.

---

*References 92, 117, 119, 133, 145.

Transmural central pressures are necessary to evaluate venous return and volume overload. Animals with cardiopulmonary abnormalities may require more invasive monitoring such as pulmonary arterial catheterization and thermodilution cardiac output determination.

Evaluating Blood Loss

Blood loss may be overestimated due to magnification of the field of view and a false perception of excessive hemorrhage during laparoscopic procedures. Conversely, tilted posture causes blood to move out of the field of view, leading to underestimation of blood loss. To estimate blood loss, the cavity is irrigated with saline and aspirated completely. The volume of blood aspirated is calculated by the following formula:

$$\frac{PCV\ (fluid) \times volume\ (fluid)}{PCV\ (animal)} = blood\ loss$$

Volume replacement therapy is similar to that in an equivalent "open" surgical procedure. However, normal insensible fluid loss is not as great because of reduced evaporative fluid loss. The clinical significance of this effect may be limited to animals in which volume load is of concern. Urine output can be used to monitor volume load but also should be monitored because of the potential for oliguria with increased IAP.

COMPLICATIONS

Complications associated with the endosurgical approach are discussed in Chapter 6. However, two critical complications demand emphasis and brief discussion: (1) gas embolism and (2) pneumothorax and pneumomediastinum.

Gas Embolism

Gas embolism is a rare but potentially fatal complication of endoscopic surgery.[146-149] Gas embolism can occur in several ways. The Veress-type insufflation needle may accidentally penetrate a large vessel or the spleen, and CO_2 may be injected directly into the venous system. Tilted posture and elevated IAP promote gas entrance into open veins. A CO_2 laser may accidentally inject CO_2 into a blood vessel.

The adverse effects of gas embolism include collection of gas bubbles in the right heart and pulmonary vasculature, reduced right heart end-diastolic volumes, increased pulmonary deadspace ventilation, reduced cardiac output and pulmonary gas exchange, and subsequent reduced blood pressure and PaO_2. A classic "mill-wheel" murmur, systemic hypotension, pulmonary hypertension, decreased $ETCO_2$, hypoxemia, and transesophageal echocardiographic evidence are indicative of gas embolism.[150] Treatment requires discontinuation of insufflation, moving the animal to left lateral recumbency, cardiac massage, and aspiration of the gas by central venous catheterization.

Pneumothorax and Pneumomediastinum

Pneumothorax and pneumomediastinum can occur in several ways.[151] With elevated IAP, the peak inspiratory pressure must be increased, which may cause air to escape from ruptured alveoli and travel down the sheaths of the pulmonary vessels into the mediastinum, thoracic cavity, pericardial space, subcutaneous tissues, or retroperitoneal spaces. During laparoscopy, gas insufflated into the abdomen can dissect around or through the diaphragm via anatomic defects. Gas may also be introduced by direct, accidental penetration of the diaphragm or dissect down retroperitoneal tracts. Pneumothorax is evident by elevated peak inspiratory pressures, hypoxemia, tachypnea, tachycardia, hypotension, and loss of breath sounds on auscultation. The attentive anesthetist can observe lung collapse and pneumothorax through the central tendon of the diaphragm by watching the video monitor. The pneumothorax is essentially a tension pneumothorax because elevated abdominal pressure continues to force air into the thoracic cavity. The elevated pressure can easily collapse both lungs, even in species with a complete mediastinum. Treatment requires immediate discontinuation of insufflation, deflation of the abdomen, placement of a chest tube with a Heimlich valve or low-pressure pleural aspiration, and ventilatory support.

Other Anesthetic Complications

Other potential complications include vasovagal reflex, intraperitoneal carbon monoxide induced by electrocautery smoke, explosion of intestinal gas presumably supported by nitrous oxide, and hyperkalemia associated with CO_2 insufflation.[89,152-156] Hyperkalemia may be of interest to equine anesthesiologists when CO_2 insufflation is used in animals known or suspected of being genetically predisposed to hyperkalemic periodic paralysis.[157]

POSTOPERATIVE MANAGEMENT

Local anesthetic infiltration of trocar sites can be performed to reduce postoperative pain. Cardiopulmonary monitoring should continue until complete recovery. Carbon dioxide absorption continues into the recovery period, and delayed embolic episodes are possible. Hypotension follows the release of IAP because of a sudden decrease in systemic vascular resistance.[26,158] Hypovolemic and cardiovascular-compromised animals will not compensate in this situation, and vasoconstrictors may be the treatment of choice. Certain laparoscopic procedures impair postoperative diaphragmatic function[7]; however, pulmonary function is often better than after an open approach.[8] Decreased PaO_2 has been noted during the recovery phase of laparoscopy of dogs, and animals should be observed and monitored for signs of hypoxemia.[26]

REFERENCES

1. Schirmer B et al: Laparoscopic cholecystectomy: treatment of choice for symptomatic cholelithiasis. *Ann Surg* 213:665-677, 1991.
2. Cigarini I et al: Pain and pulmonary dysfunction after cholecystectomy under laparoscopy and laparotomy. *Anesthesiology* 75:A122, 1991.
3. McAnena O et al: Laparoscopic versus open appendectomy. *Lancet* 338:693, 1991.
4. Messina MJ et al: Laparoscopy-assisted vaginal hysterectomy: cost analysis and review of initial experience in a community hospital. *JAOA* 95:31-36, 1995.
5. Group OLS: Postoperative adhesion development after operative laparoscopy: evaluation at early second-look procedures. *Fertil Steril* 55:700-704, 1991.
6. Nezhat C et al: Adhesion reformation after reproductive surgery by videolaseroscopy. *Fertil Steril* 53:1008-1011, 1990.
7. Erice F et al: Diaphragmatic function before and after laparoscopic cholecystectomy. *Anesthesiology* 79:966-975, 1993.
8. Frazee R et al: Open versus laparoscopic cholecystectomy: a comparison of postoperative pulmonary function. *Ann Surg* 213:651-653, 1991.
9. Lewis R et al: One hundred consecutive patients undergoing video-assisted thoracic operations. *Ann Thorac Surg* 54:421-426, 1992.
10. Joris J et al: Metabolic and respiratory changes after cholecystectomy performed via laparotomy or laparoscopy. *Br J Anaesth* 69:341-345, 1992.
11. Barnes G et al: Cardiovascular responses to elevation of intra-abdominal hydrostatic pressure. *Am J Physiol* 248:R208-R213, 1985.
12. Cullen D et al: Cardiovascular, pulmonary, and renal effects of massively increased intra-abdominal pressure in critically ill patients. *Crit Care Med* 17:118-121, 1989.
13. Richardson J, Trinkle J: Hemodynamic and respiratory alterations with increased intra-abdominal pressure. *J Surg Res* 20:401-404, 1976.
14. Obeid F et al: Increases in intra-abdominal pressure affect pulmonary compliance. *Arch Surg* 130:544-547, 1995.
15. Oikkonen M, Tallgren M: Changes in respiratory compliance at laparoscopy: measurements using side stream spirometry. *Can J Anaesth* 42:495-497, 1995.
16. Leighton T et al: Effectors of hypercarbia during experimental pneumoperitoneum. *Am Surg* 58:717-721, 1992.
17. Gross M et al: Effects of abdominal insufflation with nitrous oxide on cardiorespiratory measurements in spontaneously breathing isoflurane anesthetized dogs. *Am J Vet Res* 54:1352-1358, 1993.
18. Gilroy R et al: Respiratory mechanical effects of abdominal distention. *J Appl Physiol* 58:1997-2003, 1985.
19. Leighton T, Liu S-Y, Bongard F: Comparative cardiopulmonary effects of carbon dioxide versus helium pneumoperitoneum. *Surgery* 113:527-531, 1993.
20. Ivankovich A et al: Cardiovascular effects of intraperitoneal insufflation with carbon dioxide and nitrous oxide in the dog. *Anesthesiology* 42:281-287, 1975.
21. Lister D et al: Carbon dioxide absorption is not linearly related to intraperitoneal carbon dioxide insufflation pressure in pigs. *Anesthesiology* 80:129-136, 1994.
22. Bongard F et al: Adverse consequences of increased intra-abdominal pressure on bowel tissue. *J Trauma* 39:519-525, 1995.

23. Ishizaki Y et al: Safe intraabdominal pressure of carbon dioxide pneumoperitoneum during laparoscopic surgery. *Surgery* 114:549-554, 1993.

24. Mullet C et al: Pulmonary CO_2 elimination during surgical procedures using intra- or extraperitoneal CO_2 insufflation. *Anesth Analg* 76:622-626, 1993.

25. Wolf J et al: Carbon dioxide absorption during laparoscopic pelvic operation. *J Am Coll Surg* 180:555-560, 1995.

26. Duke T, Steinacher S, Remedios A: Cardiopulmonary effects of using carbon dioxide for laparoscopic surgery in dogs. *Vet Surg* 25:77-82, 1996.

27. Reich D et al: Do Trendelenburg and passive leg raising improve cardiac performance? *Anesth Analg* 67:S184, 1988.

28. Smith I et al: Cardiovascular effects of peritoneal insufflation of carbon dioxide for laparoscopy. *Br Med J* 14:410-411, 1971.

29. Moffa S, Quinn J, Slotman G: Hemodynamic effects of carbon dioxide pneumoperitoneum during mechanical ventilation and positive end-expiratory pressure. *J Trauma* 35:613-618, 1993.

30. Diamant M, Benumof J, Saidman L: Hemodynamics of increased intra-abdominal pressure: interaction with hypovolemia and halothane anesthesia. *Anesthesiology* 48:23-27, 1978.

31. Toomasian J et al: Hemodynamic changes following pneumoperitoneum and graded hemorrhage in dogs. *Surg Forum* 29:32-33, 1978.

32. Eisenhauer D et al: Hemodynamic effects of argon pneumoperitoneum. *Surg Endosc* 8:315-321, 1994.

33. Kashtan J et al: Hemodynamic effects of increased abdominal pressure. *J Surg Res* 30:249-255, 1981.

34. Caldwell C, Ricotta J: Changes in visceral blood flow with elevated intraabdominal pressure. *J Surg Res* 43:14-20, 1987.

35. Harman P et al: Elevated intra-abdominal pressure and renal function. *Ann Surg* 196:594-597, 1982.

36. Lynch F et al: Cardiovascular effects of increased intra-abdominal pressure in newborn piglets. *J Pediatr Surg* 9:621-626, 1974.

37. Diebel L, Saxe J, Dulchavsky S: Effect of intra-abdominal pressure on abdominal wall blood flow. *Am Surg* 58:573-576, 1992.

38. Diebel L et al: Effect of increased intra-abdominal pressure on hepatic arterial, portal venous, and hepatic microcirculatory blood flow. *J Trauma* 33:279-283, 1992.

39. Ho H, Gunther R, Wolfe B: Intraperitoneal carbon dioxide insufflation and cardiopulmonary functions: laparoscopic cholecystectomy in pigs. *Arch Surg* 127:928-933, 1992.

40. Robotham J, Wise R, Bromberger-Barnea B: Effects of changes in abdominal pressure on left ventricular performance and regional blood flow. *Crit Care Med* 13:803-809, 1985.

41. Shimizu M et al: Acute effect of intra-abdominal pressure on liver and systemic circulation. *Vasc Surg* 24:677-682, 1990.

42. Diebel L, Dulchavsky S, Wilson R: Effect of increased intra-abdominal pressure on mesenteric arterial and intestinal mucosal blood flow. *J Trauma* 33:45-49, 1992.

43. Richards W et al: Acute renal failure with increased intra-abdominal pressure. *Ann Surg* 197:183-187, 1983.

44. Probst C, Webb A: Postural influence on systemic blood pressure, gas exchange, and acid/base status in the term-pregnant bitch during general anesthesia. *Am J Vet Res* 44:1963-1965, 1983.

45. Southorn P, Rehder K, Hyatt R: Halothane anesthesia and respiratory mechanics in dogs lying supine. *J Appl Physiol* 49:300-305, 1980.

46. Nyman G, Funkquist B, Kvart C: Postural effects on blood gas tension, blood pressure, heart rate, ECG and respiratory rate during prolonged anesthesia in the horse. *Zentralbl Veterinarmend [A]* 35:54-62, 1988.

47. Schatzmann U et al: Effect of postural changes on certain circulatory and respiratory values in the horse. *Am J Vet Res* 43:1003-1005, 1982.

48. Case E, Stiles J: The effect of various surgical positions on vital capacity. *Anesthesiology* 7:29-31, 1946.

49. Henschel A et al: Posture as it concerns the anesthesiologist: a preliminary study. *Anesth Analg* 36:69-76, 1957.

50. Jones J, Jacoby J: The effect of surgical positions on respirations. *Surg Forum* 5:686, 1955.

51. Chiang S, Lyons H: The effect of postural change on pulmonary compliance. *Resp Physiol* 1:99-105, 1966.

52. Wood-Smith F, Horne G, Nunn J: Effects of posture on ventilation of patients anaesthetized with halothane. *Anaesthesia* 16:340-345, 1961.

53. Scott D, Slawson K: Respiratory effects of prolonged Trendelenburg position. *Br J Anaesth* 40:103-107, 1968.

54. Fahy B et al: Effects of Trendelenburg and reverse Trendelenburg postures on lung and chest wall mechanics. *J Clin Anesth* 8:236-244, 1996.

55. Guyton A: Circulatory shock and physiology of its treatment. In Textbook of medical physiology, ed 9, Philadelphia, 1996, WB Saunders.

56. Tomaselli C et al: Cardiovascular dynamics during the initial period of head-down tilt. *Aviat Space Environ Med* 58:3-8, 1987.

57. Sibbald W et al: The Trendelenburg position: hemodynamic effects in hypotensive and normotensive patients. *Crit Care Med* 7:218-224, 1979.

58. Abel F, Pierce J, Guntheroth W: Baroreceptor influence on postural changes in blood pressure and carotid blood flow. *Am J Physiol* 205:360-364, 1963.

59. Guntheroth W, Abel F, Mullins G: The effect of Trendelenburg's position on blood pressure and carotid flow. *Surg Gynecol Obstet* 119:345-348, 1964.

60. Slinker B et al: Arterial baroreceptor control of heart rate in horse, pig and calf. *Am J Vet Res* 43:1926-1933, 1982.

61. Shenkin H et al: Effect of change in position upon cerebral circulation of man. *J Appl Physiol* 2:317-326, 1949.

62. Hainsworth R, Al-Shamma Y: Cardiovascular responses to upright tilting in healthy subjects. *Clin Sci* 74:17-22, 1988.

63. Matalon S, Farhi L: Cardiopulmonary readjustments in passive tilt. *J Appl Physiol* 47:503-507, 1979.

64. Bagshaw R, Cox R: Nitrous oxide and the baroreceptor reflexes in the dog. *Acta Anaesthesiol Scand* 26:31-38, 1982.

65. Duke P, Fownes D, Wade J: Halothane depresses baroreflex control of heart rate in man. *Anesthesiology* 46:184-187, 1977.

66. Ebert T et al: Halothane anesthesia attenuates cardiopulmonary baroreflex control of peripheral resistance in humans. *Anesthesiology* 63:668-674, 1985.

67. Kotrly K et al: Baroreceptor reflex control of heart rate during isoflurane anesthesia in humans. *Anesthesiology* 60:173-179, 1984.

68. Morton M, Duke P, Ong B: Baroreflex control of heart rate in man awake and during enflurane and enflurane-nitrous oxide anesthesia. *Anesthesiology* 52:221-223, 1980.

69. Weiskopf R et al: Comparison of cardiopulmonary responses to graded hemorrhage during enflurane, halothane, isoflurane, and ketamine anesthesia. *Anesth Analg* 60:481-491, 1981.

70. Weiskopf R, Bogetz M: Cardiovascular actions of nitrous oxide or halothane in hypovolemic swine. *Anesthesiology* 63:509-516, 1985.

71. Joris J et al: Hemodynamic changes during laparoscopic cholecystectomy. *Anesth Analg* 76:1067-1071, 1993.

72. Goertz A et al: Effect of phenylephrine bolus administration on left ventricular function during postural hypotension in anesthetized patients. *J Clin Anesth* 5:408-413, 1993.

73. Witherspoon D, Kraemer D, Seager S: Laparoscopy of horses. In Harrison R, Wildt D, editors: Animal laparoscopy. Baltimore, 1980, Williams & Wilkins.

74. Maxwell D, Kraemer D: Laparoscopy of cattle. In Harrison R, Wildt D, editors: Animal laparoscopy. Baltimore, 1980, Williams & Wilkins.

75. Hendrickson D, Wilson D: Laparoscopic cryptorchidectomy in standing horses. ACVS Veterinary Symposium 10, San Francisco, 1996.

76. Fischer A, Vachon A, Klein S: Laparoscopic inguinal herniorrhaphy in two stallions. *J Am Vet Med Assoc* 207:1599-1601, 1995.

77. Galuppo L, Snyder J, Pascoe J: Laparoscopic anatomy of the equine abdomen. *Am J Vet Res* 56:518-531, 1995.

78. Palmer S: Standing laparoscopic laser technique for ovariectomy in five mares. *J Am Vet Med Assoc* 203:279-283, 1993.

79. Naoi M et al: Laparoscopic-assisted serial biopsy of the bovine kidney. *Am J Vet Res* 46:699-702, 1985.

80. Fischer A, Vachon A: Laparoscopic cryptorchidectomy in horses. *J Am Vet Med Assoc* 201:1705-1708, 1992.

81. Fischer A et al: Diagnostic laparoscopy in the horse. *J Am Vet Med Assoc* 189:289-292, 1985.

82. Mackey V, Wheat J: Reflections on the diagnostic approach to multicentric lymphosarcoma in an aged Arabian mare. *Equine Vet J* 17:467-469, 1985.

83. Fulton I, Brown C, Yamini B: Adenocarcinoma of intestinal origin in a horse: diagnosis by abdominocentesis and laparoscopy. *Equine Vet J* 22:447-448, 1990.

84. Anderson D, Gaughan E, St-Jean G: Normal laparoscopic anatomy of the bovine abdomen. *Am J Vet Res* 54:1170-1176, 1993.

85. Witherspoon D, McQueen R: Development of equine peritoneal fistula device. *Am J Vet Res* 31:387-391, 1970.

86. Parry B, Gay C, McCarthy M: Influence of head height on arterial blood pressure in standing horses. *Am J Vet Res* 41:1626-1631, 1980.

87. Fahy B et al: The effects of increased abdominal pressure on lung and chest wall mechanics during laparoscopic surgery. *Anesth Analg* 81:744-750, 1995.

88. Drummond G, Martin L: Pressure-volume relationships in the lung during laparoscopy. *Br J Anaesth* 50:261-269, 1978.

89. Brown D et al: Ventilatory and blood gas changes during laparoscopy with local anesthesia. *Am J Obstet Gynecol* 124:741-745, 1976.

90. Alexander G, Noe F, Brown E: Anesthesia for pelvic laparoscopy. *Anesth Analg* 48:14-18, 1969.

91. Cunningham A et al: Transoesophageal echocardiographic assessment of haemodynamic function during laparoscopic cholecystectomy. *Br J Anaesth* 70:621-625, 1993.

92. Ferguson D et al: Intra-abdominal CO_2 insufflation in the pregnant ewe: uterine blood flow, intra-amniotic pressure and cardiopulmonary effects. ACVS Veterinary Symposium 4, Chicago, Ill., Oct 29-Nov 1, 1995.

93. Baratz R, Karis J: Blood gas studies during laparoscopy under general anesthesia. *Anesthesiology* 30:463-464, 1969.

94. Peroni J, Fischer A: Effects of carbon dioxide insufflation and body position on blood gas values and cardiovascular parameters in the anesthetized horse undergoing laparoscopy. ACVS Veterinary Symposium 30, Chicago, Ill., Oct 29-Nov 1, 1995.

95. Hodgson C, McClelland R, Newton J: Some effects of the peritoneal insufflation of carbon dioxide at laparoscopy. *Anaesthesia* 25:382-390, 1970.

96. Desmond J, Gordon R: Ventilation in patients anaesthetized for laparoscopy. *Can Anaesth Soc J* 17:378-387, 1970.

97. Tang C et al: The hemodynamic and ventilatory effects between Trendelenburg and reverse Trendelenburg position during laparoscopy with CO_2-insufflation. *Ma Tsui Hsueh Tsa Chi* 31:217-224, 1993.

98. Marshall R et al: Circulatory effects of carbon dioxide insufflation of the peritoneal cavity for laparoscopy. *Br J Anaesth* 44:680-684, 1972.

99. Motew M et al: Cardiovascular effects and acid-base and blood gas changes during laparoscopy. *Am J Obstet Gynecol* 115:1002-1012, 1973.

100. Seed R, Shakespeare T, Muldoon M: Carbon dioxide homeostasis during anaesthesia for laparoscopy. *Anaesthesia* 25:223-231, 1970.

101. El-Minawi M et al: Physiologic changes during CO_2 and N_2O pneumoperitoneum in diagnostic laparoscopy. *J Reprod Med* 26:338-346, 1981.

102. Alexander G, Brown E: Physiologic alterations during pelvic laparoscopy. *Am J Obstet Gynecol* 105:1078-1081, 1969.

103. Sfez M GA, Desruelle P: Cardiorespiratory changes during laparoscopic fundoplication in children. *Paediatr Anaesth* 5:89-95, 1995.

104. Tan P, Lee T, Tweed W: Carbon dioxide absorption and gas exchange during pelvic laparoscopy. *Can J Anaesth* 39:677-681, 1992.

105. Marshall R et al: Circulatory effects of peritoneal insufflation with nitrous oxide. *Br J Anaesth* 44:1183-1187, 1972.

106. Lenz R, Thomas T, Wilkins D: Cardiovascular changes during laparoscopy: studies of stroke volume and cardiac output using impedance cardiography. *Anaesthesia* 31:4-12, 1976.

107. Johannsen G, Andersen M, Juhl B: The effect of general anaesthesia on the haemodynamic events during laparoscopy with CO_2 insufflation. *Acta Anaesthesiol Scand* 33:132-136, 1989.

108. Windberger U, Siegl H, Woisetschager R: Hemodynamic changes during laparoscopic surgery. *Eur Surg Res* 26:1-9, 1994.

109. Kelman G et al: Cardiac output and arterial blood-gas tension during laparoscopy. *Br J Anaesth* 44:1155-1162, 1972.

110. Williams M, Murr P: Laparoscopic insufflation of the abdomen depresses cardiopulmonary function. *Surg Endosc* 7:12-16, 1993.

111. Josephs L et al: Diagnostic laparoscopy increases intracranial pressure. *J Trauma* 36:815-819, 1994.

112. Mutoh T et al: Abdominal distension alters regional pleural pressures and chest wall mechanics in pigs in vivo. *J Appl Physiol* 70:2611-2618, 1991.

113. Pelosi P et al: Effects of carbon dioxide insufflation for laparoscopic cholecystectomy on the respiratory system. *Anaesthesia* 51:744-749, 1996.

114. Kendall A, Oh T: Pulmonary consequences of carbon dioxide insufflation for laparoscopic cholecystectomies. *Anaesthesia* 50:286-289, 1995.

115. Mäkinen M-T, Yli-Hankala A: The effect of laparoscopic cholecystectomy on respiratory compliance as determined by continuous spirometry. *J Clin Anesth* 8:119-122, 1996.

116. Fox L et al: Physiologic alterations during laparoscopic cholecystectomy in ASA III & IV patients. *Anesthesiology* 79:A55, 1993.

117. Wittgen C et al: Analysis of the hemodynamic and ventilatory effects of laparoscopic cholecystectomy. *Arch Surg* 126:997-1001, 1991.

118. Puri G, Singh H: Ventilatory effects of laparoscopy under general anaesthesia. *Br J Anaesth* 68:211-213, 1992.

119. Wahba R, Mamazza J: Ventilatory requirements during laparoscopic cholecystectomy. *Can J Anaesth* 40:206-210, 1993.

120. Liu S-Y et al: Prospective analysis of cardiovascular responses to laparoscopic cholecystectomy. *J Laparoendosc Surg* 1:241-246, 1991.

121. Dorsay D, Greene F, Baysinger C: Hemodynamic changes during laparoscopic cholecystectomy monitored with transesophageal echocardiography. *Surg Endosc* 9:128-133, 1995.

122. McLaughlin J et al: The adverse hemodynamic effects of laparoscopic cholecystectomy. *Surg Endosc* 9:121-124, 1995.

123. Breton G et al: Clinical and hemodynamic evaluation of cholecystectomies performed under laparoscopy. *Ann Chir* 45:783-790, 1991.

124. Loder W, Minnich M, Brotman S: Hemodynamic effects of laparoscopic cholecystectomy. *Am Surg* 60:322-325, 1994.

125. Critchley L, Critchley J, Gin T: Haemodynamic changes in patients undergoing laparoscopic cholecystectomy: measurement by transthoracic electrical bioimpedance. *Br J Anaesth* 70:681-683, 1993.

126. O'Leary E et al: Laparoscopic cholecystectomy: haemodynamic and neuroendocrine responses after pneumoperitoneum and changes in position. *Br J Anaesth* 76:640-644, 1996.

127. Felber A et al. Plasma vasopressin in laparoscopic cholecystectomy. *Anesthesiology* 79:A32, 1993.

128. Iwase K et al: Haemodynamic changes during laparoscopic cholecystectomy in patients with heart disease. *Endoscopy* 24:771-773, 1992.

129. Jones D et al: Effects of insufflation on hemodynamics during thoracoscopy. *Ann Thorac Surg* 55:1379-1382, 1993.

130. Benumof J: One-lung ventilation and hypoxic pulmonary vasoconstriction: implications for anesthetic management. *Anesth Analg* 64:821-833, 1985.

131. Drew J, Dripps R, Comroe J: Clinical studies on morphine: II. The effect of morphine upon the circulation of man and upon the circulatory and respiratory responses to tilting. *Anesthesiology* 7:44-61, 1946.

132. Kissin I: Preemptive analgesia: terminology and clinical relevance. *Anesth Analg* 79:809-810, 1994.

133. Fitzgerald S et al: Hypercarbia during carbon dioxide pneumoperitoneum. *Am J Surg* 163:186-190, 1992.

134. Ekman L et al: Hemodynamic changes during laparoscopy with positive end-expiratory pressure ventilation. *Acta Anaesthesiol Scand* 32:447-453, 1988.

135. Burchard K et al: Positive end-expiratory pressure with increased intra-abdominal pressure. *Surg Gynecol Obstet* 161:313-318, 1985.

136. Bidani A et al. Permissive hypercapnia in acute respiratory failure. *J Am Med Assoc* 272:957-962, 1994.

137. Wagner A, Bednarski R, Muir W: Hemodynamic effects of carbon dioxide during intermittent positive-pressure ventilation in horses. *Am J Vet Res* 51:1922-1929, 1990.

138. Walley K, Lewis T, Wood L: Acute respiratory acidosis decreases left ventricular contractility but increases cardiac output in dogs. *Circ Res* 67:628-635, 1990.

139. Scott D, Julian D: Observations on cardiac arrhythmias during laparoscopy. *Br Med J* 12:411-413, 1972.

140. Rasmussen J et al: Cardiac function and hypercarbia. *Arch Surg* 113:1196-1200, 1978.

141. Inque H et al: Hypoxic pulmonary vasoconstriction supports the safety of one-lung ventilation in the dog. *Researches-MA J* 7:10-14, 1986.

142. Smith G, Hirsch N, Ehrenwerth J: Placement of double-lumen endobronchial tubes. *Br J Anaesth* 58:1317-1320, 1986.

143. ACVA: Anesthesiology guidelines developed. *J Am Vet Med Assoc* 206:936-937, 1995.

144. ACVA: http://a.cvm.okstate.edu/~ACVA: Oklahoma State University's College of Veterinary Medicine, 1996.

145. Liem T, Applebaum H, Herzberger B: Hemodynamic and ventilatory effects of abdominal CO_2 insufflation at various pressures in the young swine. *J Pediatric Surg* 29:966-969, 1994.

146. Lew T, Tay D, Thomas E: Venous air embolism during cesarean section: more common than previously thought. *Anesth Analg* 77:448-452, 1993.

147. Lowenwirt I, Chi D, Handwerker S: Nonfatal venous air embolism during cesarean section: a case report and review of the literature. *Obstet Gynecol Surv* 49:72-76, 1994.

148. Lantz P, Smith J: Fatal carbon dioxide embolism complicating attempted laparoscopic cholecystectomy-case report and literature review. *J Forensic Sci* 39:1468-1480, 1994.

149. Gilroy B, Anson L. Fatal air embolism during anesthesia for laparoscopy in a dog. *J Am Vet Med Assoc* 190:552-554, 1987.

150. Couture P et al: Venous carbon dioxide embolism in pigs: an evaluation of end-tidal carbon dioxide, transesophageal echocardiography, pulmonary artery pressure, and precordial auscultation as monitoring modalities. *Anesth Analg* 79:867-873, 1994.

151. Glauser F, Bartlett R: Pneumoperitoneum in association with pneumothorax. *Chest* 66:536-540, 1974.

152. Brantley J, Riley P: Cardiovascular collapse during laparoscopy: a report of two cases. *Am J Obstet Gynecol* 159:735-737, 1988.

153. Beebe D et al: High levels of carbon monoxide are produced by electro-cautery of tissue during laparoscopic cholecystectomy. *Anesth Analg* 77:338-341, 1993.

154. Neuman G et al: Laparoscopy explosion hazards with nitrous oxide. *Anesthesiology* 78:875-879, 1993.

155. Swain J: The case for abandoning the Trendelenburg position in pelvic surgery. *Med J Australia* 2:536-537, 1960.

156. Pearson M, Sander M: Hyperkalemia associated with prolonged insufflation of carbon dioxide into the peritoneal cavity. *Br J Anaesth* 72:602-604, 1994.

157. Bailey J, Pablo L, Hubbell J: Hyperkalemic periodic paralysis episode during halothane anesthesia in a horse. *J Am Vet Med Assoc* 208:1859-1865, 1996.

158. Shelly M et al: Haemodynamic effects following surgical release of increased intra-abdominal pressure. *Br J Anaesth* 59:800-805, 1987.

159. Bongard F, Pianim N, Leighton T: Helium insufflation for laparoscopic operation. *Surg Gynecol Obstet* 177:140-146, 1993.

160. Ishizaki Y, Bandai Y, Shimomura K: Changes in splanchnic blood flow and cardiovascular effects following peritoneal insufflation of carbon dioxide. *Surg Endosc* 7:420-423, 1993.

161. Kobori M et al: Influence of posture changes on hemodynamics under fentanyl-diazepam anesthesia—effects of nitrous oxide. *Masui* 42:1587-1591, 1993.

CHAPTER 3

ACCESS, PORT PLACEMENT, AND BASIC ENDOSURGICAL SKILLS

Ronald J. Kolata, Lynetta J. Freeman

The basic procedures in minimally invasive surgery are the same as for open surgery: access, exploration, retraction, dissection, hemostasis, tissue apposition, tissue removal, and closure. Specialized methods for accomplishing each task have been developed. In this chapter, we describe the skills necessary to perform key surgical activities and suggest ways for a veterinary surgeon to improve his or her expertise. Many of the surgical instruments described in this book will become obsolete. However, we believe that the underlying principles and surgical techniques will endure.

Access

In minimally invasive surgery, access must be adequate to see and reach internal structures and perform diagnostic and therapeutic surgical maneuvers. An optical cavity, which is created by enlarging and maintaining a potential space, makes this possible. Endoscopists use air to insufflate the esophagus, stomach, intestine, and colon. Laparoscopists insufflate the abdominal cavity with carbon dioxide (CO_2), air, helium, or nitrous oxide (N_2O). Thoracoscopists take advantage of the rigid chest wall and the ability to collapse one lung to create a working space in the thorax. Arthroscopists use a liquid medium, such as saline solution, to create and maintain an optical cavity within a joint. Other techniques are used to gain access to the preperitoneal or retroperitoneal space, the subcutaneous tissue, and the area around the trachea.

PNEUMOPERITONEUM

The peritoneum lines the abdominal, pelvic, inguinal, and scrotal cavities and covers the surfaces and supporting structures of the organs within them. *Pneumoperitoneum* exists when a gas enters the potential space between the parietal peritoneum that lines the walls of the cavities and the visceral peritoneum that covers the organs contained by the cavity and creates a true space there.

Normal intraperitoneal pressure varies from −5 to 7 mm Hg and averages 2 mm Hg.[1] As gas is introduced into the peritoneal space, the abdominal wall and diaphragm are distended. Because of the elasticity of the peritoneum and the abdominal wall musculature, a considerable volume of gas may be introduced before intraperitoneal pressure increases beyond the upper extreme of the physiologic range. As the limits of compliance of the abdominal wall and diaphragm are reached, pressure rises sharply. As distention occurs, the diaphragm intrudes on the thoracic cavity. This results in decreased lung capacity and increased intrathoracic pressure. If not managed, this can lead to atelectasis and hypoventilation, resulting in hypoxemia, hypercapnia, and acidemia (see Chapter 2).

The physiologic effects are pressure-related. For most animals, an acceptable optical cavity is created with 12 to 14 mm Hg pressure. Studies have shown that intraabdominal pressures between 8 and 20 mm Hg result in mild hemodynamic changes that are within tolerable physiologic limits.[2,3] Pressures above 25 mm Hg result in detrimental hemodynamic changes. As pressure is increased to 40 mm Hg, a shocklike state with tachycardia, hypotension, decreased central venous pressure, and decreased cardiac output develops.[4]

Body position during pneumoperitoneum also has physiologic consequences. A head-up position results in pooling of blood in the caudal parts of the body, with a concomitant decrease in venous return and cardiac output. A head-down position increases venous return to the heart and augments cardiac output but puts weight of the abdominal organs on the diaphragm and accentuates the adverse ventilatory effects of pneumoperitoneum (see Chapter 2).

Gas Selection

The ideal insufflation gas is transparent, colorless, non-explosive, physiologically inert, readily available, and is either not absorbed or is eliminated by the pulmonary system. CO_2, N_2O, air, nitrogen, helium, xenon, and argon have been used as insufflation gases. Each has advantages and disadvantages. CO_2 has been used to create pneumoperitoneum in human laparoscopic surgical procedures for more than 20 years. It is readily available, inexpensive, and does not support combustion when laser or electrosurgery is used. CO_2 is a physiologic end product that is readily absorbed and excreted. The disadvantages of CO_2 are that it may irritate visceral surfaces by forming carbonic acid and it is absorbed into the blood, possibly leading to hypercapnia, stimulation of the sympathetic nervous system, vasodilation, hypertension, tachycardia, and arrhythmias.

The second favored choice, N_2O, is readily available, augments anesthesia, and is rapidly absorbed and excreted without contributing to acidemia or hypercapnia. Although less irritating, it may support combustion, leads to distention of hollow viscera, and may cause diffusion hypoxemia on recovery. N_2O is of increasing interest because of a move in human surgery to more day surgery and office-based procedures, which may benefit from the analgesic effects of N_2O.

The inert gases (argon, helium, and xenon) have advantages similar to N_2O. They have the disadvantages of relatively greater cost and less availability. A further drawback is that insufflators designed for these gases are not readily available. Oxygen and nitrogen are readily available and relatively inexpensive, but they are relatively slowly absorbed and excreted, with an accompanying greater risk of embolization. Oxygen, in addition, supports combustion. Air, although readily available and inexpensive, may promote air embolus.

The insufflation pressure is regulated by an automatic insufflator. The function of an automatic insufflator is described in Chapter 1.

Methods of Establishing Pneumoperitoneum

Methods for establishing pneumoperitoneum are simple and can be used with minor modifications in a number of species. As with all surgical procedures, it is necessary to become familiar with the instruments, equipment, and methods used to establish pneumoperitoneum so it can be done safely and optimally.

Closed Technique with the Veress Needle

The Veress needle contains a spring-loaded, hollow, blunt obturator and a stopcock (Fig. 3-1). The blunt obturator protrudes past the sharp, cutting tip of the needle once it has penetrated the peritoneum. The blunt obturator springs forward to protect abdominal organs from being injured by the tip of the needle. The gas supply is attached to the needle or stopcock, and pneumoperitoneum is established by gas passing through the obturator into the peritoneal space.

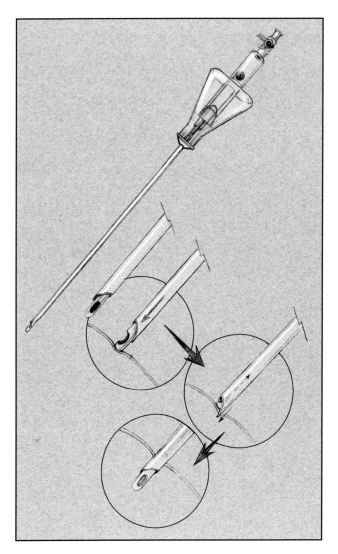

Fig. 3-1   Veress needles have an obturator that springs forward when resistance is no longer present.

TECHNIQUE Before using a Veress needle, check it for patency by flushing saline through it. Occlude the tip of the needle and check for leakage from the plastic hub. Push the obturator against a blunt object to make certain that it retracts and springs forward properly. Some needles have a red indicator that appears when the obturator retracts. Connect the needle to the insufflator and ensure that the needle and insufflator are functioning properly.

In humans the Veress needle is inserted near the umbilicus because that is where the abdominal wall is consistently thin. The primary (camera) port is usually placed at this location. The same is true in most nonhuman species when a ventral approach is used. In dogs and cats the Veress needle is inserted caudolateral to the umbilicus and directed toward the pelvis to avoid the fatty falciform ligament and avoid injuring the spleen (Fig. 3-2). Placing the animal in a slightly head-down

(Trendelenburg) position also helps avoid injuring the spleen. It is good practice to empty the urinary bladder before inserting the Veress needle and trocars.

Make a small stab incision through the skin. Tense and lift the abdominal wall by picking it up with towel clamps or by hand. Insert the needle perpendicular to the surface of the abdominal wall. With experience, one can feel the tip of the needle pass through fascial layers and peritoneum. Ensure that the tip of the needle is in the abdominal cavity by using one of the following techniques:

1. Close the stopcock on the Veress needle during insertion. When the tip of the needle is within the peritoneal cavity, return the abdominal wall to its normal position. Attach the gas tubing from the insufflator and open the stopcock. Lift the abdominal wall. If the tip of the needle is in the peritoneal cavity, the manometer on the insufflator will register a small negative pressure (Fig. 3-3).

2. Close the stopcock on the Veress needle during insertion. After the needle is inserted, open the stopcock and elevate the abdominal wall. If the tip of the needle is in the abdominal cavity, air will be

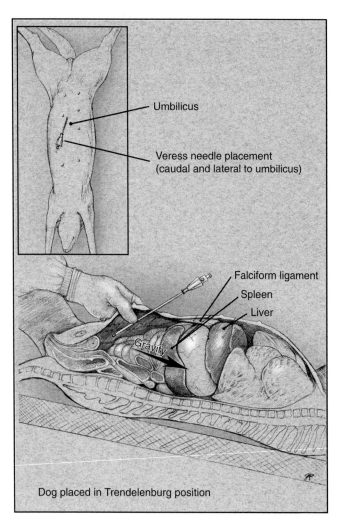

Fig. 3-2 Insertion of Veress needle to avoid injuring the spleen.

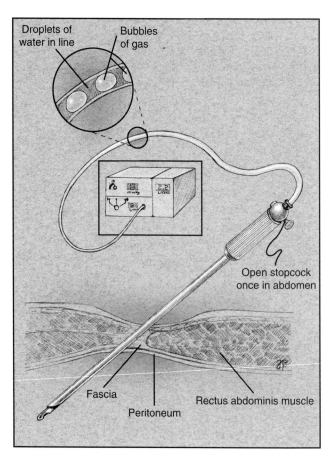

Fig. 3-3 Tests for correct needle placement. The pressure reading on the insufflator is negative or zero, and the CO_2 flow is high.

heard hissing though the stopcock as the abdomen is elevated and released (Fig. 3-4).

3. After insertion attach a syringe partially filled with sterile saline to the Veress needle. Aspirate the syringe and check for blood, mucus, or other body fluid. If none is detected, inject a small amount of saline. It should flow freely. Detach the syringe from the Veress needle and lift the abdominal wall. The saline in the hub of the needle will sink if the tip of the needle is in the peritoneal cavity and is not obstructed by omentum or bowel. This is known as the *hanging drop technique* (Fig. 3-5).

4. At the onset of insufflation, the pressure recorded by the insufflator should be low (2 to 3 mm Hg) while the flow rate is greater than 1 L/min. If the pressure is high and the flow rate is zero, the tip of the needle may be occluded. It may be lying against bowel or omentum, or it may not be in the abdominal cavity (Fig. 3-6). Lift the abdominal wall to move the tip of the needle from contact with bowel or omentum, reestablishing the low pressure and adequate flow. If the tip of the needle is not in the peritoneal cavity, the pressure will remain high and the flow rate zero. Avoid swinging the needle to determine if it is in the peritoneal cavity, because that may injure mesentery or other underlying structures.

5. The definitive indication of proper placement is that during insufflation the abdominal wall becomes distended uniformly and separation of the abdominal wall and viscera can be detected by ballottement. If insufflation is localized and the

entire abdominal wall does not bounce freely during ballottement, stop insufflation and insert the needle at another site.

When the desired pressure is reached, insert the primary trocar.

Open Technique for Placing a Hasson Trocar

Open laparoscopy was developed by Harrith Hasson in 1974 to avoid injury to intraabdominal organs encountered in the closed (blind) method. Hasson designed a

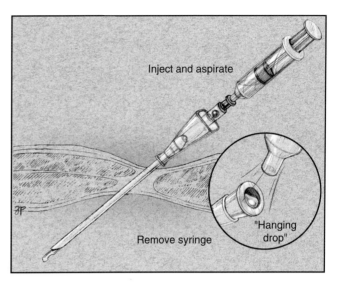

Fig. 3-5 Inject a small amount of fluid and aspirate to check for blood, mucus, or bowel contents. The hanging drop test for correct needle placement uses a drop of saline on the hub of the needle. When the abdominal wall is elevated, the drop is pulled into the abdominal cavity.

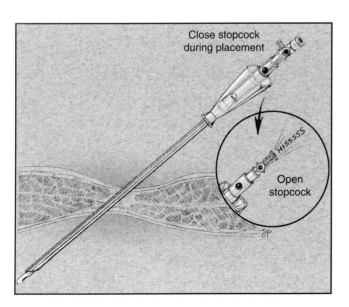

Fig. 3-4 Open the stopcock and listen for a hissing noise.

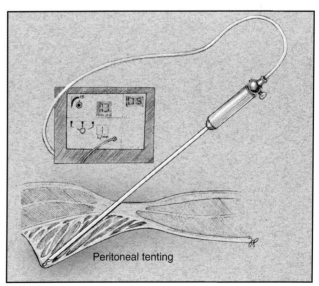

Fig. 3-6 If the needle is in the preperitoneal space, the pressure will be high (~8 mm Hg) and the flow will be low (~0.2 L/min).

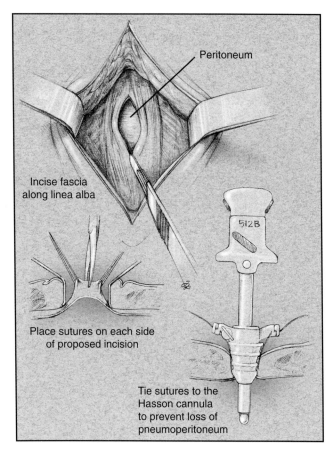

Peritoneum

Incise fascia
along linea alba

512B

Place sutures on each side
of proposed incision

Tie sutures to the
Hasson cannula
to prevent loss of
pneumoperitoneum

Fig. 3-7 Placement of a Hasson trocar. An incision is made through the fascia and linea alba. A suture is placed on each side of the fascia. The peritoneum is opened. The trocar is inserted, and the sutures are tied to the olive.

cone to fit over the cannula of a 10-mm trocar, with flanges for attaching sutures. The cone is commonly referred to as an *olive*.[5] An incision is usually made near the umbilicus because the anatomy is familiar, and bleeding and trauma to abdominal musculature are minimized. After opening the peritoneal cavity under direct vision, a blunt obturator is used to insert the trocar. A gas-tight seal is obtained by tying stay sutures from the fascia to the olive to hold the trocar firmly in place.

TECHNIQUE Make an incision through the skin and subcutaneous fat down to the linea alba. Dissect the subcutaneous fat laterally to facilitate placing a suture on each side of the proposed incision (Fig. 3-7). The sutures will be used to hold the cannula in place and close the wound at the end of surgery. Place a purse-string suture around the fascial incision to ensure a gas-tight seal if a Hasson-type cannula is not available.

Make an incision through the linea alba large enough to allow a finger or instrument to be inserted to ensure that the peritoneal cavity has been entered. In dogs and cats grasp the falciform ligament with forceps and exteriorize it. Remove as much of the ligament as possible.

Control bleeding with electrocautery. Pass two sutures, one through each fascial edge, and tag them. Insert the trocar and sleeve with the olive positioned on the outside of the cannula approximately 2 cm from the tip of the trocar sleeve. Wrap the sutures snugly around the suture tie posts on the olive. Remove the obturator. Connect the insufflator to the stopcock on the trocar cannula and establish the pneumoperitoneum.

Optical Trocar
An alternative way to create pneumoperitoneum, similar to the open approach, is to use an optical trocar.[6] Optical trocars have a hollow obturator with a lens at the distal tip. One type has a conical lens and lateral tissue-separating blades. Another type has a hemispheric lens and a cutting blade that moves forward when activated by a trigger. The laparoscope is inserted through the obturator to make contact with the lens. As the trocar is inserted, penetration of the tissue layers of the abdominal wall and the peritoneum is visible on the video monitor (Fig. 3-8). Being able to see the tissue layers allows a controlled entry into the abdominal cavity. Once the trocar is inserted, the obturator with the laparoscope is removed and the insufflation tubing is connected to establish pneumoperitoneum. The laparoscope is reinserted. Although the technique provides controlled entry and helps avoid blood vessels or adhesions to the peritoneum, surgeons must practice the technique to gain experience in identifying the tissue layers.

PRIMARY PORT PLACEMENT
If the open (Hasson) technique or an optical trocar is used to establish pneumoperitoneum, that .cannula serves as the primary port. If the Veress needle is used for insufflation, the first trocar inserted is the primary port. Usually the primary port is placed at the umbilicus; however, if the animal had a previous midline abdominal incision, placement may be moved to avoid adhesions to the incision site.

If the closed technique is used to establish pneumoperitoneum, a trocar with a safety shield is usually used to reduce the chance of injury to intraabdominal organs and vessels. The safety shield is a plastic outer covering that retracts when the trocar meets resistance and springs forward upon penetration of the abdominal cavity (Fig. 3-9). The safety shield acts in the same manner as the obturator in a Veress needle. Once the safety shield springs forward, it locks in place to cover the tip of the obturator and prevent injury to the underlying viscera.

Shielded trocars are usually disposable and therefore have single or limited-use blades that are consistently sharp. Nonshielded trocars are usually reusable and therefore have blades of variable sharpness. Differences in clinical performance have not been demonstrated, although the force required to penetrate the abdomen is lower with disposable trocars.[7]

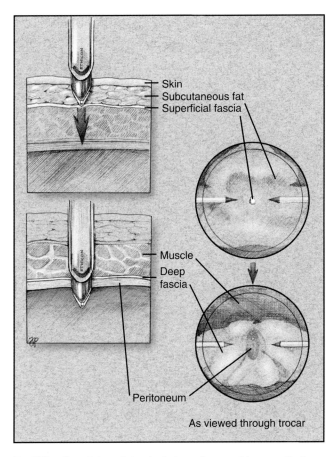

Fig. 3-8 Examining abdominal tissue layers with an optical trocar. The subcutaneous tissue is white or light yellow, with small blood vessels. The superficial fascia is white and glistening. The muscle fibers are reddish brown. As the deep fascia and peritoneum are penetrated, a small hole at the tip of the trocar gradually enlarges.

Technique

A blind primary puncture must be performed carefully. If the abdomen is not insufflated enough to become taut, the body wall will be depressed during trocar insertion, moving the tip of the trocar dangerously close to the abdominal viscera. Some surgeons use a slightly higher insufflation pressure for insertion of the trocar and then reduce the pressure during the surgical procedure.

Make a skin incision appropriate for the size of the trocar. If the skin incision is too small, the skin may prevent the safety shield from functioning properly and the force required to penetrate the abdominal wall will be increased. Excessive force also depresses the abdominal wall, moving the trocar tip closer to viscera.

Set the safety shield mechanism ("arm the trocar") and grasp the trocar firmly with the dominant hand. In a controlled manner, insert the trocar with a thrusting and twisting motion directed perpendicular to the abdominal wall. The action is similar to driving a Steinmann pin. In dogs and cats direct the trocar caudad to avoid the spleen.

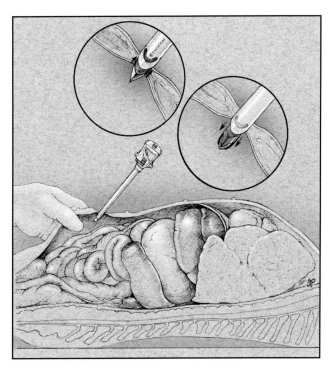

Fig. 3-9 The safety shield is pushed back as tissue provides resistance to insertion. When the abdominal wall is penetrated, the safety shield springs forward to cover the tip of the trocar.

After the trocar and cannula penetrate the abdominal wall, remove the trocar and pass the laparoscope through the cannula into the peritoneal cavity (Fig. 3-10). Keeping the cannula in the same position in which it was inserted makes it easier to see injuries that may have occurred during the insertion. Examine the abdominal cavity for the positions of organs, adhesions, and other abnormalities.

SECONDARY PORTS

Secondary ports are inserted in locations that provide optimal access to the organs of interest and facilitate the proposed surgery. To avoid paradoxical movement, place ports so that the laparoscope and instruments are pointed toward the video monitor (Fig. 3-11). Paradoxical movement occurs because the trocar cannula acts as a fulcrum. When the laparoscope and instruments are pointed toward the monitor, the instrument tip moves to the left on the monitor when the instrument handle is moved to the right. If the laparoscope is pointed toward the monitor and the instruments are pointed away from the monitor, the tip appears to move right on the monitor as the instrument handle is moved right (Fig. 3-12).

Ports should be separated enough to create angles of about 30° to 60°, to allow manipulation of instruments without interference ("sword-fighting"). Placing ports too close to an organ allows little room for manipulation. Placing them too far away prevents the instruments from

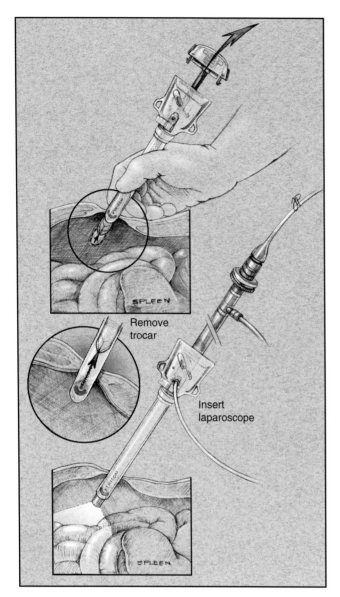

Fig. 3-10 After the trocar is inserted, the cannula is pointed in the same direction during trocar removal and laparoscope insertion to make it easier to identify iatrogenic tissue injury.

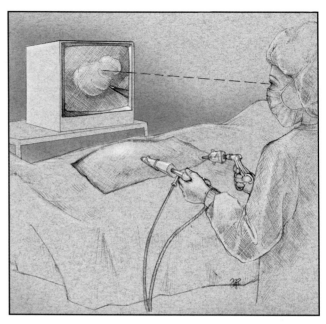

Fig. 3-11 The laparoscope and operating instruments should point toward the video monitor.

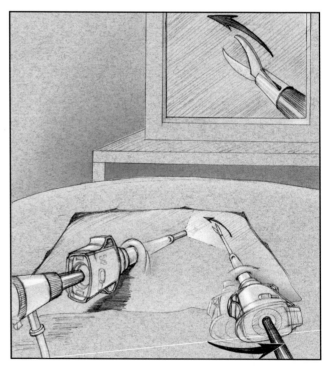

Fig. 3-12 Paradoxical movement. Moving the hand to the right causes the tip of the instrument to move to the left on the video monitor.

reaching the intended site. To plan a port location, pass the instrument through the cannula and position it over the abdomen in the plane in which it will be used. Remember that instruments have a reach that falls in the plane of an arc. To reach the extreme lateral ranges of the operative site, instruments must be closer to center.

Transilluminate the proposed trocar site to help identify vessels in the abdominal wall so they can be avoided during trocar insertion. Depress the abdominal wall and watch on the video monitor to localize the site. Make a skin incision appropriate for the size of the trocar. Use the laparoscope to monitor entry of the trocar into the abdominal cavity (Fig. 3-13).

Trocar Stabilization

During a laparoscopic procedure, the trocar cannula frequently becomes dislodged. This can be an especially difficult problem when working in a small abdominal cavity and when the abdominal wall is very thin. Dislodgment

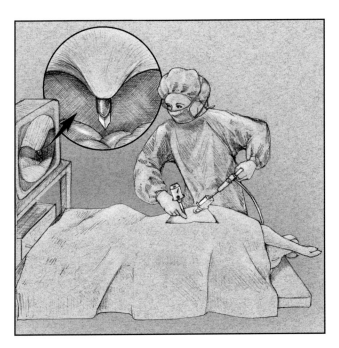

Fig. 3-13   The surgeon observes trocar insertion on the video monitor.

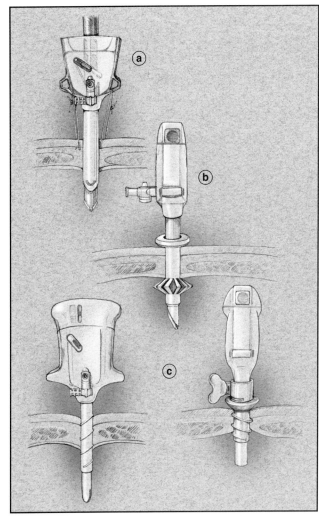

Fig. 3-14   Methods to secure the trocar to the abdominal wall: sutures (*a*), expandable sleeve (*b*), stability threads (*c*).

causes a loss of pneumoperitoneum and delays the operation. In addition, CO_2 dissects into the layers of the abdominal wall, causing subcutaneous emphysema and further complicating the procedure. On the other hand, inserting trocars too deep leads to intertrocar interference during surgery and prevents instruments from opening. Use trocars with threaded cannulas, stability screw threads, sticky pads, balloon-tipped or toggle-bolt–type trocars, or sutures secured to the skin to stabilize the cannula in the body wall (Fig. 3-14). Trocar stabilization is especially important if the surgeon is working with both hands. When planning to use electrocautery, do not use a plastic stability thread with a metal sheath, because the plastic sheath acts as an insulator between the metal trocar cannula and the body wall. If an instrument with faulty insulation is inserted and electrocautery is used, energy can be transferred to viscera rather than the body wall, and an unrecognized burn lesion of the intestine could occur.

Exchange Rod Technique

Pneumoperitoneum cannot be maintained with damaged trocar gaskets, leaky valves, or damaged stopcocks. It may be necessary to replace the trocar with a cannula of the same or larger size. An exchange rod facilitates replacement of a trocar cannula through an existing incision (Fig. 3-15). Insert the exchange rod through the trocar into the abdomen. Remove the damaged trocar cannula. Slide the new cannula over the exchange rod into the abdomen. Remove the exchange rod.

Use the exchange rod technique for inserting large (18 or 33 mm) disposable trocars. Insert the exchange rod and remove the smaller trocar. Position the obturator of the larger trocar over the exchange rod and advance the obturator to the skin surface. Enlarge the skin incision. Advance the obturator over the exchange rod into the peritoneal cavity. Secure the sleeve of the larger trocar. Remove the obturator and exchange rod.

Dilating Obturator Technique

In the dilating obturator technique, a needle with a radially expandable sleeve* is used to establish entry into the abdominal cavity. A tapered blunt obturator is passed through the expandable sleeve to progressively dilate the tissue layers to receive a 5-, 10-, or 12-mm cannula. Potential benefits of this technique are firm anchoring of

---

*Step, InnerDyne Medical, Sunnyvale, Calif. 94089.

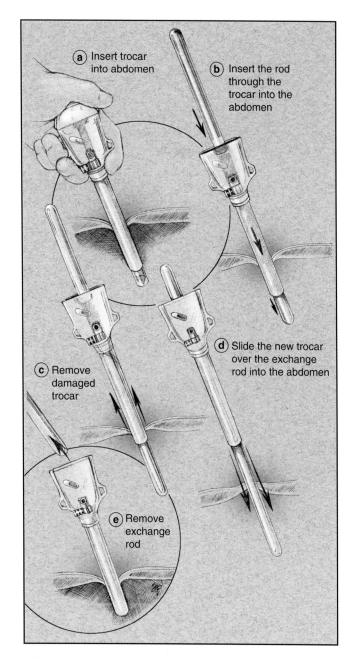

Fig. 3-15   Use of an exchange rod to replace a damaged trocar.

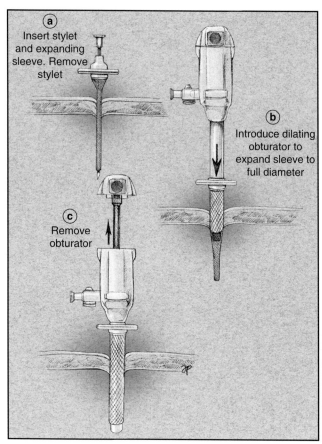

Fig. 3-16   Insertion of an obturator with a radially expanding sleeve.

the cannula in the body wall, a less traumatic insertion because the tissues are dilated rather than cut, and ease of conversion from smaller to larger ports (Fig. 3-16).

THORACIC TROCARS

Thoracic trocars prevent intercostal artery, vein, and nerve injuries during thoracoscopic procedures. Rigid and flexible trocars are available. Rigid thoracic trocars, which have a blunt conical obturator, are inserted as the primary port for the thoracoscope. To place a rigid trocar, make a generous skin incision, bluntly dissect through the intercostal space, and penetrate the parietal pleura with

Kelly forceps. Allow pneumothorax to collapse the superior lung until it falls away from the thoracic wall.

Flexible trocars are usually used as operating ports. Their flexible sleeves (cannulas) conform to the shape of the intercostal space and can provide room for two 5-mm instruments to be inserted through one port (Fig. 3-17). Make a skin incision, bluntly dissect through the intercostal space, and penetrate the parietal pleura with Kelly forceps. Measure and cut the length of flexible sleeve to the thickness of the thoracic wall. This step eliminates unnecessary sleeve length in the thoracic cavity, which interferes with visibility. Insert and expand the obturator by pressing the activating handle. Insert the trocar through the incision. Depress the sleeve release button and remove the obturator. Secure the cannula to the skin with sutures or staples.

BALLOON DISSECTOR

In humans laparoscopic surgeons use a balloon dissector* to make a preperitoneal approach for hernia repair and treatment of urinary stress incontinence (Fig. 3-18).

---

*Preperitoneal Balloon Dissector, Origin Medsystems, Inc., Menlo Park, Calif. 94025.

The balloon bluntly dissects the space between the peritoneum and the internal fascia of the rectus abdominis muscle (Fig. 3-19).

As in the Hasson approach, an incision is made through the skin, subcutaneous tissue, and external fascia of the rectus muscle. The fibers of the rectus abdominis muscle are separated bluntly down to, but not through, the internal fascia of the rectus muscle. The internal fascia is not penetrated. The balloon dissector is placed between the rectus abdominis muscle and the internal fascia. When the internal fascia disappears at the arcuate line, the balloon is correctly located between the peritoneum and the rectus muscle. The surgical telescope is inserted inside the balloon, and the balloon is filled with either saline solution or air. The surgeon observes progressive dissection with the telescope through the wall of the balloon. When dissection is complete, the balloon is deflated and removed. A cannula is inserted for the laparoscope. The optical cavity in the preperitoneal space is maintained by insufflation with CO_2 at 12 to 14 mm Hg pressure.

GASLESS LAPAROSCOPY

Methods of creating an optical cavity by mechanically lifting the abdominal wall have been developed. Abdominal wall lifts are retractors inserted through an incision in the abdominal wall and connected to a device that is raised to stretch the abdominal wall and create a working space. With this method, it is not necessary to maintain pneumoperitoneum. Therefore, sealed cannulas are not required and the physiologic effects of CO_2 pneumoperitoneum are avoided. In addition, long standard surgical instruments can be used. A severe disadvantage of mechanical wall lift is the smaller working space and limited visibility resulting from the localized tension of the retractor, rather than the more uniform and omnidirectional tension supplied by gas insufflation. Because the retractors are mounted on table rails, examination of the entire abdomen requires repositioning the retractor. Because of these disadvantages, gasless laparoscopy has limited application.

SUBCUTANEOUS RETRACTION

An optical cavity can be created and maintained with a subcutaneous lift device. One such device was designed for minimally invasive harvest of the saphenous vein (see Fig. 1-32). The retractor is designed to hold a 30° telescope and position the light cord to maintain the operative field. An incision is made on the medial aspect of the thigh or calf. A dissector is inserted and advanced along the vein. The subcutaneous retractor is used to elevate the skin and view the surgical site. Scissors are used to mobilize the vein. A 5-mm clip applier is inserted beside the retractor to ligate side branches. The vein is ligated distally and removed.

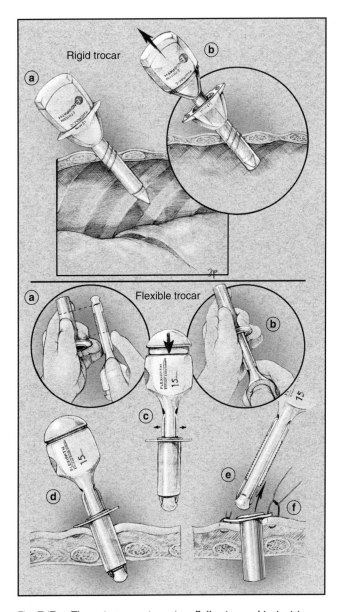

Fig. 3-17 Thoracic trocar insertion. Following a skin incision and blunt dissection through the intercostal space and pleura, a pneumothorax allows the lung to fall away from the thoracic wall. *Top view.* Rigid trocar. Insert the rigid trocar containing a blunt obturator through the intercostal space (*a*). Remove the blunt obturator (*b*). Threads on the outside of the cannula stabilize the trocar in the intercostal space. *Bottom view.* Flexible trocar. Measure the thickness of the thoracic wall and cut the flexible sleeve to the desired length (*a*). Place the cut edge of the flexible sleeve on the solid obturator (*b*). Press the activation handle to deploy the expanding sleeve grip until the flexible sleeve is secure on the obturator (*c*). Insert the mechanical obturator and flexible sleeve through the intercostal space (*d*). Press the sleeve release button to remove the obturator (*e*). Secure the sleeve to the skin with sutures or staples (*f*).

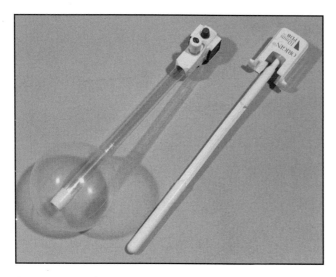

Fig. 3-18 The Origin PDB trocar system consists of a balloon on the outside of the trocar cannula and an obturator for inserting the device into the preperitoneal space. The obturator is removed and replaced with the laparoscope. The balloon is inflated to perform the dissection. Progress is observed with the laparoscope through the wall of the balloon.

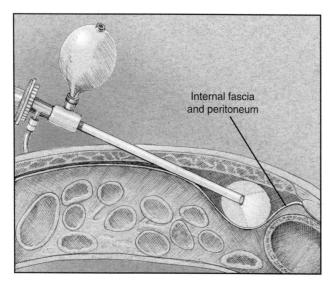

Internal fascia and peritoneum

Fig. 3-19 Lateral view of preperitoneal space dissection with a balloon and trocar system.

Endosurgical Skills

After the optical cavity and a means of access are established, additional skills are needed to perform surgical procedures.

PASSING INSTRUMENTS

Blindly passing instruments through a cannula into the abdomen or thorax is dangerous. To pass an instrument, stabilize the trocar cannula to avoid pushing it deeper.

Use a reducer cap to match the external trocar gasket to the instrument being inserted. Close the instrument during insertion. Position the telescope so the end of the cannula is visible inside the optical cavity. Watch the instrument as it enters the abdomen or thorax and follow the movement to the operative site. To improve depth perception, touch the tissue with the instrument closed. When the instrument reaches the operative site, open the jaws and gently grasp the tissue.

HANDLING TISSUE

Just as a surgeon uses both hands to perform surgery, so too should an endoscopic surgeon learn to use both hands to perform minimally invasive surgery. The additional tactile input from the second hand, the focus on a two-dimensional field, and the ability to apply tension and countertension are reasons to become ambidextrous.

In introductory surgery, students learn how much force is transmitted from thumb forceps to tissue. In laparoscopic surgery, it is difficult at first to determine how tightly to grasp tissue. Techniques for handling tissue are learned by trial and error. One learns that if the tissue is grasped with too little force, it is displaced during manipulation. Too much force results in injury. Some tissues respond differently to similar forces. Initially it is a good idea to avoid using instrument ratchets until the user gains an appreciation for tactile feedback and tissue friability.

RETRACTION

Retraction improves visibility of the operative site. Simply tilting the table or rotating the animal slightly to shift the viscera may be the best method of retraction (Fig. 3-20). As in open procedures, bowel clamps and lung forceps applied directly to the tissue aid in retraction and exposure of the operative site. Specialized retractors are available.

Intraluminal devices serve as retractors. In human gynecologic procedures, surgeons retract the uterus with a uterine manipulator inserted through the cervix. Flexible endoscopes are used to manipulate the esophagus, stomach, or colon in laparoscopic procedures. Vaginal and rectal probes improve visibility in the pelvis.

DISSECTION

Grasping forceps and scissors are the most commonly used instruments for dissection, although electrosurgical devices, lasers, and the ultrasonic scalpel are also used. As in open surgery, an ideal dissection follows tissue planes. The technique depends on traction and countertraction. Grasp and elevate the tissue with grasping forceps in the nondominant hand. Insert scissors or dissecting forceps with the dominant hand and open the jaws beside the structure being dissected. Take care to avoid electrical

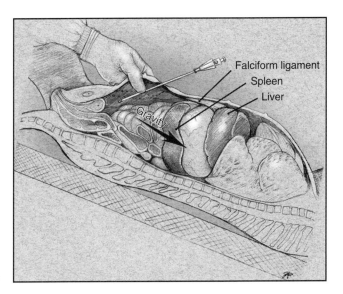

Fig. 3-20   Gravity is used to retract abdominal viscera.

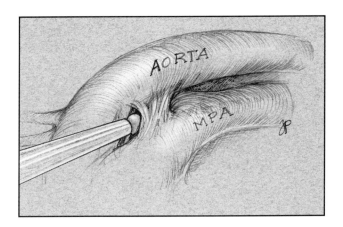

Fig. 3-21   Cherry dissectors are used for blunt dissection near vascular structures.

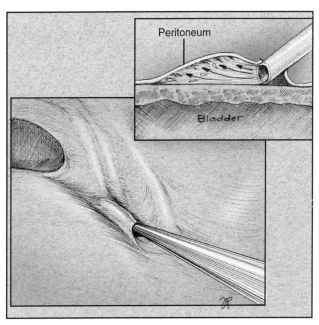

Fig. 3-22   Aquadissection is used to separate tissue layers.

arcing or conducting energy to adjacent structures if electrosurgical devices are used. Blunt dissection is performed in relatively avascular areas. "Peanut" or "cherry" dissectors are most useful in avascular areas and close to major blood vessels (Fig. 3-21).

Aquadissection, also called *hydrodissection*, is a technique of instilling fluid under pressure into tissue planes (Fig. 3-22). The tissue plane becomes thicker and better defined, which allows the surgeon to dissect more quickly with less chance of tissue injury. To instill fluids, place a pressure cuff around a saline bag to raise the pressure to 250 mm Hg. One system uses CO_2 to pressurize fluid up to 700 mm Hg.* Aquadissection is very useful for displacing fatty tissue.

*Nezhat-Dorsey Hydro-dissection Pump, Storz Veterinary Endoscopy, Goleta, Calif. 93117.

HEMOSTASIS

Anticipation, recognition, and control of bleeding are essential in endoscopic surgery. It may be more difficult to anticipate bleeding in minimally invasive surgery than in open surgery because the surgeon is not able to palpate or easily reposition the tissue. Ideally, minimally invasive surgery should be virtually bloodless. Even small amounts of hemorrhage obscure the tissue planes and absorb light, making it more difficult to identify the plane of dissection.

Endoscopic surgeons must select hemostatic techniques *in anticipation* of bleeding because severed vessels retract into the tissue and are more difficult to identify and isolate during endoscopic surgery. Vascular tissue planes can be dissected with monopolar and bipolar electrosurgery devices, laser dissectors, argon beam coagulators, and ultrasonic surgery devices.

Once bleeding begins, small amounts of blood can obscure the operative field. Try to identify and control the bleeding vessel quickly. Remove the scissors and insert an irrigation and suction device. After identifying the site, work quickly because during the subsequent instrument exchange the site may again become covered with blood. If arterial bleeding obscures the lens of the scope, remove, clean, and defog the scope and reinsert it.

Unlike open surgery, using pressure packs to control hemorrhage is difficult in laparoscopic procedures. Temporary control can be achieved by clamping the tissue with grasping forceps. Alternatively, apply pressure with forceps holding a 2-inch × 2-inch sponge. After the bleeding site is identified, use clips, suture, electrosurgery, or staples to control the bleeding (Fig. 3-23).

Application of Hemostatic Clips

Hemostatic clips are available in small, medium, large, and extra large sizes. Clamped tissue should fill approximately three fourths of the internal diameter of a clip. If necessary, replace a small trocar with a larger one

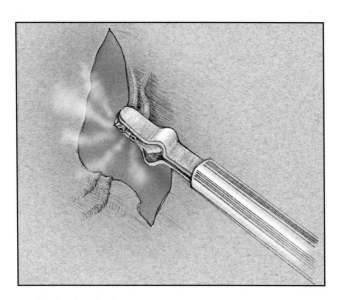

Fig. 3-23 Bipolar forceps are used to coagulate tissue between the jaws of the instrument.

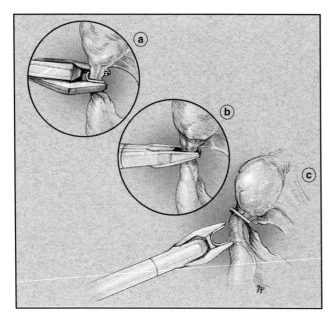

Fig. 3-24 Sequence of ligating clip application. The jaws are positioned around the vessel (a) and rotated slightly so the tips of the applier are visible before the clip is closed (b). The clip is applied and inspected (c).

to introduce the clip applier. For proper positioning, both tips of the clip applier must be around the vessel (Fig. 3-24). Squeeze the handle of the applier to close the clip completely. Observe the clip to evaluate its security and effectiveness. The ideally placed clip completely surrounds the bleeding tissue and is not placed over another clip. The clip jaws are aligned and closed completely.

Ligation with Pre-tied Loops

Pre-tied loop ligatures* facilitate ligating free pedicles (Fig. 3-25). Pass the suture loop through the trocar to the operative site. Grasp the free pedicle through the

---

*Endoloop, Ethicon, Inc., Somerville, N.J. 08876.

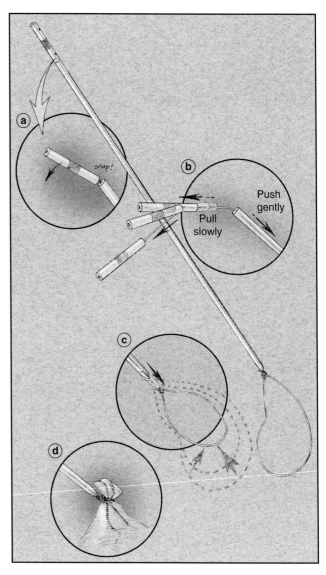

Fig. 3-25 Sequence of Endoloop application. The nylon cannula is advanced (a) while the suture is withdrawn (b), closing the loop and advancing the knot (c) to the surgical site (d).

loop and pull the tissue through the ligature loop. Break the plastic shaft at the score. Cinch the loop by simultaneously pulling the suture and advancing the plastic shaft outside the suture. The plastic shaft pushes the knot to the surgical site. Release the tissue from the grasper and apply additional tension to the shaft to tighten the knot more securely. Remove the plastic cannula. Introduce the scissors along the suture. Cut the suture, leaving a 3- to 4-mm tail.

TISSUE APPOSITION
Endoscopic Stapling
When used properly, vascular staplers are effective in achieving both hemostasis and tissue apposition. To use a stapler for hemostasis, select a cartridge according to the thickness of the tissue (Table 3-1). Load a cartridge and close the stapler for insertion through the trocar. Open the instrument and position its jaws on the tissue to be stapled and transected. Close the instrument and fire it to activate the staples and cut the tissue (Fig. 3-26). Open the stapler and remove it from the tissue. Close the stapler for withdrawal from the trocar.

For tissue apposition, endoscopic staplers save time and minimize tissue trauma. Tissue is apposed with four or six rows of B-shaped staples. A knife simultaneously cuts the tissue between the middle rows. Select a blue or green cartridge to transect, resect, or perform an anastomosis of most tissues (Fig. 3-27).

Box-shaped staples maintain tissue in apposition. They have been used successfully to close colotomy incisions in pigs and are very useful for closing mesentery after an intestinal anastomosis.[8] Hold the tissue in apposition with two grasping forceps. Apply the staples where the tissue edges just touch each other. Apply additional staples until the tissue is completely apposed (Fig. 3-28).

TISSUE REMOVAL
Isolated or diseased tissue that must be removed is often much larger than the trocar cannula or any of the incisions through the body wall. Several techniques have been developed to solve this problem in human laparoscopic surgery. An incision between two trocars can be enlarged to remove the large bowel during laparoscopic low anterior resection. An umbilical incision is enlarged to remove a stone-filled gallbladder. Large uterine fibroids are often morcellated to avoid increasing the incision size. In-

		TABLE 3-1		
		Cartridge Selection for Endoscopic Staplers		
COLOR	NUMBER OF ROWS	STAPLE LINE LENGTH	STAPLE LEG LENGTH	INDICATED TISSUE THICKNESS
Gray	6	32.5 mm	2.0 mm	0.75 mm
White	6	32.5-60 mm	2.5 mm	1.0 mm
Blue	4-6	32.5-60 mm	3.5 mm	1.5 mm
Green	4-6	45-60 mm	4.8 mm	2.0 mm

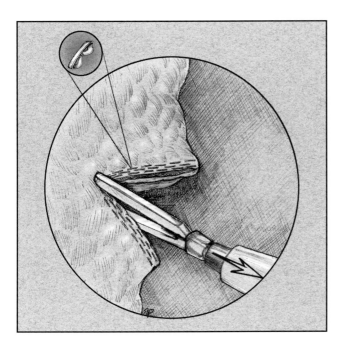

Fig. 3-26 Endoscopic linear cutters place four to six rows of B-shaped staples and cut between the middle rows.

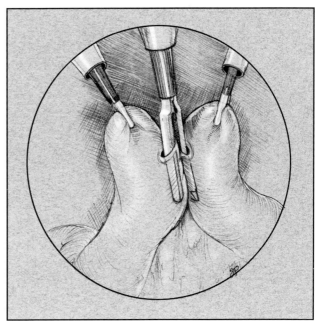

Fig. 3-27 A side-to-side anastomosis performed with an endoscopic linear stapler.

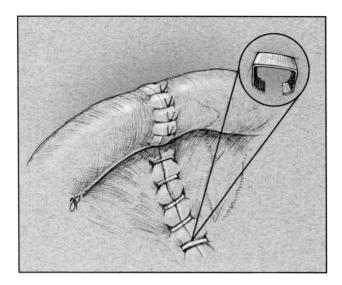

Fig. 3-28 Use of box-shaped staples for tissue apposition.

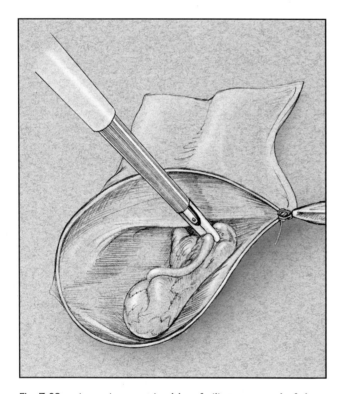

Fig. 3-29 A specimen retrieval bag facilitates removal of the testis after cryptorchid castration.

fected or noninfected tissue may be removed in specimen retrieval bags during laparoscopic procedures (Fig. 3-29).

The finger of a surgical glove or a sterile condom can be used to collect, transport, and deliver materials safely from the peritoneal cavity. The neck of a specimen retrieval bag can be brought through the trocar cannula and opened outside the body. An instrument is inserted into the bag to crush and extract tissue until the bag is small enough to be removed.

When choosing the exit site for a tissue specimen, consider the umbilicus for most small specimens. If a larger port is used during the procedure at another site, the larger port is usually preferable. In some cases, tissue is delivered by another route. A resected colon can be brought externally through the remaining colon, rectum, and anus. In gynecologic surgery, the uterus or an enlarged ovary can be removed through the vagina if it is large enough. In each case the surgeon should choose a site that provides the least resistance to delivery of the specimen, is least painful for the animal, and does not compromise aseptic or other good surgical techniques.

IRRIGATION AND INSPECTION

Before closure the surgeon should irrigate and examine the body cavity. During aspiration keep the side holes on the suction tip submerged beneath the fluid level to prevent rapid loss of pneumoperitoneum and decreased visibility of the operative site. If extensive blood clots are present, use a 10-mm suction device to keep the shaft from becoming obstructed with tissue or fat. Examine ligated sites under reduced pressure of insufflation (4 to 6 mm Hg) to ensure adequate hemostasis. Sites that were hemostatic at 12 to 14 mm Hg have begun bleeding when the abdominal pressure was relieved.[9]

Examine the secondary port sites for bleeding. Treat bleeding from trocar incision sites with electrocoagulation or suture pressure. Use a Keith needle to place a through-and-through suture from outside the abdomen to the inside and out again, compressing the bleeding site (Fig. 3-30). If sutures do not control the bleeding, remove the cannula and insert a Foley catheter with a 30-cc balloon through the trocar site into the peritoneal cavity. Inflate the balloon and apply traction to the catheter to compress the balloon against the body wall. Use a clamp to anchor the catheter at the skin level overnight and remove the Foley catheter the next day (Fig. 3-31).

CLOSURE

When using traditional sutures, use Senn retractors to expose the external sheath of the rectus abdominis muscle after removal of the insufflation gas. Place sutures through the fascia, taking care not to incorporate omentum or bowel in the closure. Close the subcutaneous tissue and skin routinely. Injecting local anesthetic agents at the port sites may reduce postoperative pain. Devices are available to facilitate port site closure in animals with a thick abdominal wall.

Techniques for Skill Development

The basic technical skills needed for endoscopic surgery are hand-eye coordination, working about a pivot point, working with loss of three-dimensional viewing, and op-

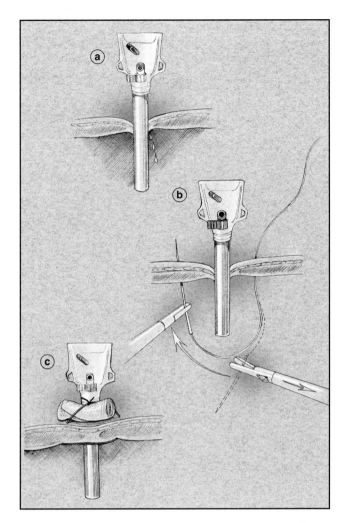

Fig. 3-30 Use of a Keith needle and suture to tamponade bleeding vessels in the abdominal wall. Injury to epigastric vessels causes blood to drip continuously into the surgical field (*a*). Pass a Keith needle and suture percutaneously through the abdominal wall. Inside the abdomen, use laparoscopic needle holders to reposition the needle so that it can be driven outside the abdomen (*b*). On the skin surface, remove the needle and tie the two suture ends over a rolled gauze pad to tamponade the bleeding vessel (*c*).

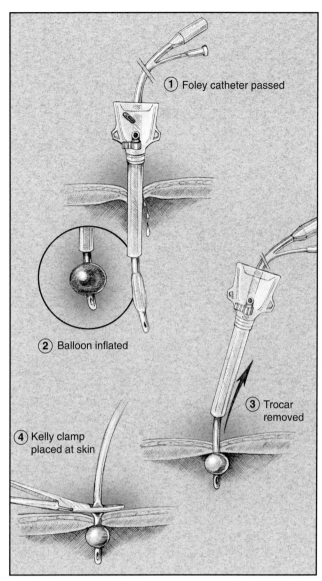

Fig. 3-31 A Foley catheter may be used temporarily to treat hemorrhage from vessels in the abdominal wall.

erating endoscopic graspers, dissectors, scissors, clip appliers, and suture devices. Perfecting the skills necessary for complicated laparoscopic surgery requires a commitment of time and work.

Several inanimate models are available (Box 3-1). Pelvi-trainer and thoraco-trainer models are available with either a clear or a dark top so a student can begin by viewing directly through a glass and progress to using the dark top with a video monitor. Very simple and inexpensive training simulators can be made from cardboard boxes and two mirrors. Endoscopic suturing techniques should be mastered in phantom trainers before they are attempted in animals.

The next level of difficulty is accomplished best with a live animal. Veterinary surgeons learn to insert a Veress needle for insufflation of the abdomen, test for correct needle placement, perform open trocar placement, insert a surgical telescope with an attached camera, insert secondary trocars under direct inspection, and manipulate tissue with instruments. Camera operators learn how to hold the camera so the image is positioned correctly and to move the telescope in and out and laterally to improve visibility of the operative site.

An exercise to improve tissue handling is called *running the bowel*. Just as this technique is used during exploratory laparotomy, so it should be used in explor-

BOX 3-1

INANIMATE MODELS FOR ENDOSCOPIC SURGERY TRAINING

Pelvi-trainer*
Thoraco-trainer
Abdominal torso with uterus
Expert hernia trainer
Expert biliary trainer
Expert suture trainer
Expert OB/GYN trainer

*Laparoscopy trainers are available from the following companies: Advanced Surgical, Inc.; Auto Suture Co.; Cabot Medical Corp.; Ethicon Endo-Surgery, Inc.; Marlow Surgical Technologies; Richard Wolf Medical Instruments Corp.

Tissue models are available from Limbs & Things Ltd., Radnor Business Centre, Radnor Road, Horfield, Bristol BS7 8QS, England, UK.

atory laparoscopy to provide an equally thorough examination. Two grasping forceps are necessary to perform this procedure efficiently. Begin at the descending colon as it enters the pelvis and trace it to the large colon. Depending on the species, it may or may not be possible to trace the large colon sequentially. Next,

identify the cecum and find the ileocecal ligament to identify the ileum. Trace the ileum proximally to the jejunum, duodenum, and stomach. By performing this exercise routinely on all laparoscopy cases, the surgeon, assistant, and camera operator will learn to work as a team and, over time, significantly improve their technical skills.

REFERENCES

1. Iberti TJ et al: A simple technique to accurately determine intra-abdominal pressure. *Crit Care Med* 15:1140-1142, 1987.
2. Ivankovich AD et al: Cardiovascular effects of intraperitoneal insufflation with carbon dioxide and nitrous oxide in the dog. *Anesthesiology* 42:281-287, 1975.
3. Liem T, Applebaum H, Herzberger B: Hemodynamic and ventilatory effects of abdominal CO_2 insufflation at various pressures in young swine. *J Pediatr Surg* 29:966-969, 1994.
4. Diebel LN et al: Effect of increased intra-abdominal pressure on hepatic arterial, portal venous, and hepatic microcirculatory blood flow. *J Trauma* 33:279-283, 1992.
5. Kadar N: Preliminaries: positioning the patient and equipment, entering the abdomen. In Kadar N, editor: Atlas of laparoscopic pelvic surgery, 1995, Cambridge, Mass., Blackwell Science.
6. Melzer A et al: Ports, trocars/cannulae, and access techniques. *Semin Laparosc Surg* 2:179-204, 1995.
7. Kolata R: Unpublished data. 1993.
8. Cohen SM et al: An initial comparative study of two techniques of laparoscopic colonic anastomosis and mesenteric defect closure. *Surg Endosc* 8:130-134, 1994.
9. Freeman LJ: Unpublished data. 1994.

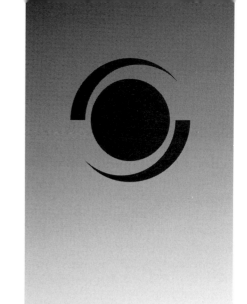

CHAPTER 4

ELECTROSURGERY, LASERS, AND ULTRASONIC ENERGY

Suzanne E. Thompson, Laura Potter

Energy technologies allow surgeons to perform operations through smaller incisions. Instruments using electrical, laser, and ultrasonic energy are superior to mechanical surgical instruments for dissecting, resecting, and controlling or preventing hemorrhage. Surgeons must understand the basic concepts of energy transfer and tissue effects to match the technology with the proposed surgical procedure correctly (Table 4-1).

Hemostasis is critical in performing minimally invasive surgery. Even minor hemorrhage complicates the performance and results of endoscopic surgical procedures because the subject is magnified, the image is two dimensional, and blood is more difficult to remove from the surgical field. The correct use of electrosurgical, laser, or other devices to manage bleeding is essential. Electrosurgical devices are the most economical and are used the most.

TABLE 4-1						
Energy Modality Comparison						
CHARACTERISTICS	MONO-POLAR ES*	BIPOLAR ES	ARGON BEAM	CO_2 LASER	KTP LASER	Nd:YAG LASER	ULTRASONIC SCALPEL
Tissue charring, destruction	Yes	Yes	Yes	Yes	Yes	Yes	Yes, minimal
Blade/tip heat generated at tissue	150° C	150° C	150° C	150° C	150° C	150° C	<150° C
Tissue damage/depth of injury	2-3 mm	2-3 mm	0.5-2.0 mm	<0.5 mm	0.5-2.0 mm	3-5 mm	0.5-2.0 mm
Tissue damage/lateral spread	2.5-3 mm	2-3 mm	0.5-1.0 mm	0.5 mm	0.5-1.0 mm	0.5-1.0 mm	0.2-3.0 mm
Cutting ability	Good	Poor	Poor	Good	Good	Good	Good
Coagulating ability	Good	Good	Good	Poor	Fair	Fair	Good
Tactile feedback	Yes	Yes	No	No	No	Yes	Yes
Blunt dissection	Yes	Yes	No	No	No	No	Yes
Smoke, fumes, odors generated	Yes	Yes	Yes	Yes	Yes	Yes	Some
Debris (eschar) accumulates on blade	Yes	Yes	No	No	No	No	No
Alternate site burns/direct coupling	Yes	No	Yes	No	No	No	No
Alternate site burns/capacitive coupling	Yes	No	Yes	No	No	No	No
Alternate site burns/stray energy	Yes	Yes	Yes	Yes	Yes	Yes	No
Alternate site burns/grounding pad	Yes	No	Yes	No	No	No	No

*ES, Electrosurgery.

Electrosurgery: Principles and Practice

TERMINOLOGY

The terms diathermy, electrocautery, and electrosurgery are often used incorrectly. *Diathermy* is the use of heat for medical purposes. Electrosurgery, electrocautery, lasers, and ultrasound are all forms of surgical diathermy. *Electrocautery* is the use of direct or alternating current to heat a metal instrument that contacts tissues. *Electrosurgery* is the use of alternating current that passes through the patient's tissues to complete the circuit.[1,2]

In *monopolar electrosurgery*, current passes through the body from the active electrode in the wound to the passive return electrode, the grounding pad (Fig. 4-1). In *bipolar electrosurgery*, the active and return electrodes are in the electrosurgical instrument in the surgical wound. Current passes only through the tissues confined between the electrodes. No grounding pad is necessary (Fig. 4-2).[3]

Electrosurgical cutting (Fig. 4-3) divides tissue by focusing current to a small area and vaporizing or exploding cells. The electrode is near, but does not touch, the tissue. Vaporization of the cells dissipates heat, a cooling effect that minimizes the heat transfer to deeper tissues. Therefore, coagulation and hemostasis are minimal. *Electrosurgical desiccation* (coagulation) occurs when the electrode touches the tissue and current is less focused. Cells are dried by the vaporization of cellular water and form a coagulum. The thermal damage is more widespread and hemostasis is improved. *Electrosurgical fulguration* coagulates and chars only the surface of the tissue over a wider area. The electrode does not touch tissue, and the energy sparks across air or argon gas to complete the circuit.

PHYSICS

The tissue effects created by electrosurgery (cutting, dessication, or fulguration) are controlled by the electrosurgical generator output (current frequency, waveforms, voltage, watts), tissue resistance to current flow, electrode shape, contact of the electrode with tissue, and time.

Frequency

Alternating current is characterized by rapid reversal of the direction of the current. The frequency of this oscillation is expressed in cycles per second, or Hertz (Hz). Current frequencies of less than 100,000 cycles per second (100 kHz) cause undesirable neuromuscular stimulation that could result in death. Electrosurgical generators convert standard 60-cycle electrical current to frequencies from 300 kHz to 3.8 MHz (3800 kHz). These frequencies are in the range of AM broadcast radio waves, hence, the term *radio frequency* or *RF current*. At these high frequencies it is difficult or impossible to contain all of the current within the wiring, switches, and connections of the electrosurgical system. "Leaky" current can be seen as interference on cardiac and video monitors and is capable of being induced into metallic instruments. This can pose hazards, which will be discussed later.

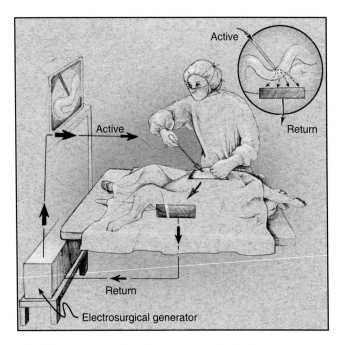

Fig. 4-1 A monopolar electrosurgical circuit. Current passes from the active electrode in the wound, through the body, to the grounding pad.

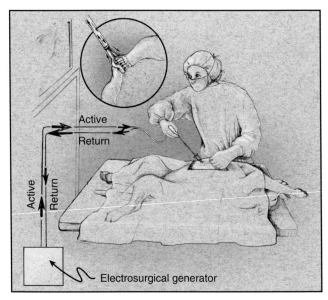

Fig. 4-2 A bipolar electrosurgical circuit. The active and return electrodes are in the electrosurgical instrument in the surgical wound.

Waveforms: Cutting and Coagulation

High-frequency current produces heat in tissues because of the tissue's inherent resistance (impedance) to current flow. The rate of temperature rise and maximum temperature generated determine whether the cells are vaporized (cutting effects), desiccated (coagulation effects), or carbonized (Table 4-2). Most electrosurgical generator systems vary their output by adjusting the amount of time the current is actually flowing. This is best understood by viewing the waveform images with an oscilloscope. For pure cutting applications, the current is "on" all the time at lower voltages and generates high temperatures rapidly. A pure sinusoidal waveform is created (Fig. 4-4, *a*). For coagulation applications the current is "off" a percentage of time so heat is generated more slowly, and lower temperatures are produced in a larger area of tissue. "Blended" waveforms vary the percentage of time that the current flows to achieve a blend between cutting and coagulation effects (see Fig. 4-4, *b* and *c*).

Current

Current is the flowing of electrons, measured in amperes. Current is limited by electrosurgical generators when the devices are used in tissues with very low impedances. The low impedance produces a short circuit and the generator current is limited to avoid melting electrodes and wiring. Generators can typically deliver 1 ampere or more.

Power

Power is measured in watts. A watt is the power developed in a circuit by a current of 1 ampere flowing

TABLE 4-2

Effect of Temperature on Tissue

TEMPERATURE (°C)	VISIBLE EFFECT	CELLULAR EFFECT
<45	None, then edema	Vasodilation, inflammation
45-50	None, then necrosis	Cell metabolism disruption
50-80	Blanching, then sloughing	Collagen denaturation
80-100	Shrinkage, then sloughing	Dessication
100-200	Steam, then ulceration	Vaporization
>200	Carbonization, then cratering	Combustion of cellular hydrocarbons

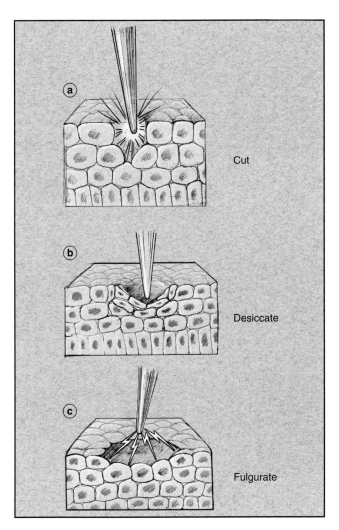

Fig. 4-3 Cutting (*a*), desiccating (*b*), and fulgurating (*c*) techniques. Cutting and fulgurating are noncontact, superficial effects. Desiccating is a contact, penetrating effect.

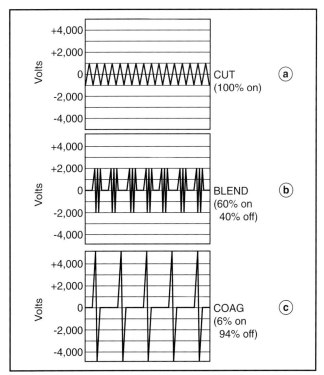

Fig. 4-4 Cut (*a*), blend (*b*), and coagulate (*c*) waveforms.

through a potential difference of 1 volt. The numbers on any generator are relative only to other settings on that generator to serve as a guide for increasing or decreasing that generator's power output. Generators typically can be set from 1 to 300 watts (cutting) and 1 to 120 watts (blend or coagulation).

Voltage

Voltage is the result of the available power and tissue resistance. The maximum voltage depends on the power and waveform selection. The highest voltages are created when the tissue resistance is high or the generator is activated while the instrument is not touching tissue (open circuit). Voltage maximums may vary from several hundred volts (cutting) to several thousand volts (blend or coagulation).

Equations and Tissue Resistance

Electrical heating of tissues obeys the basic laws of electrical physics. Current is measured in amps (I), voltage (electron force) is measured in volts (V), and resistance is measured in ohms (R). Ohm's law, $V = I \times R$, and the power formula, P (watts) $= I \times V$, can be useful when studying the basics of current flow and heating in tissue.[1]

Tissue resistance varies inversely with the water content of the tissue. The higher the water content of the tissue, the lower the resistance (blood < nerve < muscle < fat < bone). As tissue is heated, water is vaporized and the water content of the tissue decreases; therefore, tissue resistance increases.

Electrode Shape and Tissue Contact

Tissue heating is also a function of the *current density*, defined as the amount of current flowing through a given area of tissue. In monopolar electrosurgical applications, a small tissue contact zone produces high current density and faster heating (the active electrode). A large contact zone has lower current density, and the tissue heats slowly or not at all (return electrode). When cutting or fulgurating, the electrode does not contact tissue, so the current density is determined by the sparking between the active electrode and the tissue. Low voltages used in cutting allow the electrode to ride on a steam layer very near the tissue. Blend or coagulation waveforms and higher power settings produce higher voltages, which allow the spark to traverse a larger distance to tissue. This is the principle of fulguration.

In bipolar electrosurgical applications, the electrodes are usually similar in size. The tissue is confined between the electrodes and desiccated by a low-voltage, continuous cutting–type current. As the tissue heats, resistance increases and current flow decreases until it eventually ceases (open circuit). The process is therefore self limit-

ing and the coagulation or tissue dessication endpoint can be detected by using a current monitor. This principle is used in some "smart generator" systems that detect coagulation endpoints. Bipolar devices are used primarily for dessication because of the impractical nature of providing cutting-shaped electrodes in the bipolar current path.[2]

Time

At any setting, the longer the generator is activated, the greater the amount of heat that is produced. As more heat is produced, the area of thermal damage increases.

SAFE PRACTICE OF ELECTROSURGERY
General Considerations

Always take precautions when using electrosurgery. In monopolar applications it is important to ensure good contact between the patient and the return electrode pad. Poor contact causes increases in current density, and enough heat may be generated to burn the skin at the site of the grounding pad. This is the most common electrosurgical injury.

High-frequency currents produced by electrosurgical generators can leak and induce electrical currents in metallic objects or instruments. Coiling the wire for an electrosurgical instrument and hooking it in the handle of a metallic towel clamp (a common practice) can induce enough current to burn the patient.

When cutting and fulgurating, the electrosurgical generator should be activated before approaching tissue with the instrument. This is an appropriate technique in noncontact applications. Touching the tissue before activating the generator causes charring and carbon build-up on the instrument tips, which degrades performance and results in unnecessary tissue damage. When desiccating tissue, the electrosurgical instrument should contact the tissue before activation of the generator.[2,3]

The argon beam coagulator* uses an argon gas jet to deliver monopolar electrosurgical energy evenly over a broad surface of tissue. This electrofulguration technique is used for rapid and effective coagulation of large parenchymal surfaces and vessels ≤4 mm, as in hepatic, splenic, or renal surgery. It should not be used on bowel because of the risk of creating full-thickness injuries.[4]

Endoscopic Procedures

Monopolar electrosurgery can be hazardous in minimally invasive surgical procedures. Because current takes the path of least resistance, the return of current from the active to the return electrode is never constant or predictable. Endoscopic procedures often involve the use

---

*Argon Beam Coagulation System, ConMed Corp., Utica, N.Y. 13501.

of access ports and a scope for imaging. Typically, only a small part of the electrosurgical instrument is visible, and most scopes and other instruments will conduct electrical current. Insulation failure, sparking, direct coupling, current concentration at a distal site, capacitive coupling, and explosions can cause unintentional and even unrecognized tissue burns.

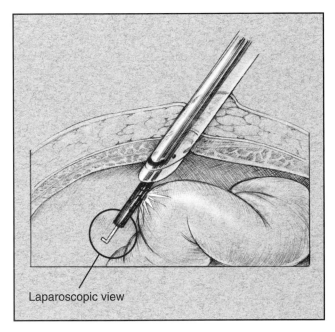

Fig. 4-5 Insulation defects can result in unintended tissue damage outside the field of view.

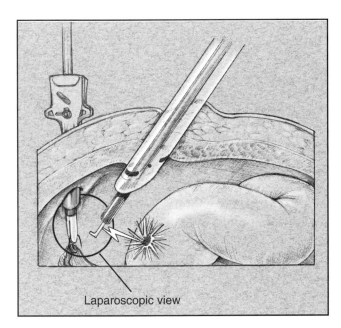

Fig. 4-6 Sparking occurs when the electrosurgical instrument is activated when not in contact with tissues and a high-voltage coagulate or fulgurate waveform is used.

Insulation failure can occur after repeated use and sterilization of reusable instruments. Pinpoint defects in insulative coatings can cause injury by creating an alternate active electrode (Fig. 4-5).

Spark injuries occur when the electrosurgical instrument is activated while not in contact with tissues or while in contact with high-resistance tissues. They are most likely to occur when higher voltage coagulate waveforms are used (Fig. 4-6).

Direct coupling injuries occur when the electrosurgical instrument comes in contact with the scope or other instrument outside the field of view (Fig. 4-7).

Distal site current concentration can occur if the tissue to which the energy is applied is not the smallest cross-sectional area of tissue in the current pathway. The tissue in the smallest area will be heated first (Fig. 4-8).

Capacitors are created when two conductors are separated by an insulator. Capacitors become better conductors at higher frequencies. At electrosurgical frequencies, the capacitors created by combinations of conductors and insulators in common surgical equipment can become the path of least resistance and channel the energy to undesirable sites. If the energy is ultimately discharged through a small contact area of tissue, a burn may result. This situation can occur when active electrosurgical cable is wound around a metal towel clamp or when active electrosurgical instruments are passed through metal cannulas. When plastic retention threads are used with metal cannulas, capacitive coupling can occur to tissues in the operating cavity. This is most likely to occur when the generator is activated without tissue

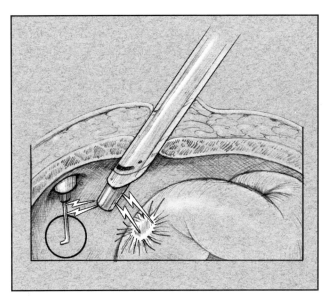

Fig. 4-7 Direct coupling injury outside the field of view.

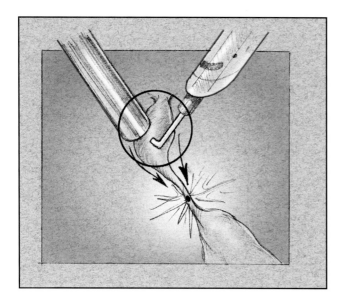

Fig. 4-8   Current concentration injury at a distal site outside the field of view.

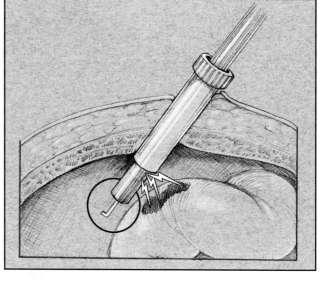

Fig. 4-9   Capacitive coupling injury occurs when a metal cannula is used with plastic (insulating) stability threads.

contact and set to the higher voltage coagulation modes (Fig. 4-9). When metal cannulas are in direct contact with the body wall, capacitively coupled energy is discharged into the body wall (large contact area of tissue) and flows to the return electrode.[2,3]

Explosions can occur when combustible gases escape from the bowel into a confined abdominal cavity and an electrosurgical device is activated. Carbon dioxide (CO_2) is the recommended insufflation gas when electrosurgical devices are used. Nitrous oxide (N_2O) is also used for insufflation, but it is potentially combustible and therefore is not used with electrosurgical instruments.

RECOMMENDATIONS

Surgeons should have a thorough understanding of the principles of electrosurgery before using the devices. Used appropriately, electrosurgery is a safe and economical means of providing hemostasis in all surgical procedures. When it is used in minimally invasive procedures, the following points should be kept in mind:

1. Bipolar techniques should be used whenever possible because the current passes only through the tissue grasped in the electrodes. This minimizes chances for tissue injury outside the field of view. Bipolar current is low-voltage cutting current and is less likely to spark to surrounding tissues than are coagulation waveforms.
2. Always select the minimum power setting that is effective. If the desired effect is not achieved, ensure a complete current pathway (especially with monopolar electrosurgery) before raising the settings. Boosting the power setting forces the current to seek alternative paths.
3. Use cutting current whenever possible. By activating cutting current at low power settings with a broad-based (large contact area) active electrode in contact with tissue, coagulation similar to bipolar techniques can be achieved. Coagulation will be slower, but safety is increased. For cutting applications, a pinpoint active electrode or one with a small area of contact is used.
4. Inspect the insulation on all instruments each time they are used.
5. Avoid metal-to-metal contact, which may cause unseen direct coupling.
6. Unless cutting, do not activate an electrode not in contact with tissue. This may cause sparking to nearby tissues.
7. Remove carbonized tissues from electrodes. Carbon has very high resistance, which increases the chance of sparking and interferes with conduction through intended tissues.
8. If metal cannulas are used, do not insulate them from the body wall with plastic retention sleeves. This can set up capacitive coupling to unintended tissues.
9. Generator systems operating at frequencies in the range of 3.8 MHz do not require intimate patient contact with the return electrode. The current is so poorly contained in wiring that a

return antenna located near the patient is used instead of a grounding pad. Because of the poor current containment, there is concern about capacitance and unintended current pathways causing injury in minimally invasive procedures.

10. When using an argon beam coagulator in laparoscopic procedures, argon gas flows may contribute to elevated intraabdominal pressures. The intraabdominal pressure should be monitored carefully.

Lasers: Principles and Practice

Laser surgery is another method of surgical diathermy. Heat is created in tissue to achieve a desired effect. At present, surgical laser systems are expensive and lack versatility. They are often appropriate for very selective applications. Personnel and patient safety issues exist, requiring training for safe usage. These factors have limited the use of lasers in veterinary surgery. Lasers are used for tissue ablation and coagulation in equine endoscopic applications. New laser technologies in development may provide the economics and versatility to allow a more widespread use in veterinary surgery.

PHYSICS

LASER is an acronym for light amplification by stimulated emission of radiation, a concept first conceived by Einstein in 1917 and perfected in the 1950s and early 1960s.[4,5]

A laser beam consists of photons of coherent light traveling in the same direction. All photons have the same wavelength and are in phase across time and space. This coherent light is created by passing light or electrons through a lasing medium. Lasing mediums include gases (CO_2, argon, helium), crystals (neodymium:yttrium-aluminum-garnet [Nd:YAG]), potassium titanyl phosphate (KTP), liquid dyes (rhodamine), and diode semiconductors.

As atoms of the lasing medium absorb energy, electrons are moved to a higher orbit. The absorbed energy is spontaneously emitted as a photon of a wavelength characteristic of the atoms of the lasing medium. These photons strike other atoms, generating many photons of coherent light traveling in random directions in the lasing medium. Using partially reflective mirrors, the photons are focused to create a laser beam with all photons traveling in the same direction. This process is inefficient, requiring laser systems to have extensive power sources and cooling systems. Lasers are typically named for their lasing mediums, each of which produces a unique wavelength of laser light (Fig. 4-10).

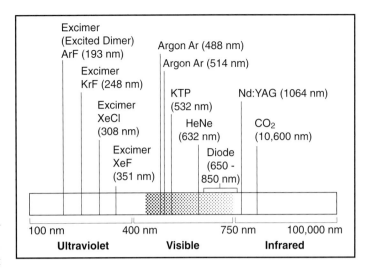

Fig. 4-10   The electromagnetic spectrum and some current lasers.

LASER-TISSUE INTERACTION

The absorption of coherent laser light is predictable. If a substance absorbs light, absorption of the laser energy generates heat. Substances in tissues that absorb light, called *chromophores*, include water, hemoglobin, melanin, hematoporphyrin, and bilirubin. Each chromophore has a specific pattern of light absorption. For example, water absorbs light in the ultraviolet and infrared portions of the electromagnetic spectrum. Lasers with these wavelengths heat or vaporize tissues with high water content. Light in the visible portion of the electromagnetic spectrum is absorbed by tissue chromophores of a color complementary to the beam of light. Thus a red lesion could be treated by a green laser such as KTP.[4]

To minimize penetration of the energy and spare the surrounding tissues, a laser should be chosen that is absorbed most by the target tissue and least by the background tissue. If deeper penetration is required for larger lesions, the laser wavelength should be poorly absorbed by tissue chromophores. This allows scattering of the light and more widespread, slower heating. The Nd:YAG laser is used for these applications because it is poorly absorbed by water and hemoglobin.

LASER USE IN ENDOSCOPY

Laser light diverges unless focused with a lens. Lenses can collimate the beam so that spot size does not change, or lenses can focus the laser at a distance beyond the lens.

CO_2 lasers are delivered through a mechanical arm containing a series of mirrors. The initial lens collimates the beam, and the distal lens focuses the beam in the handpiece. The handpiece is used through the working channel of an operating laparoscope. These lasers provide

TABLE 4-3

Laser Characteristics

LASER TYPE	WAVE-LENGTH (MICRONS)	FLUID PENE-TRATION	USES FLEXIBLE FIBERS	EYE PRO-TECTION	CUT-TING	COAG-ULA-TION
CO_2	10.6	No	No	Yes	Very good	Poor
KTP	0.532	Good	Yes	Yes	Good	Fair
Nd: YAG	1.064	Very good	Yes	Yes	Poor	Very good

precise cutting and vaporization of surface lesions but do not penetrate fluids or coagulate bleeding vessels well.

Lasers with wavelengths between 250 and 2500 nm (KTP, Nd:YAG) transmit through extruded quartz crystal fibers. In minimally invasive procedures, the fibers are used in contact or noncontact applications. Noncontact fibers focus the laser light at a predetermined distance (usually 3 to 5 mm) from the fiber tip. Contact laser fibers have a sapphire crystal or frosted conical tip that is heated by absorbing the laser. The fibers are typically passed through instruments such as suction-irrigators. Table 4-3 characterizes the principal lasers currently used in endoscopy.[6]

Filters are used between the scope and camera lens to prevent image distortion during laser use. If no video camera is used, an in-line filter is necessary for eye protection. Protective eyewear should be used by all operating room personnel.

The ideal laser system would be tunable to different wavelengths in response to desired tissue absorption effects. Such a system would have spectrophotometric capabilities to analyze the target and background tissues, select a waveform that heats target tissue and spares surrounding tissue, and control depth and rate of tissue heating. It should be inexpensive and safe to use. Obviously, this state of the technology is not yet available. New diode laser systems under development may eventually allow many of these ideals to be met.

Ultrasonic Energy: Principles and Practice

Sound is mechanical energy that is transmitted by longitudinal pressure waves through matter. As a sound wave moves through matter, molecules vibrate and collide but maintain the same relative position to one another. Because the molecular motion is coordinated, a wave is produced and energy is transmitted in the absence of bulk matter displacement.[7] Audible sound waves have frequencies in the range of 20 to approximately 20,000 cycles per second. Sound waves above the audible range are called *ultrasonic waves*.

Ultrasonic waves are produced by applying electromagnetic energy to a piezoelectric transducer. The transducer converts the electrical field to mechanical (ultrasonic) energy. Diagnostic ultrasound imaging uses low-power ultrasonic waves, which cause no appreciable tissue effect. At higher power levels and densities, ultrasonic energy can dissect, coagulate, and cut tissue.

GENERATOR, FOOT SWITCH, AND HANDPIECE

An ultrasonic surgical unit* consists of a high-frequency generator controlled by a microprocessor, a foot switch, a handpiece that houses the ultrasonic transducer, an adaptor, and a selection of interchangeable blades.

The generator converts 115V AC power to an electric drive signal when the foot switch pedal is depressed. The ultrasonic transducer, housed in the handpiece, receives the electric signals from the generator and converts them into ultrasonic mechanical vibration. Piezoelectric ceramics, stacked like coins in the transducer, begin to vibrate at their natural frequency when stimulated by the electric signals. The vibration is transferred to the blade. The blade vibrates longitudinally at 55,500 cycles per second (ultrasonic motion). The blade tip moves 50 to 100 μ per cycle, depending on the generator energy setting (Fig. 4-11).

Ultrasonic energy application permits controlled hemostatic coagulation and cutting of tissue. No electric current is passed through the tissue. Tissue effects are produced by the mechanical vibration of the blade.

BLADE SYSTEMS

A blade is selected based on the procedural application and the surgeon's preference. The principal difference between open and endoscopic blades is the shaft length. Longer shafts facilitate minimally invasive surgical procedures.

Ultrasonically activated blades with sharp edges cut tissues rapidly with minimal coagulation (Table 4-4). Blunt edges and flat surfaces coagulate tissue more and cut less rapidly. Most blade designs provide multiple functions, depending on how they are applied to tissue. For example, the broad surface of the hook blade is used to compress and coagulate blood vessels. The hook blade is then rotated 90° and the concave cutting surface transects the vessel (Fig. 4-12). This reduces the total number of instruments and instrument exchanges required to complete a surgical procedure (see Table 4-4).

The most versatile of the blade designs is the laparosonic coagulating shears, which consists of a blade with a Teflon clamp pad. The blade can be rotated into any of three positions relative to the pad (Fig. 4-13).

---

*UltraCision, Ethicon Endo-Surgery, Inc., Cincinnati, Ohio 45242.

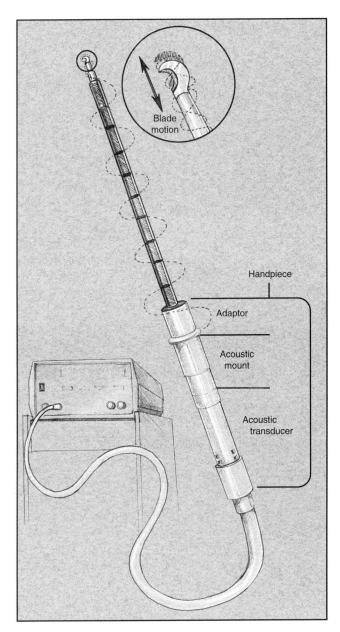

Fig. 4-11   The UltraCision Generator, the handpiece containing the transducer and acoustic mount, the adaptor, and an attached blade. The dotted line represents energy transmission from the transducer through the ultrasonic blade. The result is 50 to 100 μ longitudinal motion of the blade tip per cycle.

The flat surface is used to grasp and coagulate large vessels (Fig. 4-14). The sharp side is used for blunt dissection and cutting avascular structures (Fig. 4-15). Medium to large vessels are coagulated with the blunt surface of the blade (Fig. 4-16). After coagulation of the vessel, the tissue is transected by increasing the grip force on the handle.

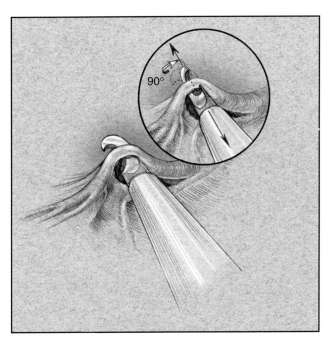

Fig. 4-12   The broad surface of the hook blade is used to compress and coagulate a blood vessel. The hook blade is rotated 90° and the vessel is transected with the concave cutting surface of the blade.

TABLE 4-4			
Blade Systems for Ultrasonic Generator			
OPEN SURGERY BLADE SYSTEM			
		PRINCIPAL FUNCTIONS	
PRODUCT	CUT	COAGULATE	DISSECT	GRASP
Sharp hook blade	X	X	X	
Coagulating shears	X	X	X	X
MINIMALLY INVASIVE SURGERY BLADE SYSTEM			
		PRINCIPAL FUNCTIONS	
PRODUCT	CUT	COAGULATE	DISSECT	GRASP
Sharp hook blade	X	X	X	
Dissecting hook blade	X	X	X	
Ball coagulator		X [broad surface]		
Laparosonic Coagulating Shears (LCS)	X	X	X	X

PRINCIPLES OF ULTRASONIC TISSUE EFFECTS

Ultrasonically activated blades are capable of simultaneously coagulating and cutting numerous tissue types. The amount of energy delivered to tissue and the resultant tissue effect vary with the generator power level, the tissue type, and factors such as blade configuration, blade surface used, amount of blade-tissue contact, pressure exerted, blade speed, and activation time.

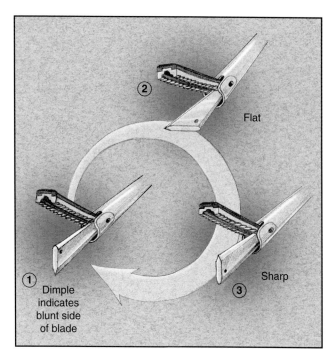

Fig. 4-13   The laparosonic coagulating shears (LCS) blade can be rotated into three different positions relative to the clamp pad.

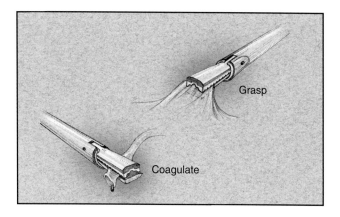

Fig. 4-14   Tissue grasping and coagulation of large bleeding vessels with the flat surface of the LCS blade.

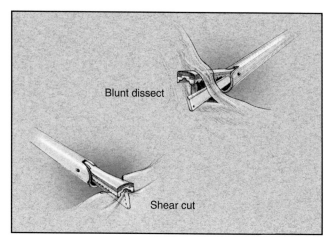

Fig. 4-15   Blunt dissection and shear cutting of avascular structures with the sharp side of the LCS blade apposed to the clamp pad.

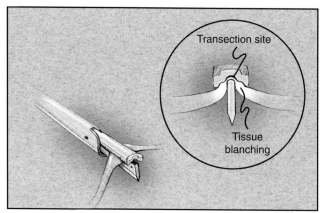

Fig. 4-16   Coagulation and cutting of medium to large vessels with the blunt surface of the LCS blade apposed to the clamp pad.

Coagulation Mechanism

An ultrasonically activated scalpel blade couples with and vibrates tissue. Mechanical energy transferred to the tissue from the blade breaks tertiary hydrogen bonds, and friction and shear stress generate a moderate amount of heat. The result is protein denaturation and the production of a sticky protein coagulum capable of sealing compressed blood vessels.[8]

Mechanical energy from the vibrating blade is propagated in tissue in the direction in which the force is applied. Very little energy effect occurs lateral to the direction of the applied force, so collateral thermal damage is minimized (Fig. 4-17). The depth of penetration of the coagulation effect is related to the power setting of the generator, the amount of pressure applied to the tissue, and the length of time the blade is in contact with the tissue. If the power setting and pressure are held constant, the depth of coagulation increases linearly with time. This is in contrast to the effect of electrosurgical energy, in which the depth of coagulation plateaus with time.

Before activating the blade, the intimal surfaces of blood vessels are brought into apposition and compressed. When energy is applied, tissue denaturation occurs, a coagulum is formed, and the endothelial surfaces of the vessel stick together to seal the vessel. The surgeon controls the balance between tissue coagulation and cutting by changing the blade configuration and varying the amount of tissue tension.

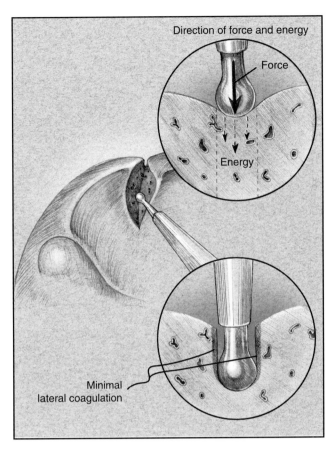

Fig. 4-17   Mechanical energy from the ultrasonic vibrating blade is propagated in tissue in the direction the force is applied. Very little energy effect occurs lateral to the direction of the applied force. Collateral thermal damage is minimized.

Cutting Mechanism

Increased generator power, increased tissue tension, and increased clamp force with the laparosonic coagulating shears act to increase the tissue cutting rate. The surgeon can transect tissue with the blunt and flat surfaces of the ultrasonic blades. However, when the sharp surface of the blade is used, tissue cutting is rapid, with less coagulative effect.

During tissue cutting, all of the ultrasonic blades deliver tactile feedback similar to that provided by conventional scalpels. The laparosonic coagulating shears can be used like scissors (see Fig. 4-15) or a scalpel blade. To use the shears as a scalpel blade, the sharp side of the blade is oriented away from the clamp pad. The tissue is held under tension, and the activated blade is drawn across the tissue to create a hemostatic incision (Fig. 4-18).

Tissue Dissection

Rapid vibration of the ultrasonic blade in tissue causes cell disruption. Intracellular water is vaporized at physi-

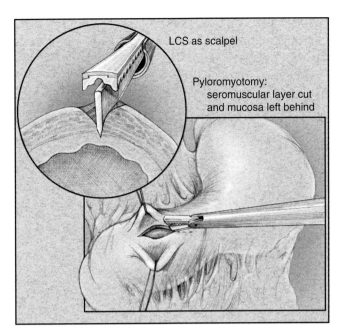

Fig. 4-18   The LCS blade is ready to be used like a scalpel blade. The sharp blade configuration is oriented away from the clamp pad. The activated blade is drawn across tissue held under tension to create a hemostatic incision.

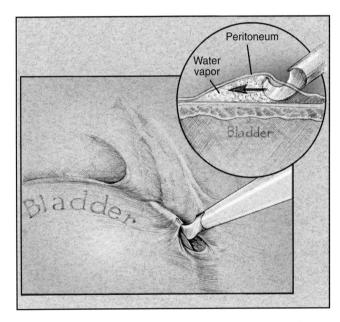

Fig. 4-19   The rapid vibration of the ultrasonic blade creates water vapor and cavitational fragmentation of cells. The cavitational effect is characterized by separation of tissue planes in advance of the blade.

ologic temperatures. As the water vaporizes, it expands and causes cavitational fragmentation of cells. This cavitational effect is characterized by separation of tissue planes in advance of the blade and is an effective method of tissue dissection (Fig. 4-19).[9]

ADVANTAGES OF ULTRASONIC ENERGY

In contrast to electrosurgery, ultrasonic surgery eliminates the potential hazards associated with passing electricity to or through a patient.[10,11] Precise cutting and controlled coagulation with minimal lateral thermal damage allow safer dissection near vital structures than does electrosurgery or laser surgery.[12,13] The ability of ultrasonic devices to coagulate and transect vessels up to 3 mm in diameter eliminates a need to clip or staple vessels in this size range.[10,12,14] Because of the vibration and low heat generation, less tissue adheres to ultrasonic blades than to electrosurgery blades.[15,16]

REFERENCES

1. Odell RC: Laparoscopic electrosurgery. In Hunter JG, Sackier JM, editors: Minimally invasive surgery, New York, 1993, McGraw-Hill.
2. Nolan LJ: Principles of electrosurgery. In Sugarbaker PH, editor: Pelvic surgery and treatment for cancer, St. Louis, 1994, Mosby.
3. Valleylab, Inc.: Principles of electrosurgery, Boulder, Colo., 1995.
4. Hunter JG: Laser physics and tissue interaction. In Hunter JG, Sackier JM, editors: Minimally invasive surgery, New York, 1993, McGraw-Hill.
5. Nolan LJ: Laser physics and safety. *Clin Podiatr Med Surg* 4(4):777-785, 1987.
6. Goldstein DS et al: Laparoscopic equipment. In Soper NJ et al, editors: Essentials of laparoscopy, St. Louis, 1994, Quality Medical Publishing.
7. Sternheim MM, Kane JW, editors: Sound. In General physics, ed 2, New York, 1991, John Wiley and Sons.
8. Amaral JF: Laparoscopic application of an ultrasonically activated scalpel. *Gastrointest Endosc Clin North Am* 3:381-392, 1993.
9. Meltzer RC et al: The ultrasonically activated scalpel vs. electrosurgery for seromyotomy: acute and chronic studies in the pig. Presented at the SAGES meeting, Nashville, Tenn., April 1994.
10. McCarus SD: Physiologic mechanism of the ultrasonically activated harmonic scalpel. *J Am Assoc Gynecol Laparoscopists* 3:601-08, 1996.
11. Miller CE, Johnston M, Rundell M: Laparoscopic myomectomy in the infertile woman. *J Am Assoc Gynecol Laparoscopists* 3:525-532, 1996.
12. Rothenberg S: Laparoscopic splenectomy using the harmonic scalpel. *J Laparoendosc Surg* 6:S61-S63, 1996.
13. Swanstrom LL, Pennings JL: Laparoscopic control of short gastric vessels. *J Am Coll Surg* 181:347-351, 1995.
14. Amaral JF: Ultrasonic energy in laparoscopic surgery. Surgical Technology Int. III, San Francisco, 1995, Universal Medical Press.
15. Amaral JF: Ultrasonic dissection. *Endosc Surg Allied Technol* 2:181-185, 1994.
16. Amaral JF: Laparoscopic cholecystectomy in 200 consecutive patients using an ultrasonically activated scalpel. *Surg Laparosc Endosc* 5:255-262, 1995.

CHAPTER 5

LAPAROSCOPIC SUTURING AND KNOT TYING TECHNIQUES

David R. Stoloff

Instrumentation

General laparoscopic equipment and specialized instrumentation facilitate laparoscopic suturing and knot tying (Box 5-1).

NEEDLE HOLDER

A needle holder with a 5-mm shaft diameter and straight or curved jaws is suitable for suturing (Fig. 5-1, *A*). Needle holders with straight jaws can be used for most laparoscopic suturing. Needle holders with curved jaws can be used effectively to create loops of suture and prevent the suture from sliding off the ends of the jaws. When the needle holders are held at angles of 45° or more from the tissue, curved needle holders provide an advantage.

Needle holder handles should be in axial alignment with the shaft of the instrument because that allows easier manipulation in various port locations. It also makes it easier to rotate the instrument 360°, facilitating knot formation. Pistol grip handles do not offer the same flexibility. The locking mechanism should be adjustable so the surgeon can vary the tightness of the grip on a needle. Minimal holding force is required for most suturing. When the needle penetrates very dense tissue, the locking mechanism must provide greater holding force (Fig. 5-2).

NEEDLES

Straight, $\frac{1}{2}$ circle, $\frac{3}{8}$ circle, and half-curved ("ski") needles are suitable for endoscopic suturing. The J needle

can be used to facilitate closure of trocar ports (Fig. 5-3). When suturing in an area with limited access, a straight needle is more difficult to work with.

GRASPING FORCEPS AND SCISSORS

Grasping forceps ("graspers") with a 5-mm shaft diameter are used to position the needle in the jaws of the needle holder, manipulate tissue during suturing, and assist in intracorporeal knot tying. The jaws of the forceps can be straight or curved. The design of the jaws should minimize trauma to tissue and suture material. Instruments with curved jaws may provide an advantage in intracorporeal knot tying. A handle lock enables the surgeon to rotate the instrument on its axis while maintaining a hold on the suture. Straight, curved, or hook-type 5-mm scissors are used to cut sutures. Microscissors are not used because cutting the suture dulls the blades.

KNOT PUSHERS

Knot pushers are used to drive an extracorporeal throw or knot along one limb of suture into the body cavity. Disposable and reusable knot pushers are manufactured for laparoscopic suturing. Knot pushers can be purchased separately or as an integral component of an extracorporeal knot-tying system (e.g., Endoloop, Endoknot, Pre-Tied Loop Suture). There are two knot-pusher designs. One is a rod with a side groove and a concavity at the tip (see Fig. 5-1, *B*). One limb of the suture is placed in the groove. The extracorporeal tie is advanced as before. With this design, care must be taken to keep

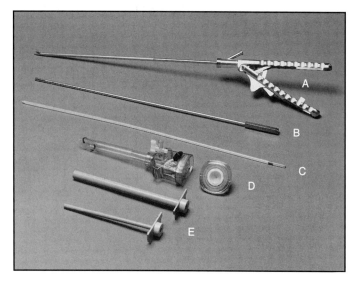

Fig. 5-1 Instruments for endoscopic suturing. Needle holder (A), reusable knot pusher (B), disposable knot pusher (C), 10/12 mm trocar and Universal Oneseal reducer cap (D), and 5- and 10-mm introducer sleeves (E).

BOX 5-1

INSTRUMENT LIST FOR LAPAROSCOPIC SUTURING AND KNOT TYING

General Equipment List

Needle holder, 5 mm
Grasping forceps, 5 mm
Endoscopic scissors, 5 mm
Trocars, 10/12 mm
Universal reducer cap
Endoscopic suture materials
Knot pusher
Introducer sleeve, 10 mm
Endoscopic Babcock forceps

Special Instrumentation

Endoloop* ligature
Pre-tied Endoknot* suture
Pre-tied loop* suture
Lapra-Ty* suture clip

---

*Trademarks of Ethicon, Inc., Somerville, N.J. 08876.

---

the suture in the groove of the rod during advancement. The other design is a conical-tipped rod with a central channel (see Fig. 5-1, C). Suture is passed through the central channel of the rod and pulled until the extracorporeal tie rests against the tip of the rod. Pushing the rod against the tie advances the tie to the site of application. The advantage of this design is that during placement

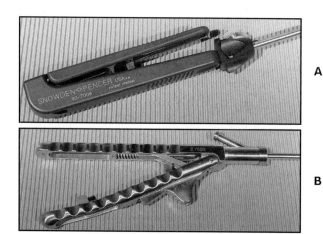

Fig. 5-2 Two types of needle holder handles. **A,** The Snowden Pencer needle holder secures the needle with a ratchet mechanism. The needle is released by squeezing the handle tighter to clear the ratchet. **B,** The Endopath reusable needle holder also secures the needle with a ratchet mechanism. The needle holder is opened by depressing a ratchet release mechanism.

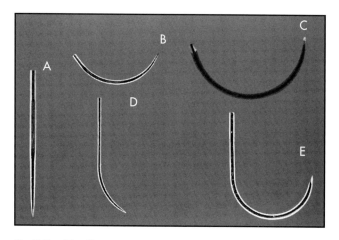

Fig. 5-3 Needles commonly used in minimally invasive surgery. Straight needle (A), 3/8 circle needle (V-4 taper cut) (B), 1/2 circle (CT-2 taper) (C), Endoski needle (EN-S, 1/2 curved) (D), and J needle (V-38) (E).

the suture is held securely within the channel of the knot pusher.

TROCARS

Three ports are usually used to perform extracorporeal knot tying and intracorporeal suturing and knot tying. One port is a viewing port; the other two ports are used to manipulate the suture or needle and suture combination. The outer diameter of the scope determines the diameter of the trocar cannula needed for the viewing port. Trocars and their cannulas are typically sized as 10-12 mm or 10/12 mm based on the smallest diameter of instrument that is sealed by the outer gasket (10 mm) and the largest diameter of instrument that the cannula will accept (12 mm) (see Fig. 5-1, D). If

10/12 mm trocars have been used earlier in the procedure, a reducer cap may be needed to prevent loss of pneumoperitoneum during suturing or ligation (see Fig. 5-1, *D*). If the endoscopic Babcock clamp technique is used, a 10/12 mm trocar will be needed.[1]

INTRODUCER SLEEVE

The introducer sleeve is a cylinder with a gasket that prevents loss of pneumoperitoneum (see Fig. 5-1, *E*). The introducer, which is inserted through a trocar, prevents damage to the needle and suture. It facilitates introduction of pre-tied ligatures and extracorporeally tied slip-knots.

Video Monitor, Port Placement, and Surgeon Positioning

The video monitor should be positioned directly in front of the surgeon and in alignment with the suture line. Place the optical port a short distance from, and in coaxial alignment with, the monitor and the wound. Position the optical port to provide an optimal view of the wound closure site. To provide the best viewing perspective, the wound site should be in the center of the field and the long axis of the wound should lie in the 12 o'clock to 6 o'clock direction.[2] Because a right-handed surgeon is most comfortable suturing in a 1 o'clock to 7 o'clock direction, rotate the wound axis to a 10 o'clock to 4 o'clock direction if suturing difficulty is experienced.[3]

Place instrument ports on each side of and equidistant from the suture site in a comfortable position for suturing (Fig. 5-4). Consider the length of the instruments when placing ports. Separate the instrument ports by at least 15 to 20 cm.[4] Place the instrument ports approximately 10 cm from the optical port.[2] This will minimize the angle between the needle holder and suture line and reduce the difficulty of suturing.

MINIMIZING DEPTH PERCEPTION PROBLEMS[2]

Unless the surgeon has three-dimensional videoimaging equipment, suturing must be performed in a two-dimensional visual field. Under this condition, depth perception is impaired. To address this problem, touch the object to be grasped with an endoscopic instrument to confirm its location before it is grasped. This eliminates haphazard grasping motions to locate an object. In a deep surgical field, operating close to the tissue surface reduces the working depth of the surgical field and improves depth perception.

Knot Tying Terminology

For the purposes of knot tying, a suture is divided into the standing part, the bight, and the end (Fig. 5-5). The *standing part* is the longest section of the suture

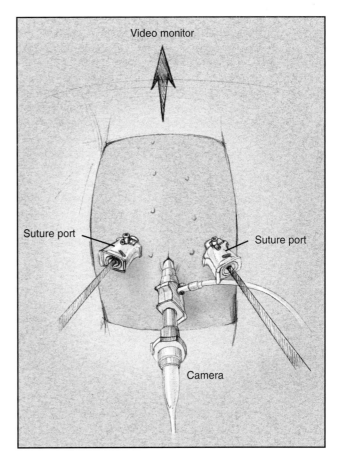

Fig. 5-4 Position the video monitor in front of the surgeon. The optical port is in coaxial alignment with the wound, and the suturing ports are on opposites sides of the wound.

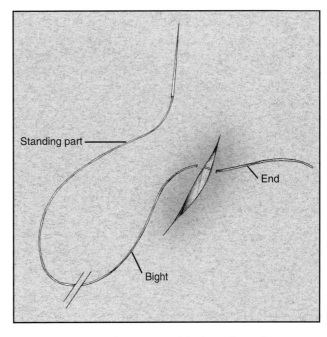

Fig. 5-5 Parts of a suture: end, bight, and standing part.

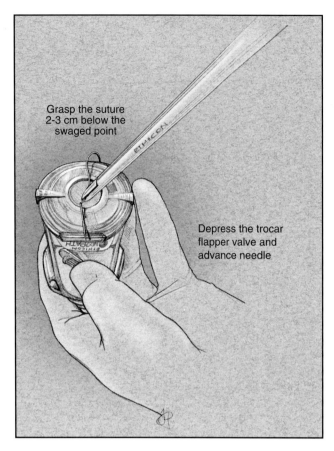

Fig. 5-6 Inserting a straight needle. Grasp the suture below the swage and insert the needle holder through the reducer cap.

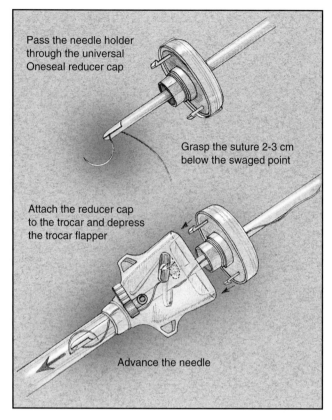

Fig. 5-7 Inserting a ½ circle needle. Insert the needle holder through the reducer cap. Grasp the suture below the swage. Attach the reducer cap and advance the needle.

or that portion swaged to the needle. The *bight* is the section of suture between the standing part and the end. The knot is formed around the loop configuration of the bight. The *end* is the portion of the suture that is used to form the knot.[5] If the suture is not attached to a plastic cannula, identify which limb of the suture will be used with the knot pusher and will be the standing part.

Placing the Suture

INTRODUCING THE NEEDLE

Straight needles and curved needles equivalent to CT-1 and smaller can be introduced through a 10/12 mm trocar. Cut the suture to the desired length (usually 10 cm). When using a straight needle, grasp the suture 2 to 3 cm below the swaged end, depress the trocar flapper valve, and advance the needle (Fig. 5-6). When inserting a curved needle, place the needle holder through the universal reducer cap.[6] Grasp the suture 2 to 3 cm below the swaged end (Fig. 5-7). Attach the reducer cap to the trocar. Depress the trocar flapper valve and advance the needle.

LOADING THE NEEDLE HOLDER
Method 1 (Pirouette Technique[7])

With a grasper, hold the suture approximately 2.5 cm from the needle. Lift the suture so that only the point of the needle is in contact with the serosa (Fig. 5-8, *a*). Rotate the body of the needle until it is correctly positioned for grasping (Fig. 5-8, *b*). If the port placement and the suture line are positioned optimally, the needle swage will be at the 1 o'clock position with the needle point directed at 7 o'clock. Grasp a ³⁄₈ circle or straight needle approximately two thirds of the length from the needle point and a ½ circle needle half the length from the needle point.[3]

Method 2

Position the needle on the serosal surface by manipulating the suture. Grasp the needle loosely in the needle holder (Fig. 5-9, *a* and *b*). Realign the needle as needed by pressing or brushing the needle tip or swage against the serosa (Fig. 5-9, *c*).

After loading the needle in the needle holder, bring the needle close to the viewing port to confirm that the needle is perpendicular to the needle holder jaws.[8]

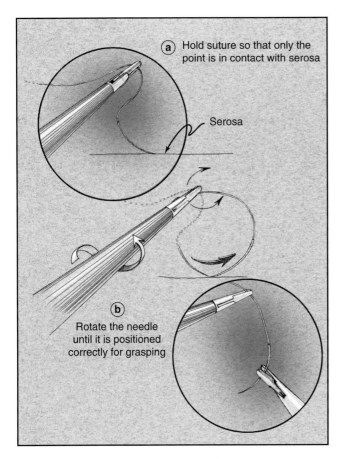

Fig. 5-8 Loading the needle—Method 1. Hold the suture so that only the point of the needle is in contact with the serosa (*a*). Rotate the needle until it is positioned correctly for grasping (*b*).

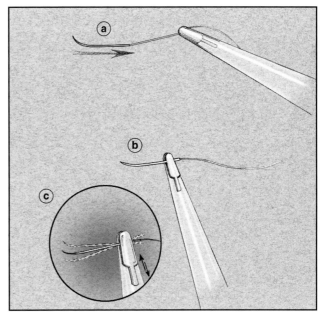

Fig. 5-9 Loading the needle—Method 2. Lay the needle on the serosal surface and position the needle by manipulating the suture (*a*). Grasp the needle loosely (*b*). Brush the needle against the serosa to position the needle (*c*).

ADJUSTING THE NEEDLE IN THE NEEDLE HOLDER

It is possible to change the orientation of the needle while keeping it in the jaws of the needle holder. One method is to anchor the tip of the needle in tissue. While gently holding the needle, apply angular forces to the needle to change its axial orientation (Fig. 5-10).[9] Re-grasp the needle firmly when it is positioned correctly. Another method is to tap the needle gently near its tip with the grasping forceps.

NEEDLE ENTRY[6,10]

Hold one edge of the wound with grasping forceps to stabilize the tissue during needle penetration (Fig. 5-11, *a*). Drive the needle perpendicular to the wound edge. As you begin to drive the needle through the tissue, look for any change in direction of the needle's path. The needle holder should apply force along the axis of the needle. The amount of force required for penetration should be appropriate to the specific tissue penetrated. Excessive force should not be required. If the needle holder applies a nonaxial or tangential force to the

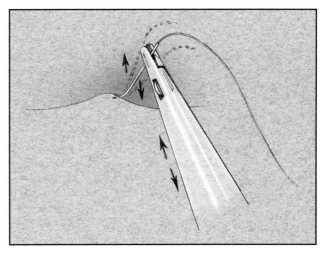

Fig. 5-10 Further positioning of the needle. Drive a portion of the needle tip into the serosa. Apply angular forces to reposition the needle.

needle, difficulty in directing the needle, needle breakage, and tissue damage can result.

Grasp the opposite wound edge adjacent to the site of needle penetration with the grasper (see Fig. 5-11, *b*) and drive the needle through the tissue. If needed to facilitate passage of the needle, place the open jaws of the grasper adjacent to the point of needle tenting and apply counterpressure. When the tip of the needle penetrates the

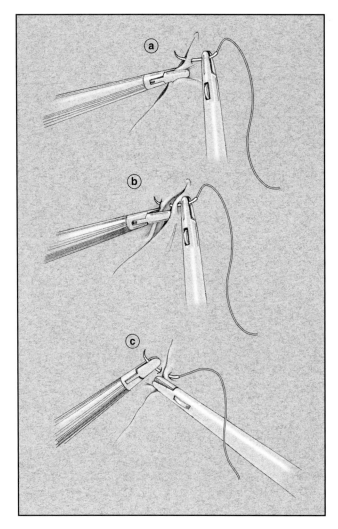

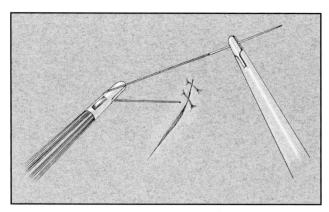

Fig. 5-12   Grasping forceps are used as a pulley to minimize tissue trauma while the suture is pulled through tissue.

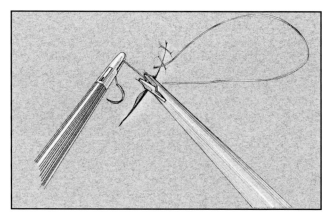

Fig. 5-13   Apply counterpressure adjacent to the emergence of the suture when pulling suture through tissue.

Fig. 5-11   Driving the needle through tissue. Grasp one edge of the wound adjacent to the site of needle penetration (*a*). Grasp the apposing wound edge and drive the needle through tissue (*b*). Apply counterpressure with the needle holder and complete needle passage (*c*).

tissue, grasp the needle with the grasping forceps. Open the jaws of the needle holder and apply counterpressure to the tissue adjacent to the needle to facilitate needle and suture passage through the tissue (see Fig. 5-11, *c*). Alternatively, regrasp the body of the needle with the needle holder and complete the needle passage.

PULLING SUTURE THROUGH TISSUE[10]
There are two ways to minimize tissue damage when pulling suture through tissue. In one technique, the needle holder pulls the suture around closed grasping forceps. The grasper serves as a pulley, keeping the suture in line with the original tissue passage (Fig. 5-12). This is especially useful while pulling a long strand of suture through tissue when tying extracorporeal knots. Any additional tension on the suture is placed on the pulley

rather than on the surrounding tissue. The other technique is to use the grasping forceps to pull the suture along the axis of the original needle passage while the open jaws of the needle holder apply counterpressure to tissue adjacent to the point of suture emergence (Fig. 5-13). The latter method is frequently used during intracorporeal suturing.

Extracorporeal Knot Tying

An *extracorporeal knot* is formed outside the body, advanced into a body cavity, and secured. Extracorporeal knots are commonly used for ligation, tissue approximation, and wound closure, especially when distraction is a problem and for surgical sites with limited access.[11]

RETRIEVING THE NEEDLE AND SUTURE
The suture must be of adequate length to enable the surgeon to tie an extracorporeal knot. With one end of the suture external to the cannula, pass the needle through the tissue. Pull sufficient suture through the tissue to exteriorize the needle and suture. Use the grasper as a

pulley to minimize tension on the tissue. Grasp the suture 2.5 cm behind the swage point, open the flapper valve, and pull the needle and suture through the port of entry.

EXTRACORPOREAL KNOTS

Extracorporeal knots are formed with specialized pre-tied sutures or clips, by tying a surgeon's knot and using a knot pusher to advance individual throws, or by tying a slipknot and using a device to advance the knot into the body cavity.

Pre-tied Sutures
Endoloop Ligature
The Endoloop ligature is a pre-tied suture with a sliding knot and disposable cannula. It can be used to ligate vascular structures, obtain biopsy specimens, temporarily close small tissue defects, and manipulate structures intraoperatively. Endoloop ligatures are available in PDS II (polydioxanone) suture, Coated Vicryl (polyglactin 910) suture, Monocryl (poliglecaprone 25) suture, and Ethibond Excel polyester suture.

TECHNIQUE Insert the introducer into a 5-mm trocar or through a universal Oneseal reducer cap on a 10/12 mm trocar (Fig. 5-14, *a*). Advance the loop ligature until the entire loop is visible within the body cavity. Insert a 5-mm grasper through an open trocar port and pass the jaws of the grasper through the loop (Fig. 5-14, *b*). Grasp the tissue pedicle to be ligated. While elevating the structure slightly with grasping forceps, guide the loop over the grasper and around the tissue pedicle (Fig. 5-14, *c*). Transfer the grasper to an assistant. To close the loop, snap the plastic cannula at its scored end (Fig. 5-14, *d*). Position the tip of the cannula and pre-tied slipknot at the exact site of ligation. Pull back on the short portion of the cannula and advance the longer portion. To tighten the ligature securely, apply additional tension by holding the tip of the cannula against the pre-tied knot and pulling on the short portion of the cannula (Fig. 5-14, *e*). The suture can be cut by inserting scissors through a secondary port or through the same port used for insertion of the Endoloop. If the scissors are inserted through the Endoloop port, cut the suture at its attachment to the small plastic cannula and withdraw the longer portion of the cannula from the trocar. Place some tension on the suture with one hand, slide a pair of 5-mm scissors through the trocar adjacent to the suture, and cut the suture 2 cm from the knot. If a biopsy specimen is taken, transect the tissue first (Fig. 5-14, *f*) and then cut the suture (Fig. 5-14, *g*). If scissors are inserted through a secondary port, then simply cut the suture and pull the long end of the suture and cannula out of the trocar cannula.
Pre-tied Endoknot Suture[12]
The Pre-tied Endoknot suture consists of a plastic cannula that is scored at one end and conical at the opposite

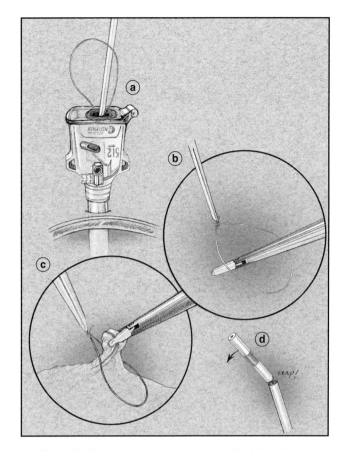

Fig. 5-14 Endoloop ligature. Introduce the Endoloop ligature through a reducer cap on a 10/12 mm trocar (*a*). Pass the grasping forceps through the Endoloop ligature (*b*). Grasp the vascular pedicle and guide the loop around the pedicle (*c*). Snap the cannula at the scored end (*d*). *Continued*

end (Fig. 5-15, *a*). The cannula has a small channel through its center. A stainless steel wire with a loop at the conical end runs through the central channel of the cannula. The pre-tied knot is available in Coated Vicryl suture and PDS II suture and comes swaged to a straight taper point needle.

TECHNIQUE Grasp the suture below the swage, introduce the needle and suture through a 10/12 mm trocar with a universal reducer cap, and place the needle at the site of application. Grasp the needle with the needle holder and drive the needle through the tissue. Pull additional suture through tissue by using the pulley technique (Fig. 5-15, *b*) and exteriorize the needle through the port of introduction. Cut the suture near the needle. Pass approximately 5 cm of the suture through the wire loop (Fig. 5-15, *c*). Snap the plastic cannula where it is scored to detach a small section (Fig. 5-15, *d*). Pull on the detached portion to pull the wire loop and suture out through the center channel of the cannula. Using one hand and applying tension, hold the long suture segment running through the cannula; with the other hand

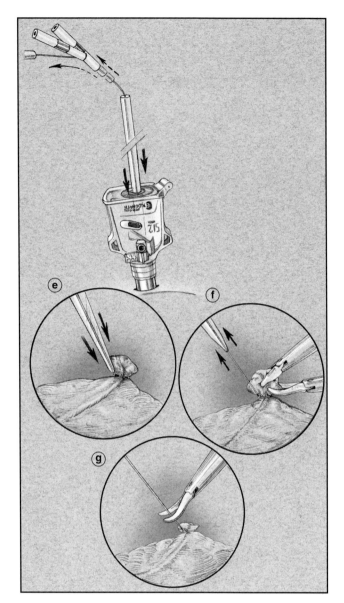

Fig. 5-14, cont'd   Advance the long portion of the cannula; hold the tip of the cannula against the tissue and tighten the ligature (*e*). Transect the tissue to obtain a biopsy specimen (*f*). Cut the suture tail (*g*).

slide the pre-tied slipknot off the cannula (Fig. 5-15, *e*). Tighten the slipknot by applying tension to the tail (end) while keeping tension on the portion of the suture passing through the plastic cannula (standing part; Fig. 5-15, *f*). Cut the tail to a length of approximately 2 cm. While holding the standing part under slight tension with one hand, advance the cannula and knot through the reducer cap to the site of application. Press the conical tip of the cannula and knot against the tissue and pull on the standing part to tighten the loop and secure the knot (Fig. 5-15, *g*). Cut the tail approximately 2 cm from the knot.

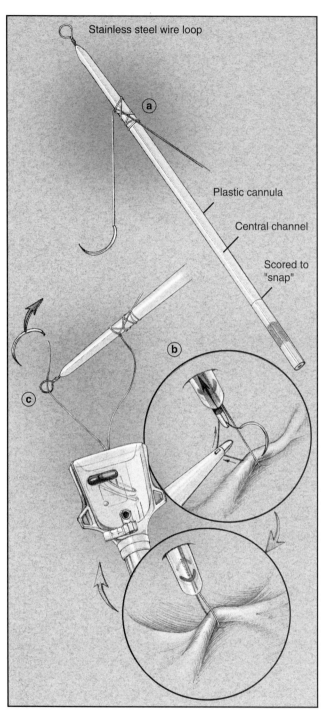

Fig. 5-15   Pre-tied Endoknot suture. Description (*a*). Pull additional suture through tissue using the pulley technique and exteriorize the needle (*b*). Pass approximately 5 cm of suture through the wire loop (*c*).

Pre-tied Loop Suture[13]

A pre-tied loop suture consists of a plastic cannula, a pre-tied loop, and a ½ curved, ½ circle, or straight taper point needle (Fig. 5-16, *a*). It is available with Ethibond Excel Suture.

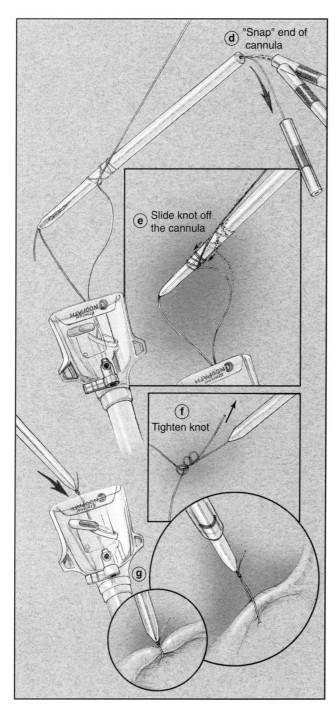

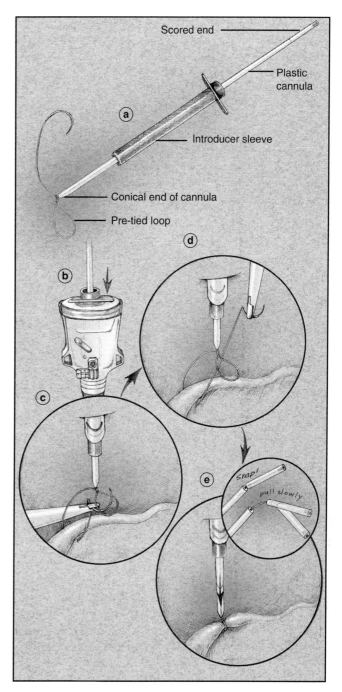

Fig. 5-15, cont'd   Snap off the small plastic cannula and pull the suture through the cannula (*d*). Slide the preformed knot off the cannula (*e*). Tighten the slipknot (*f*). Press the conical tip against the tissue and tighten the loop (*g*).

Fig. 5-16   Pre-tied loop suture. Description (*a*). Back load the pre-tied loop suture into the introducer sleeve and insert through a 10/12 mm trocar with reducer cap (*b*). After passing the needle through tissue, position the loop for easy passage of the needle holder. Pass the needle holder through the loop (*c*). Pull the needle through the loop (*d*). Place the tip of the cannula against the tissue. Snap the cannula and pull on the detached portion to tighten the knot (*e*).

TECHNIQUE Back load the plastic cannula into the introducer until the suture loop and needle are completely covered by the shaft of the introducer. Insert the introducer through a 10/12 mm trocar (see Fig. 5-16, *b*). Advance the plastic cannula to expose the needle and loop suture in the body cavity. Grasp the needle with the needle holder and pass it through the edges of the wound. Position the preformed loop so the needle holder can be passed through the loop (Fig. 5-16, *c*). Pass the needle holder through the preformed loop, grasp the needle, and pull the needle and suture through the loop (Fig. 5-16, *d*). Place the conical tip of the plastic cannula and pre-tied knot against the tissue. Place tension on the suture by pulling the needle suture combination in the direction of the cannula. Snap the scored end of the plastic cannula. Tighten the loop by pulling on the detached portion of the plastic cannula while maintaining tension, using the grasping forceps, on the segment of the needle or suture adjacent to the swage and keeping the tip of the cannula against the knot (Fig. 5-16, *e*). Cut the suture passing through the cannula approximately 2 cm from the knot.

Absorbable Suture Clip[14]

The Lapra-Ty suture clip provides an alternative to tying intracorporeal or extracorporeal knots when soft tissue approximation is needed for 14 days or less. The Lapra-Ty suture clip is an absorbable clip made of polydioxanone polymer. The clip can be applied to a single strand of size 2/0 to 4/0 polyglactin 910 suture.

Technique

Withdraw one suture clip from the clip cartridge with the Lapra-Ty suture clip applier. Place the clip over the suture approximately 5 mm from the end (Fig. 5-17, *a*). Avoid positioning the suture near the latch of the clip. Squeeze the handle of the applier to lock the clip in place. Introduce the needle holder through a universal Oneseal reducer cap on a 10/12 mm trocar. Pass the needle through the edges of the wound and pull the suture until the absorbable suture clip is resting against the tissue at the point of suture penetration (see Fig. 5-17, *b*). After placing an interrupted or continuous suture pattern, load a second suture clip into the applier and insert the applier through a trocar. Apply tension on the suture with a grasper and slide the clip along the suture (Fig. 5-17, *c*). Apply additional force on the clip at the suture-tissue interface to increase suture tension and improve wound edge approximation. Close the jaws of the applier to close the suture clip. Confirm that the suture clip is secure. Cut the suture approximately 2 cm from the suture clip.

EXTRACORPOREAL SURGEON'S KNOT

Single or double half hitches are advanced with a knot pusher or endoscopic Babcock forceps.

Using a Standard Knot Pusher[15]

Introduce the suture or suture-needle combination through a universal reducer cap on a 10/12 mm trocar cannula. Keep one limb of the suture external to the can-

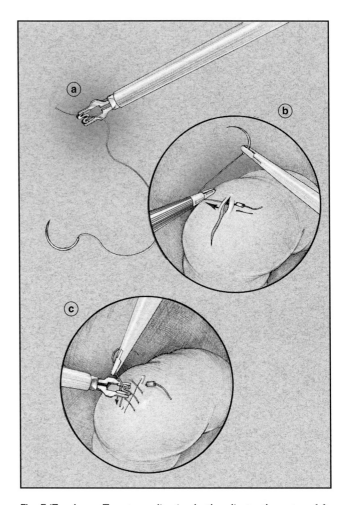

Fig. 5-17 Lapra-Ty suture clip. Apply the clip to the suture (*a*). Pass the needle through the edges of the wound and pull the suture until the Lapra-Ty clip rests against the tissue (*b*). Slide a second clip along the suture. With the wound edges under modest tension apply the clip to the suture (*c*).

nula. Pass the suture through the tissue to be apposed or around the tissue to be ligated and exteriorize the suture (Fig. 5-18, *a*). Create a double half hitch, that is, the end of the suture is passed through the loop twice instead of once. Use the knot pusher to advance the double half hitch to the tissue while applying slight tension to both limbs of the suture (Fig. 5-18, *b*). Convert the double half hitch to an overhand knot (the first throw of a surgeon's knot) by exerting corrective tension on the suture. Withdraw the knot pusher and make a single half hitch. Use the knot pusher to advance what will become the second half of a surgeon's knot (Fig. 5-18, *c*). Additional throws are placed in a similar fashion, as needed. Cut both tails approximately 2 cm from the knot.

Using Endoscopic Babcock Forceps[1,16]

This technique can be performed through a 10/12 mm trocar cannula. After passing the suture through the tissue to be apposed or around the tissue to be ligated,

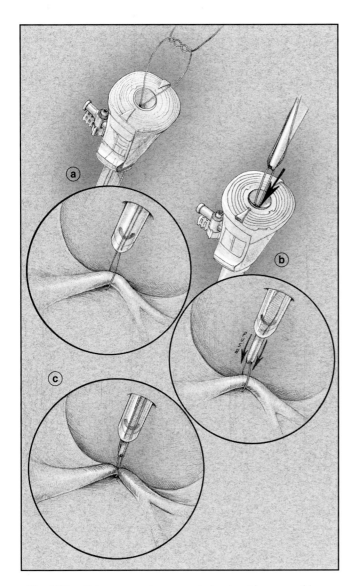

Fig. 5-18 Extracorporeal surgeon's knot with a reusable knot pusher. Both limbs of the suture are external to the trocar cannula in preparation for extracorporeal tying (*a*). Advance a double half hitch through the cannula with a knot pusher (*b*). Advance the second throw of the surgeon's knot (*c*).

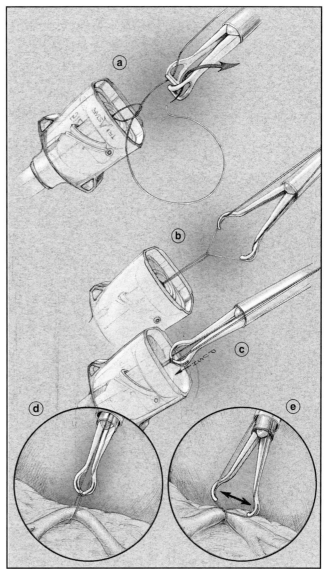

Fig. 5-19 Extracorporeal surgeon's knot with an endoscopic Babcock forceps. After tying a single or double half hitch, thread one end of the suture through one jaw of the endoscopic Babcock forceps from its convex to its concave surface. Feed the opposite end through the other jaw in a similar fashion (*a*). Hold the suture in tension (*b*). Close the jaws of the Babcock forceps, hold both suture ends, and advance through the trocar cannula (*c, d*). Spread the jaws of the forceps to seat the first portion of the knot (*e*). *Continued*

exteriorize both ends of the suture. Create a single or double half hitch. Insert one end of the suture through one jaw of an endoscopic Babcock grasping forceps. Direct the suture through the open jaw from the outer convex surface to its inner concave surface. Feed the opposite end of the suture through the other jaw in a similar manner (Fig. 5-19, *a*). Grasp both suture ends in one hand and hold the suture under tension parallel and adjacent to the longitudinal axis of the Babcock forceps

(Fig. 5-19, *b*). Close the jaws of the forceps and push the tie through the cannula to the site of application (Fig. 5-19, *c* and *d*). Open and close the jaws of the forceps as needed to advance the tie. While maintaining slight tension on both suture ends, spread the jaws of the forceps to apply horizontal tension to the suture to seat the first portion of the knot (Fig. 5-19, *e*). Remove the Babcock forceps from the cannula. Free one suture end from the jaw of the forceps (Fig. 5-19, *f*) and tie the

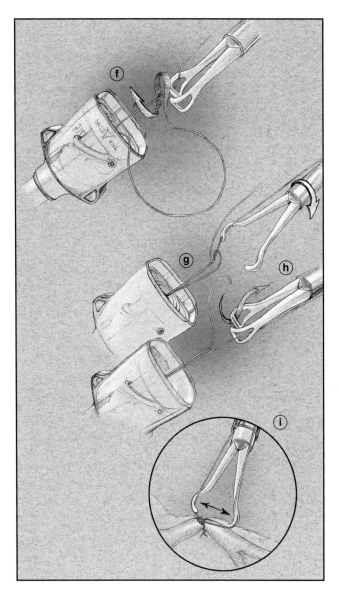

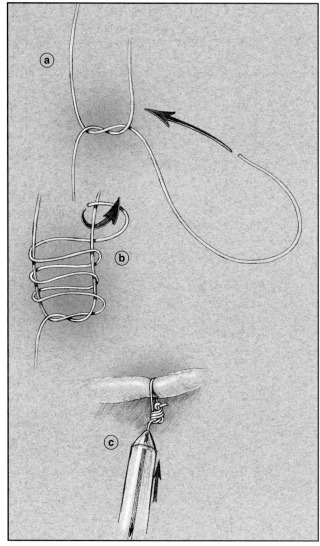

Fig. 5-19, cont'd   Exteriorize the forceps and free one suture end. Throw the second single or double half hitch. Rotate the forceps (f, g). Reinsert the free suture in the jaw of the forceps (h). Advance the ligature and secure the knot (i).

Fig. 5-20   Roeder knot. Create a half hitch (a). Wrap the end three and a half times around the limbs of the loop. Bring the end back between the last half wrap and complete the third wrap (b). Apply traction on the standing part and push on the knot pusher to lock and secure the knot (c).

second portion of the knot. Rotate the forceps to properly position the throw (Fig. 5-19, g). Reinsert the free suture through the jaw of the forceps (Fig. 5-19, h). Hold both suture ends in tension and in axial alignment with the Babcock forceps when advancing the ligature and securing the knot (Fig. 5-19, i). If needed, additional half hitches are placed in the same manner. Cut the suture approximately 2 cm from the knot.

SLIPKNOTS

The Roeder, Modified Roeder (Meltzer), and Weston knots are extracorporeal slipknots that can be used effec-

tively in laparoscopic surgery. Slipknots are advanced into the body with a knot pusher.

Roeder Knot[16,17]

Create a half hitch and hold this throw between the thumb and index finger of the left hand (Fig. 5-20, a). Wrap the end three and a half times over and around the limbs of the loop, bring the end back between the last half wrap, and complete a third wrap (Fig. 5-20, b). Compress the loosely constructed knot by pulling the end back and sliding the initial half hitch and last half wrap closer together. While maintaining tension on the standing part,

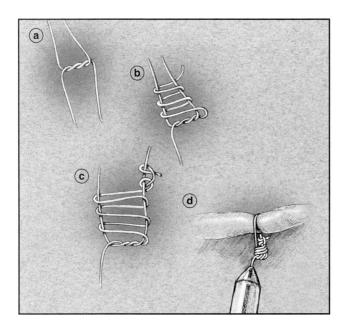

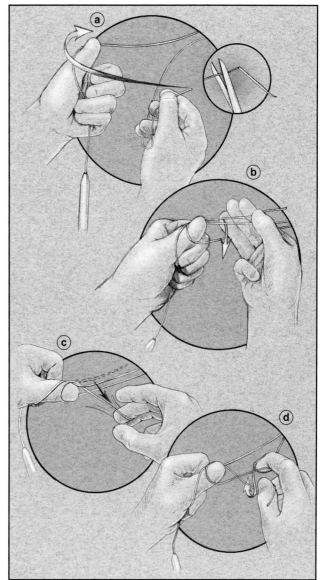

Fig. 5-21 Modified Roeder knot. Create a double half hitch (*a*). Wrap the end three times around the limbs of the loop (*b*). Throw two half wraps and pull the end between the first and second half wrap (*c*). Tighten by pushing on the knot pusher to secure the knot (*d*).

use the knot pusher to advance the Roeder knot onto the tissue. To tighten and lock the knot, apply traction on the standing part of the suture while pushing on the knot with the knot pusher (Fig. 5-20, *c*). Cut the tail of the suture to 2 cm.

Modified Roeder Knot (Meltzer Knot)

The modified Roeder knot provides additional resistance to slippage when suturing with synthetic absorbable materials such as polydioxanone suture.[18] This knot should not be used with natural suture materials, such as catgut, in which resistance to sliding and premature locking may pose problems.[11] Create a double half hitch (Fig. 5-21, *a*) and hold the hitch between the thumb and index finger. Wrap the short end three times around the limbs of the loop (Fig. 5-21, *b*). Throw two additional half wraps, pulling the end between the half wrap and the previous full or halp wrap (Fig. 5-21, *c*). Tighten and apply as previously described (Fig. 5-21, *d*).

Clinch Knot (Weston Knot)[19]

Grasp the standing part of the suture in the palm of the left hand with the suture passing over the back (dorsal aspect) of the thumb. Hold the end with the thumb and index finger of the right hand (Fig. 5-22, *a*). Pass the end around the thumb (Fig. 5-22, *b*). Pass the third and fourth fingers of the right hand under the standing part, grasp the end and pull it under the standing part to form the first half hitch (Fig. 5-22, *c*). Grasp the end with the

Fig. 5-22 Weston knot. Hold standing part in palm of left hand and end in right hand. Pass the end around the thumb (*a, b*). With the third and fourth fingers of the right hand pull the end under the standing part to form the first half hitch (*b, c*). Grasp the end with the thumb and third finger of the right hand and place the index finger over one limb of the loop (*d*).

Continued

thumb and third finger of the right hand and place the index finger over one limb of the loop (Fig. 5-22, *d*). Hook the end and bring it through the loop to form the second hitch (Fig. 5-22, *e*). Grasp the end between the index and middle finger of the left hand and wrap it around both limbs of the loop (Fig. 5-22, *f*). Hold the end between the left thumb and index finger (Fig. 5-22, *g*). Pull the two strands over the thumb and index finger and bring the end through the second loop

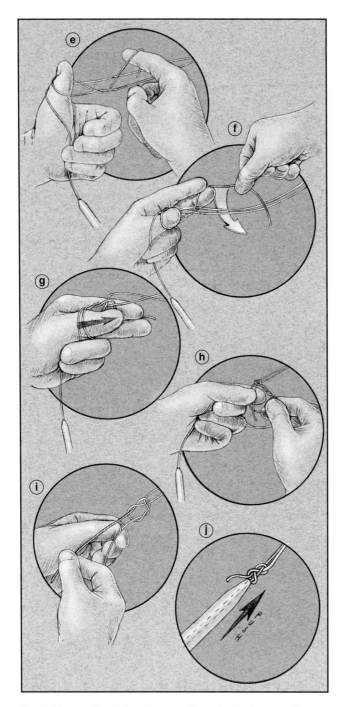

Fig. 5-22, cont'd   Bring the end through the loop to form the second hitch (*e*). Grasp the end between the index and middle fingers of the left hand and wrap the end around both limbs of the loop (*f*). Hold the end between the left thumb and index finger (*g*). Pull the two strands over the thumb and index finger and bring the end through the second loop (*h*). Apply tension to the end and standing part to tighten the knot (*i*). Push on the knot and apply tension to the end to secure the knot (*j*).

(Fig. 5-22, *h*). Grasp the end with the right hand and apply tension to the end and the standing part to tighten the knot (Fig. 5-22, *i*). Push on the knot with the knot pusher and apply traction to the end to lock the knot at the site of application (Fig. 5-22, *j*).

Intracorporeal Knot Tying

Knots fashioned entirely within the abdominal or thoracic cavity are called *intracorporeal knots*. A simple interrupted or continuous suture pattern or ligature may be secured with these knots.

The suture is passed through the trocar cannula and through or around the tissue to be sutured or ligated, and the knot is tied inside the body cavity.

Extracting the Needle
To extract the needle before tying, grasp the suture approximately 2.5 cm from the swaged needle and cut the suture adjacent to the needle holder on the side opposite the needle. Withdraw the needle into the cannula, depress the trocar flapper valve, and extract the needle.

INTRACORPOREAL KNOTS
Square Knot
An intracorporeal square knot is similar to a conventional instrument tie made with two instruments. Three basic techniques can be used to tie a square knot.
Classic Microsurgical Technique[8]
To tie a simple interrupted suture with an intracorporeal square knot, cut the suture to a length of approximately 15 to 20 cm.[20] Limiting the length of suture reduces operating time. Lay the suture on the tissue in the shape of a C (Fig. 5-23, *a*). With the animal in dorsal recumbency and the scope inserted through the ventral abdominal wall and directed cranially, the terminal portion of the bight lies caudal to the end.

With the left hand, place grasping forceps ventral to the bight and direct the instrument jaws toward the end of the suture in preparation for grasping. With the needle holder in the right hand, grasp the bight at its junction with the standing part. Loop the bight once around the grasping forceps (see Fig. 5-23, *b*) and pull the loop to the tips of the grasping forceps. This loop can be made more easily if the jaws of the instruments are kept close to each other. Simultaneously advance both instruments toward the end. Grasp the end with the grasping forceps and pull it through the loop (see Fig. 5-23, *c*). Complete the first overhand knot by pulling the end and the bight in opposite directions and parallel to the suture passing through the tissue (Fig. 5-23, *d*). Open the jaws of the grasping forceps and release the end. Using the needle holder, move the portion of the bight adjacent to the standing part to the left of the field, caudal and parallel to the end, to create a reverse C. Hold the bight adjacent to the standing part with the grasping forceps. Place the needle holder ventral to the bight and direct its jaws toward the end (Fig. 5-23, *e*). With the grasping forceps, place a single suture loop around the needle holder and pull the loop toward the tip of the needle holder. Simultaneously advance both instruments toward the end. Grasp the end with the needle holder and pull it through the loop (see Fig. 5-23, *f*). Pull the end and the bight in opposite directions and parallel to the first half of the knot to complete the second overhand knot of the square knot (see Fig. 5-23, *g*). Additional throws are fashioned in a similar manner.

Endoski Needle Technique[21]

An Endoski ("ski") needle is a half-curved needle used in endoscopic surgery that resembles a snow ski. The configuration of the Endoski needle can be used to advantage in tying knots. Position the suture in a C configuration as previously described. With the needle holder held in the right hand, grasp the Endoski needle near the juncture of its straight and curved portions. Place the grasping forceps held with the left hand ventral to the bight with the grasper's point directed toward the end. Hold the straight shaft of the needle parallel to the shaft of the grasping forceps and the swage of the needle adjacent to the grasping forceps (Fig. 5-24, *a*).

In this technique the half hitch is formed primarily by the instrument holding the needle. Loop the bight once around the grasping forceps by rotating the swage around the jaws of the grasping forceps (see Fig. 5-24, *b*). Pull the loop toward the jaws of the grasping forceps. Simultaneously advance both instruments toward the end. Grasp the end with the grasping forceps and pull it through the loop (see Fig. 5-24, *c*). Complete the overhand knot by pulling the end and the Endoski needle in opposite directions, parallel to the suture passing through the tissue (see Fig. 5-24, *d*). Open the jaws of the grasping forceps and release the end. Grasp the Endoski needle with the grasping forceps held in the left hand and create a reverse C configuration by moving the needle to the left of the field, caudal and parallel to the end. Place the needle holder held in the right hand ventral to the bight. Hold the straight shaft of the needle parallel to the shaft of the needle holder and the swage of the needle adjacent to the needle holder (see Fig. 5-24, *e*). Loop the bight once around the needle holder by rotating the swage around the jaws of the needle holder. Pull the loop toward the jaws of the needle holder. Grasp the end with the needle holder (see Fig. 5-24, *f*) and pull it through the loop. Pull the end and the Endoski needle in opposite directions parallel to the first overhand knot

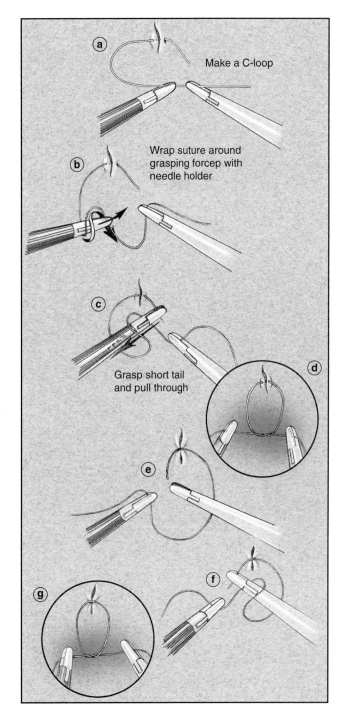

Fig. 5-23 Square knot—classic microsurgical technique. Lay the suture in a C configuration (*a*). Loop the bight once around the grasping forceps (*b*). Grasp the suture end with the grasping forceps and pull it through the loop (*c*). Pull the end and bight in opposite directions to complete the first half hitch (*d*). Create a reverse C. Place the needle holder ventral to the bight with its jaws directed toward the end (*e*). Place a single loop around the needle holder. Grasp the end with the needle holder and pull it through the loop (*f*). Tighten the square knot (*g*).

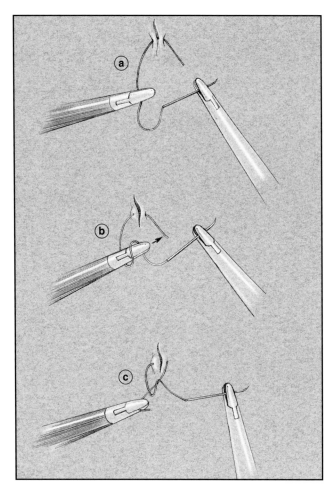

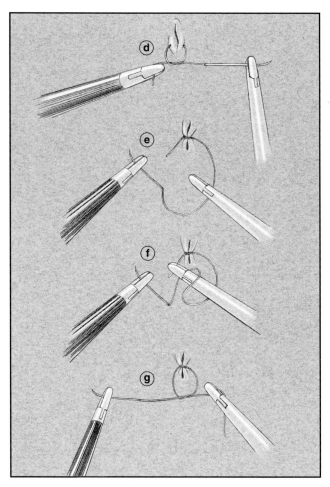

Fig. 5-24   Square knot—Endoski needle. Create a C configuration (*a*). Using the Endoski needle, loop the bight once around the grasping forceps (*b*). Grasp the end with the grasping forceps and pull it through the single loop (*c*).

Fig. 5-24, cont'd   Pull the end of the suture and the Endoski needle in opposite directions to complete the first half hitch (*d*). Reverse the C suture configuration. Hold the shaft of the ski needle parallel to the needle holder (*e*). With the Endoski needle, loop the bight once around the needle holder. Pull the end through the loop with the needle holder (*f*). Tighten to complete the square knot (*g*).

to complete the square knot (see Fig. 5-24, *g*). Additional throws are fashioned in a similar manner.

Modified "Smiley Face" (based on Curved Needle Technique)[22]

The curve of a ½ circle or ⅜ circle needle can be used to advantage in tying knots. After passing the suture through the tissue, create the C configuration with the suture and grasp the curved needle with the needle holder (right hand). Grasp the needle at mid-body with the needle radius (concave surface) directed ventrad and the swaged end directed toward the grasping forceps (left hand). The needle will have the profile of a smile and the suture near the swage will have a slight anterior bow (Fig. 5-25, *a*).

In this technique the overhand knot is formed primar-

ily by the instrument that does not hold the needle. Place the jaws of the grasping forceps ventral to the suture near the swage (see Fig. 5-25, *b*). Rotate the jaws of the grasping forceps around the suture, through the radius of the needle, and back to the starting point (see Fig. 5-25, *c*). Slide the loop of suture above the jaws of the grasping forceps by pulling the needle up along the shaft of the grasping forceps. Grasp the end with the grasping forceps and pull it through the loop (see Fig. 5-25, *d*). Pull the end and the needle in opposite directions to tighten the first overhand knot (see Fig. 5-25, *e*).

To create the second overhand knot, reverse the C configuration. Hold the curved needle in the profile of a "smiley face," with the grasping forceps (left hand). Direct the swaged end toward the needle holder (right

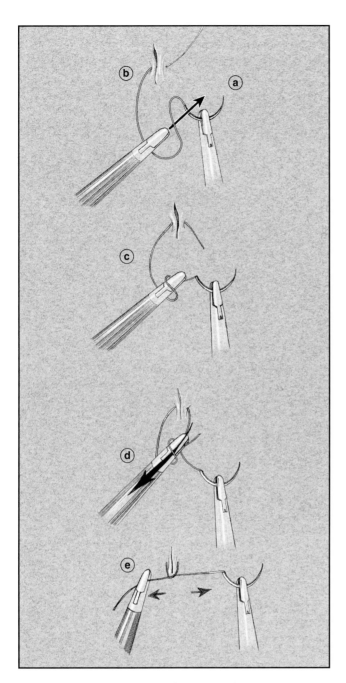

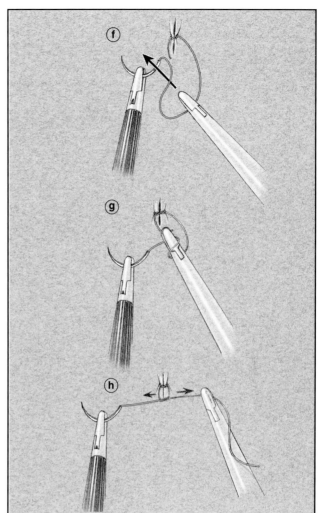

Fig. 5-25, cont'd Reverse the C configuration. Hold the curved needle with the grasping forceps (*f*). Rotate the jaws of the needle holder around the suture, through the radius of the needle, and back to the starting point. Grasp the end with the needle holder and pull it through the loop (*g*). Tighten the square knot (*h*).

Fig. 5-25 Curved needle modified "smiley face" technique. Grasp the curved needle in the profile of a smiley face (*a*). Place the jaws of the grasping forceps ventral to the suture near the swage (*b*). Rotate the jaws of the grasping forceps around the suture, through the radius of the needle, and back to the starting point (*c*). Pull the end through the loop (*d*). Tighten the first half hitch (*e*).

hand; see Fig. 5-25, *f*). Place the jaws of the needle holder ventral to the suture near the swage. Rotate the jaws of the needle holder around the suture, through the radius of the needle to the starting point. Slide the loop of suture above the jaws of the needle holder by pulling

the needle up the shaft of the needle holder. Grasp the end with the needle holder (see Fig. 5-25, *g*) and pull it through the loop. Tighten the second throw by pulling the end and the needle in opposite directions (see Fig. 5-25, *h*).

Double Knot with a Straight Needle[23]

A double knot is a modified surgeon's knot in which both component overhand knots have an extra wrap. After passing the suture through the tissue, grasp the needle with the needle holder so the swage of the needle is directed toward the grasping forceps. While holding the straight needle, wrap two suture loops counterclockwise around the jaws of the grasping forceps (Fig. 5-26, *a*) and pull the two loops up the shaft of the grasping

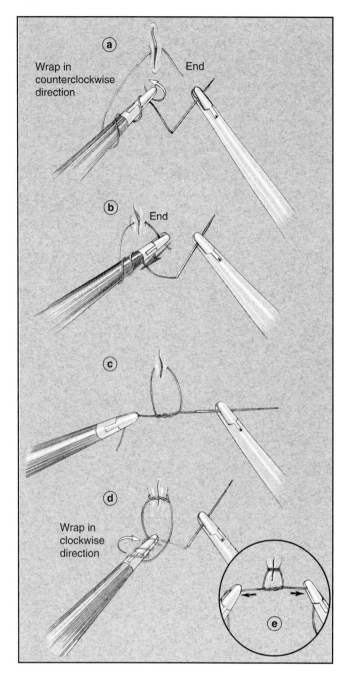

Fig. 5-26 Double knot with straight needle. With the straight needle, wrap two loops counterclockwise around the grasping forceps (*a*). Pull the loops up the shaft of the grasping forceps (*b*). With the grasping forceps pull the end through the double loops and tighten the double hitch (*c*). Wrap a double loop of suture clockwise around the grasper (*d*). Grasp the end of the suture and pull it through the double loop (*e*). Tighten the double knot.

forceps. Grasp the end of the suture with the grasping forceps and pull the end through the double loops (Fig. 5-26, *b*). Tighten this first half of the knot by pulling the end and the needle in opposite directions (Fig. 5-26, *c*). With the needle wrap a double loop of

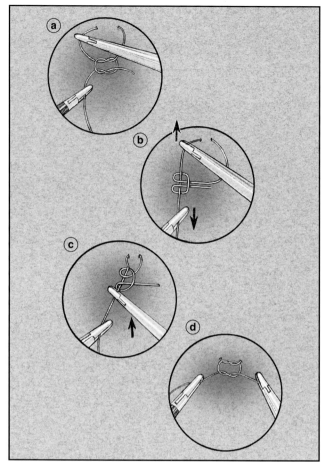

Fig. 5-27 Conversion of a square knot to a half hitch. Grasp the left half loop adjacent to the knot and left tail (*a*). Distract the two instruments to convert the square knot to a slipknot (*b*). Straddle the suture with the needle holder and push against the knot to tighten the loop (*c*). Grasp both tails and apply equal and opposite tension to convert the slipknot to a square knot (*d*).

suture clockwise around the grasper. Grasp the end of the suture with the grasping forceps and pull the suture through the double loop (Fig. 5-26, *d*). Pull the end and the needle in opposite directions and parallel to the first half of the knot, to tighten the double knot (Fig. 5-26, *e*). Tie additional throws similarly.

Conversion of a Square Knot to a Half Hitch[7]
A square knot can be converted to two half hitches to tighten a ligature or improve tissue apposition. Conceptually, divide the square knot into left and right halves. Each half consists of a half loop and tail. To convert the square knot into two half hitches, grasp the left tail with the grasping forceps (left hand) and grasp the left half loop adjacent to the knot with the needle holder (right hand; Fig. 5-27, *a*). Place tension on the square knot by separating the grasper and needle holder. When appro-

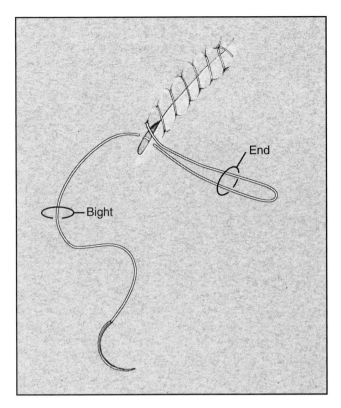

Fig. 5-28 Surgeon's knot. Use the double loop as the end and the single strand as the bight when ending a simple continuous suture pattern.

priate tension is applied, the square knot will convert into two half hitches (Fig. 5-27, *b*). Release the grasp on the loop but continue to hold the tail. With the needle holder straddle the suture adjacent to the knot. Push the jaws of the needle holder against the knot to slide the knot and tighten the loop (Fig. 5-27, *c*). When appropriate tissue apposition or ligature size is reached, convert the half hitches to a square knot by grasping both suture tails and applying equal and opposite tension (Fig. 5-27, *d*).

CONTINUOUS SUTURE PATTERN

The same manipulations for placing a simple interrupted suture are used for placing a continuous suture pattern. The knot used to begin a continuous suture pattern can be tied intracorporeally or extracorporeally before introduction of the suture. A simple continuous suture pattern can be ended with a square knot or surgeon's knot by using the loop of suture between the last two suture passes as the end. The knot is tied as previously described (Fig. 5-28).

REFERENCES

1. Topel HC: Endoscopic suturing and knot tying. 1996, Ethicon, Inc. and Endo-surgery, Inc., Somerville, N.J.
2. Cuschieri A, Szabo Z: Tissue approximation in endoscopic surgery. Oxford, UK, 1995, Isis Medical Media, Ltd.
3. Szabo Z: Endoscopic suturing and knotting. In Braverman MH, Tawes RL, editors: Surgical technology international II. San Francisco, Calif., 1993, University Medical Press.
4. Szabo S, Patton Jr. GW: Microsurgical laparoscopy. In Behrman SJ, Patton GW, Holtz G, editors: Progress in infertility, ed 4, Boston, 1994, Little, Brown & Co.
5. Weston PV: Instruments and methods: a new clinch knot. *Obstet Gynecol* 78(1):144-147, 1991.
6. Topel HC: Endoscopic suturing and knot tying. Ethicon Endo-Surgery, Inc., 1996.
7. Szabo Z, Bowyer DW: Laparoscopic suturing: principles and techniques. In Das S, Crawford ED, editors: Urologic laparoscopy. Philadelphia, 1994, WB Saunders.
8. Szabo Z et al. Analysis of surgical movements during suturing in laparoscopy. *Endosc Surg* 2:55-61, 1994.
9. Szabo Z: Laparoscopic suturing and tissue approximation. In Hunter JG, Sackier JM, editors: Minimally invasive surgery. New York, 1993, McGraw-Hill.
10. Szabo Z: Laparoscopic suturing and tissue approximation. In Hunter JG, Sackier JM, editors: Minimally invasive surgery. New York, 1993, McGraw-Hill.
11. Cuschieri A, Szabo Z: Tissue approximation in endoscopic surgery. Oxford, UK, 1995, Isis Medical Media Ltd.
12. Instructions for use of pre-tied Endoknot suture made with coated Vicryl (Polyglactin 910) suture coated with polyglactin 370 and calcium stearate dyed (violet) braided synthetic absorbable suture. Ethicon, Inc., Somerville, N.J.
13. Follow the path to pre-tied loop sutures. 1993, Ethicon, Inc., Somerville, N.J.
14. Now, you can be nimble and be quick with endoscopic suturing: exclusive Lapra-Ty absorbable clips and suture clip applier. 1994, Ethicon, Inc., Somerville, N.J.
15. Cuschieri A, Nathanson LK, Buess G: Basic surgical procedures. In Cuschieri A, Buess G, Perissat J, editors: Operative manual of endoscopic surgery. Berlin Heidelberg, 1992, Springer-Verlag.
16. Sanfilippo JS: Instrumentation and knot-tying. In Vitale GC, Sanfilippo JS, Perissat J, editors: Laparoscopic surgery: an atlas for general surgeons. Philadelphia, 1995, JB Lippincott.
17. Roeder H: Die tecknik der mandelgesundungvestrebungen. *Aertzl Rundschau: Munchen* 57:169-171, 1918.
18. Cuschieri A, Nathanson LK, Buess G: Basic surgical procedures. In Cuschieri A, Buess G, Perissat J, editors: Operative manual of endoscopic surgery. Berlin Heidelberg, 1992, Springer-Verlag.
19. Weston PW: A method of tying the Weston knot. Presentation. 1991.
20. Topel HC: Endoscopic suturing and knot tying. 1996, Ethicon, Inc. and Endo-Surgery, Inc., Somerville, N.J.
21. Cuschieri A, Szabo Z: Tissue approximation in endoscopic surgery. Oxford, UK, 1995, Isis Medical Media Ltd.
22. McDougall EM, Soper NJ: Laparoscopic suturing and knot tying. In Soper NJ et al, editors: Essentials of laparoscopy. St. Louis, 1994, Quality Medical Publishing.
23. Topel HC: Endoscopic knot tying manual. 1991, Ethicon, Inc. Somerville, N.J.

CHAPTER 6

COMPLICATIONS

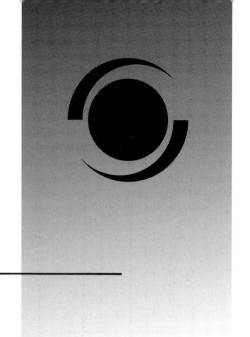

Lynetta J. Freeman

"Laparoscopy is an innocuous, rapid, and elegant procedure in the hands of well-trained specialists. It can also be a source of errors and accidents if put in the hands of physicians without proper training and the proper spirit of continuous attention to all the technical details, indispensable for total safety."

R. Palmer, Paris 1974[1]

In veterinary medicine, minimally invasive surgery is an emerging field and the frequency of various complications has not yet been documented. Most procedures have been performed in healthy animals to develop human endoscopic surgical procedures, train surgeons, and develop endoscopic instrumentation. Morbidity rates of approximately 4% and mortality rates of less than 0.1% have been documented in retrospective studies of tubal sterilization in women.[2-5] The most common complications were related to pneumoperitoneum, hemorrhage, and organ perforation. Infection, intestinal burns from electrocautery, and cardiac arrest also occurred.[6] We may anticipate that veterinary surgeons will encounter the same types of complications as those seen in human surgery.

In any activity, avoiding complications starts with knowing how and why they occur. Some complications in endoscopic surgery are common to all surgery, but others are specific to minimally invasive procedures. Complications associated with specialized instruments and equipment are discussed along with instructions for their use in Chapters 2 and 3 and other appropriate sections of the book. In this chapter complications are considered in the order in which one might encounter them during any minimally invasive procedure.

Anesthesia

Hypercapnia and acidosis are the most common anesthetic complications to occur during laparoscopy. Their severity is correlated with the amount of pressure and length of time the peritoneal cavity is insufflated with carbon dioxide (CO_2). Hypercapnia from CO_2 absorption can result in tachycardia, hypertension, and cardiac arrhythmias. Monitoring the abdominal pressure, increasing ventilation, and monitoring the depth of anesthesia help prevent hypercapnia.

Hypotension occurs because of decreased venous return from increased abdominal pressure, positioning, or inadequate blood volume. To maintain venous return, maintain circulating blood volume with intravenous fluids and limit the pressure of insufflation to 12 to 14 mm Hg. Positioning the animal with the head down can result in hypoxemia caused by pressure of the abdominal contents on the diaphragm, migration of the endotracheal tube into the mainstem bronchus, or reflux of gastric contents into the esophagus. Hypoxemia is controlled by increasing the rate and pressure of ventilation. Care should be taken to place the endotracheal tube properly and avoid dislodging it while positioning the animal. Gastric reflux with aspiration is common in ruminants used in our studies. Reflux esophagitis has not been identified.

In thoracoscopy the most serious anesthetic complications result from physiologic changes caused by one-lung ventilation and CO_2 insufflation of the thoracic cavity. Hypotension, hypercapnia, and shunting should be managed. See Chapters 2 and 9 for details.

Veress Needle and Trocar Insertion

Complications of Veress needle and trocar insertion include injury to abdominal or thoracic wall vasculature, injury to intraabdominal or intrathoracic vessels, penetration of solid organs, and perforation of a hollow viscus.

INJURY TO ABDOMINAL OR THORACIC WALL VASCULATURE
Abdominal wall penetration often injures the superficial epigastric artery or vein and the deep epigastric vessels. In the chest, subcutaneous vessels, lateral thoracic vessels, the thoracodorsal artery and vein, intercostal vessels, and internal thoracic vessels are the most frequently injured. In most instances, self-limiting hemorrhage is the only detectable result. If a large vein or artery is injured, corrective action must be taken.

Superficial hemorrhage and hemorrhage from intercostal vessels are addressed by removing the trocar cannula and identifying the source. The bleeding vessel is ligated with suture or clips, or coagulated with electrocautery. The cannula is reinserted, and the procedure is continued. The deep epigastric vessels can be controlled by passing a suture with a Keith needle through the abdominal wall and, with the aid of the laparoscope and a needle holder, redirecting the needle to exit the abdominal wall. The suture is tied to compress the vessel (see Fig. 3-30). A suture can also be passed through the layers of the abdominal wall by using a Semm needle or a small crochet hook with a sharp tip. The needle or crochet hook is passed from the skin surface through the abdominal wall. The suture is placed in the hook and brought externally and tied on the skin surface or over a "roll-over" bandage or stent. Removal of the suture within 72 hours is recommended to avoid necrosis of the skin under the ligature.[7]

An alternative means of applying pressure to a deep vessel is to pass a Foley catheter through the trocar. The trocar is removed and the balloon is inflated inside the abdominal cavity (see Fig. 3-31). The balloon is pulled up against the abdominal wall, and the catheter is secured externally with forceps at the trocar site. After 24 to 48 hours, the balloon is deflated and the Foley catheter is removed.

Prevention is the best treatment for injuries resulting from Veress needle and trocar insertion. Transillumina-

ting the body wall before each secondary trocar insertion helps identify and avoid superficial abdominal wall vessels.[8] Transillumination is performed by placing the telescope lens close to the proposed trocar insertion site and dimming the room lights. The subcutaneous vessels are easily seen in the darkened room. In addition to transillumination, all secondary port insertions should be made under direct inspection. If the trocar tip appears to be very close to an epigastric artery or vein during insertion, the tip can be redirected.

Some trocar designs may reduce the risk of vessel injury. Trocars with tips that cut less and dilate the tissue to accommodate the cannula include a dilating tip trocar* and a radially expanding access system.† An optical trocar allows identification of the tissue layers during insertion.‡ The surgeon can redirect the tip of the trocar during insertion to avoid vessels in the subcutaneous tissue, muscle, or fascia.

INJURY TO INTRAABDOMINAL OR INTRATHORACIC VESSELS
Vascular injuries in humans occur in 1 to 2 per 1000 patients.[9] Injuries occur equally frequently with Veress needles and trocars. An animal's smaller size may make it more vulnerable to intraabdominal injury, and anatomic differences may cause a different distribution of injuries.

In humans the aorta, vena cava, and right common iliac vessels have the greatest potential for life-threatening injuries because they are very close to the abdominal wall. The lumbar spine of domestic mammals does not have a lordotic curve, so the aorta and iliac vessels are relatively farther from the abdominal wall. Nevertheless, depending on the size of the abdominal cavity, a Veress needle or trocar may be able to reach the major vessels (Fig. 6-1).

Prevention of injuries by careful technique is the best practice. A controlled trocar insertion is essential. Some surgeons advocate placing the middle finger of the hand holding the trocar on the outside of the cannula to act as a brake to prevent sudden deep insertion of the trocar (Fig. 6-2). Others advocate using the opposite hand as a stop. Trocars requiring very little force to insert can be controlled by using the pencil-grip method and resting the palm of the same hand on the animal's abdomen (Fig. 6-3). Trocars with a safety shield protect the tip as soon as the abdominal wall is penetrated. Ensuring adequate pneumoperitoneum and stability of the abdominal wall during insertion are two

*Endopath Dilating Tip Surgical Trocar, Ethicon Endo-Surgery, Inc., Cincinnati, Ohio 45242.
†Step Blunt Obturator/Cannula with Radially Expanding Sleeve, InnerDyne Medical, Sunnyvale, Calif. 94089.
‡Endopath Optiview Optical Surgical Obturator and Sleeve, Ethicon Endo-Surgery, Inc., Cincinnati, Ohio 45242.

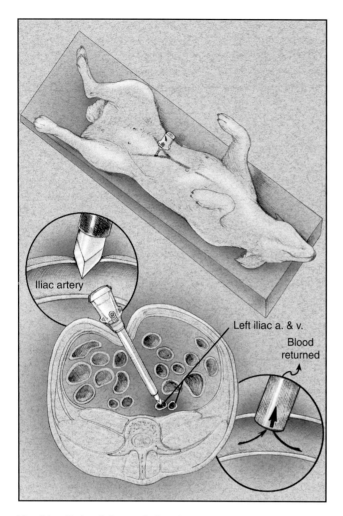

Fig. 6-I If the abdomen lacks adequate insufflation during trocar insertion, the pressure of the trocar displaces the abdominal wall, causing it to move closer to vital structures. Insertion of the right lower abdominal port may be associated with damage to the left iliac artery and vein (*a* & *v*).

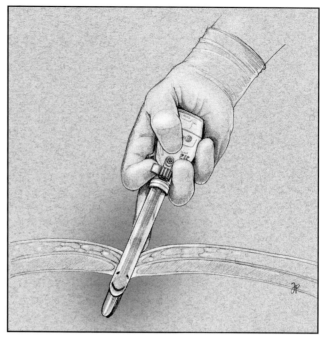

Fig. 6-2 Using the middle finger as a "stop" during trocar insertion.

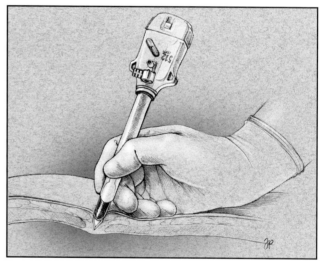

Fig. 6-3 The pencil-grip technique for trocar insertion.

more steps that can be taken to minimize the risks of improper trocar insertion.

If signs of significant hemorrhage are seen after initial entry into the abdomen, conversion to open laparotomy is indicated. Any vascular injury that results in hypotension or rapid accumulation of blood in the abdominal cavity requires an open surgical repair. If the trocar cannula is placed inside a major blood vessel, it should be left in place to stem the bleeding.

Early detection is the next best thing to prevention. As soon as the primary port is established and the laparoscope inserted, explore the abdomen underlying the site where the Veress needle and trocars have been inserted. Keep in mind that injuries in the retroperitoneal space may be hidden by loops of bowel or omentum. Be alert to hemodynamic changes during surgery that are not accounted for by the procedure being performed. At the

end of the procedure, inspect the abdomen for signs of injury. Pay particular attention to blood pooling in the dependent body position (i.e., in the pelvis or near the diaphragm). If signs of injury are found at the end of surgery and the animal is stable, perform a detailed laparoscopic exploration. If the lesion is located and repair is feasible, it may be performed laparoscopically (Fig. 6-4). If any question exists regarding an injury or its repair, conversion to open laparotomy is indicated.

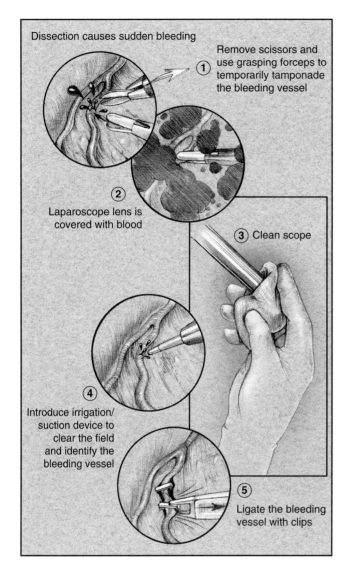

Fig. 6-4   Arterial bleeding spurts onto the lens of the telescope. Use a grasping forceps to temporarily tamponade the bleeding vessel (*1*). Remove the telescope, clean the lens, and reinsert it, avoiding the bleeding vessel (*2* and *3*). Introduce an irrigation and suction device to clear the field. Isolate and identify the bleeding vessel (*4*). Ligate the vessel with sutures, clips, or an energy source (*5*).

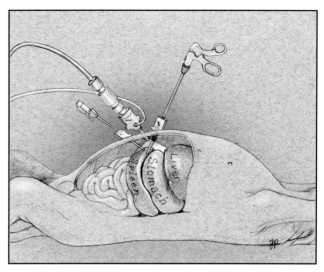

Fig. 6-5   Injury to abdominal viscera occurs when instruments are inserted without directly viewing the entry.

PENETRATION OF SOLID ORGANS

Injuries to the spleen are uncommon in humans. In dogs and cats, splenic injuries may be more common because of the organ's size and position (Fig. 6-5). Controlled trocar and Veress needle insertions will limit the incidence of splenic injury. Inserting the Veress needle caudal and lateral to the umbilicus and directing the needle toward the pelvis avoids injuring the spleen at the level of the umbilicus. The open approach to primary trocar placement is the safest approach. Placing the animal in a slightly head-down (Trendelenburg) position moves the spleen closer to the diaphragm and away from the umbilicus. During passage of a Veress needle and trocars, towel clips can be used on each side of the needle and trocars to elevate the body wall slightly away from the spleen. Splenic bleeding can be electrocoagulated with an argon beam coagulator* or controlled by laparoscopic application of Gelfoam,† Avitene,‡ or oxycellulose sheets alone or in combination with thrombin. If significant injury has occurred, open surgery may be necessary to repair the injury or to perform splenectomy or partial splenectomy.

The lung can be injured during thoracic trocar placement. Careful dissection through the parietal pleura, creation of pneumothorax, and digital palpation to identify pleural adhesions reduce the occurrence of pulmonary trauma during initial port placement. All secondary ports should be placed under direct inspection. One-lung ventilation facilitates creation of the largest optical cavity and operating space. Lung injuries are treated best by enlarging the intercostal incision, exteriorizing the injured tissue, and repairing it with sutures or staples.

PERFORATION OF A HOLLOW VISCUS

Injuries to the stomach, intestine, and bladder are probably as likely to occur in animals as in humans because of their similar positions in the abdominal cavity (see

---

*Argon Beam Coagulation System, ConMed Corp., Utica, N.Y. 13501-1203.
†The Upjohn Co., Kalamazoo, Mich. 49001-0102.
‡MedChem Products, Inc., Woburn, Mass. 01801-6346.

Fig. 6-5). Aspiration of intestinal contents, gastric contents, or urine is readily apparent. Gastric dilation can occur with mask induction of anesthesia, accidental esophageal intubation, upper gastrointestinal endoscopy, or as a result of ileus. Inserting an orogastric tube facilitates decompressing the stomach. A full bladder predisposes to bladder injury. Inserting a urinary catheter decreases the risk of bladder perforation. Penetration of the stomach, bowel, or bladder with a Veress needle is usually apparent during the aspiration and irrigation step for assessing correct Veress needle placement. Perforating a hollow viscus with a Veress needle is usually not serious unless there is a continuing leak; however, trocar-induced injuries must be repaired. Unless the surgeon is a skilled laparoscopist, an open laparotomy is indicated.

Insufflation

If the tip of the Veress needle is not placed in the peritoneal cavity or if it is dislodged from that position, subcutaneous, preperitoneal, or subfascial emphysema develops during insufflation. Emphysema is not usually a dangerous problem. If CO_2 is the insufflation gas, emphysema is resolved in 48 hours or less, depending on the volume instilled and the capillary distribution in the area insufflated. Insufflation of the preperitoneal space creates a special problem for insertion of the trocar or reinsertion of the Veress needle. The emphysematous space may be so large that the tip of the needle or trocar cannot reach and penetrate the peritoneum, and pneumoperitoneum cannot be established (Fig. 6-6). Resorting to the open technique for trocar placement can salvage the situation.

SUBCUTANEOUS EMPHYSEMA
Subcutaneous emphysema is considered a minor complication. It results from dissection by CO_2 gas along the trocar tract and may prolong the surgical procedure if not prevented or not addressed as soon as it occurs. In the early part of our learning curve, we observed subcutaneous emphysema extending to the periorbital region in dogs when the insufflation pressures were not automatically regulated and they exceeded 14 mm Hg.[10] The CO_2 is rapidly absorbed. Transitory postoperative respiratory acidosis has been noted in pigs with CO_2 subcutaneous emphysema.[11] The most extensive occurrences of subcutaneous emphysema were resolved within 24 hours. If an insoluble gas, such as helium, is used, subcutaneous emphysema may take weeks to be resolved.[12]

Subcutaneous emphysema results from gas dissection between the trocar cannula and the layers of the abdominal wall. The trocar should be inserted in the direction in which it will be used. If it is not, the cannula acts as a fulcrum at the body wall and external movement of the cannula results in opposite internal movement. The in-

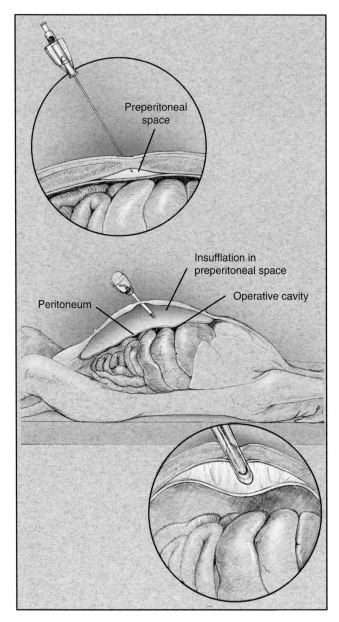

Fig. 6-6 Insufflation of the preperitoneal space results in collapse of the operative cavity, inadequate cannula length, and difficulty in manipulating instruments inside the abdominal cavity.

ternal movement enlarges the opening in the peritoneum and muscle, creating a path for gas dissection (Fig. 6-7). Subcutaneous emphysema may also occur around the site of open trocar insertion if the olive plug is not properly sealed to the abdominal wall with sutures. The condition may be more likely to occur in obese animals or in large animals with muscular abdominal walls, in which the trocar tract is longer. Emphysema is also more likely to occur with high insufflation pressures.

Proper surgical technique includes maintaining the trocar cannula in its correct position. Devices are available to enhance trocar security. Inserting an adequate

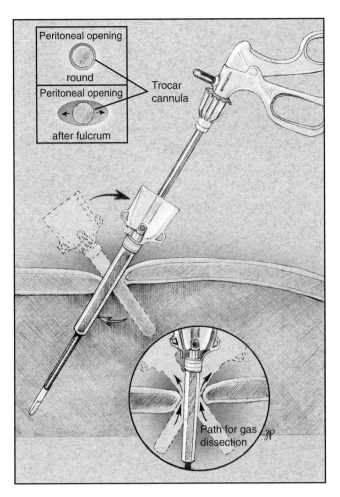

Fig. 6-7 Trocar cannula acts as a fulcrum and can enlarge a hole in the peritoneum as the cannula is manipulated during the surgical procedure.

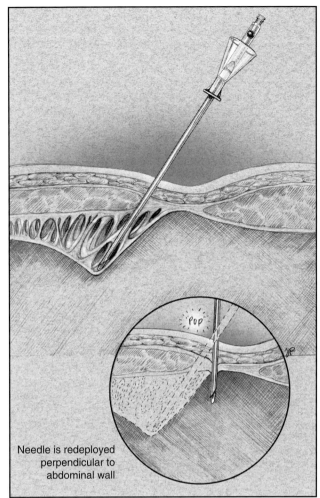

Fig. 6-8 Peritoneal tenting occurs when the tip of the insufflation needle fails to penetrate the peritoneum.

length of cannula into the abdomen is critical. If the cannula is too short, the trocar is easily dislodged. If too much of the cannula is inside the abdomen, too little space may be available to open and manipulate instruments. If subcutaneous emphysema occurs during an operative procedure, a purse-string suture incorporating the skin and external abdominal fascia can be placed around the trocar site. If one trocar site is a continuing source of gas loss, the site should be closed and another port inserted.

PERITONEAL TENTING

Peritoneal tenting occurs when the peritoneum is not penetrated by the Veress needle or trocar and the distal end of the needle or cannula does not communicate with the abdominal cavity (Fig. 6-8). Peritoneal tenting is unlikely in animals with tightly adherent peritoneum, such as dogs and goats. It is common in pigs and in animals with a large amount of fat in the preperitoneal space.

Peritoneal tenting occurs more commonly when dull, reusable trocars are used, and when a safety-shielded trocar or Veress needle is inserted obliquely. The safety shield locks out or the obturator springs forward before the tip of the blade or needle penetrates the peritoneum. If peritoneal tenting is suspected when using the Veress needle, the needle is withdrawn to the level of the rectus fascia and inserted more perpendicular to the abdominal wall (see Fig. 6-8). A distinct "popping" sensation is noted when the Veress needle penetrates the peritoneum. Needle placement is evaluated by one of the methods described in Chapter 3. If peritoneal tenting occurs during trocar placement, the cannula is withdrawn to the level of the fascia. The trocar is replaced in the cannula, and the safety shield is reactivated. The trocar is reinserted into the abdomen. If the peritoneum tents deeper than the shaft length of the cannula, the trocar is removed, leaving the cannula in place. Endoscopic scissors are inserted through the cannula to cut the peritoneum directly under its tip. The cannula is advanced through the peritoneal opening into the abdominal cavity.

INAPPROPRIATE INSUFFLATION

Insufflation of the omental bursa, falciform ligament, or mesentery can develop if the tip of the Veress needle is inserted into those potential spaces (Fig. 6-9). The laparoscopic appearance of the abdominal cavity is unusual. When the omental bursa is insufflated, the abdominal cavity appears as a white, fat-lined, uniformly pale, relatively featureless cavity. If this occurs, remove the primary trocar and allow the abdomen to desufflate. Reinsert the cannula, using a blunt obturator or a locked-out safety shield. For insufflation of the falciform ligament, desufflate and reposition the Veress needle more laterally or use an open approach in a lateral position to complete the procedure.

Occasionally the Veress needle tip is positioned between layers of the omentum or mesentery when it is first inserted. If the abdomen is insufflated before the Veress needle has been positioned properly, the omentum or the mesentery may be insufflated slightly. When this occurs, the omentum or mesentery may appear to have bubbles in it (Fig. 6-10). No treatment is necessary.

PNEUMOTHORAX

Pneumothorax, pneumomediastinum, and pneumopericardium have been reported as complications of pneumoperitoneum and pneumoretroperitoneum. These conditions may also occur with accidental penetration of the diaphragm during a laparoscopic surgical procedure, or in the presence of a diaphragmatic hernia (Fig. 6-11). Fatal pneumothorax occurred in one animal when the diaphragm was penetrated with a needle during a laparoscopic surgical procedure.[13] Pneumothorax is frequently observed during mobilization of the esophagus when performing laparoscopic Nissen fundoplications. The positive pressure of pneumoperitoneum creates a tension pneumothorax. Prompt recognition and treatment are necessary for a successful outcome. Caudal bulging of the diaphragm and progressive loss of pinkness of the tissues are visual clues to this condition. The anesthetist will detect a decrease in tissue oxygenation and a change in the ventilatory pattern. Tachycardia or bradycardia may occur. When pneumothorax is recognized, the abdomen should be desufflated immediately

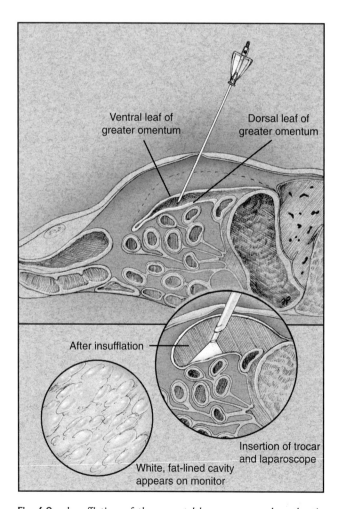

Fig. 6-9 Insufflation of the omental bursa occurs when the tip of the Veress needle is placed between the dorsal and ventral leaves of the greater omentum.

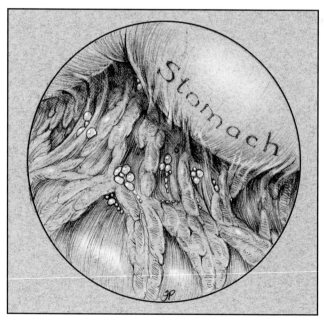

Fig. 6-10 Bubbles appear in the omentum if the tip of the Veress needle partially penetrates the omental bursa. The needle may be repositioned to ensure insufflation of the abdominal cavity.

and a chest tube inserted. Occasionally, bilateral chest tubes are necessary. If the pneumothorax cannot be managed while maintaining an adequate optical cavity for the laparoscopic procedure, conversion to open surgery is indicated. Our laboratory has successfully managed numerous pneumothorax cases in swine. It was possible to evacuate the thorax, maintain an adequate optical cavity, and complete the procedure laparoscopically.[14,15] Others have shown that the physiologic effects of CO_2 pneumothorax in swine can be reversed without a chest tube by desufflating the abdomen, increasing the minute ventilation, and repairing the rent in the diaphragm.[16]

GAS EMBOLISM

Venous gas embolism is a potentially fatal complication of peritoneal insufflation. Gas embolism can occur if a Veress needle is inserted into a blood vessel or a vascular arcade and CO_2 is infused into the vascular system. Fatal gas embolism occurred during insufflation for laparoscopy in one dog when the insufflation needle was accidentally placed in the spleen. Gas bubbles were observed in the spleen, blood vessels, and stomach.[17] Misdirecting a Veress needle into lung parenchyma during thoracoscopy can also result in air embolism. Using an open approach for the initial trocar placement or carefully placing and aspirating the Veress needle before insuffla-

tion reduces the risk of embolism. Gas emboli can also occur through venous structures because the peritoneum is under positive pressure.[12] The condition is less likely to occur during thoracoscopy because when insufflation is used, pressures are low.[18]

Large amounts of embolized gas may travel to the right ventricle and cause an outflow obstruction, resulting in cardiovascular collapse. Auscultation reveals a classic "mill wheel" murmur. The animal should be placed in left lateral recumbency with the head down (Durant's maneuver) to help alleviate the outflow obstruction (Fig. 6-12).[12-19] Hyperventilation with 100% oxygen (O_2) is indicated. If CO_2 or nitrous oxide (N_2O) is used, the high blood solubility of these gases will allow the embolus to dissolve rapidly.

Miscellaneous Problems

UNRECOGNIZED ANATOMIC STRUCTURES

Two examples from human surgery demonstrate the types of difficulties that veterinary surgeons may encounter when learning endoscopic surgery. When general surgeons were learning to perform laparoscopic cholecystectomy, several injuries to the common bile duct occurred during dissection of the cystic duct and artery. Laparoscopic cholangiography was developed to elucidate anatomic variations in the cystic duct and

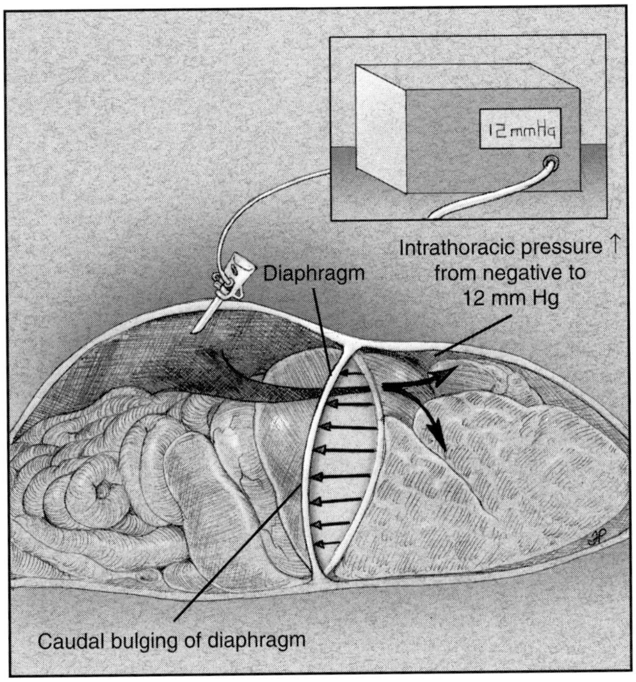

Fig. 6-11   The increased pressure of insufflation takes a path of least resistance. A small hole in the diaphragm may allow gas to move from the abdominal to the thoracic cavity, resulting in a tension pneumothorax.

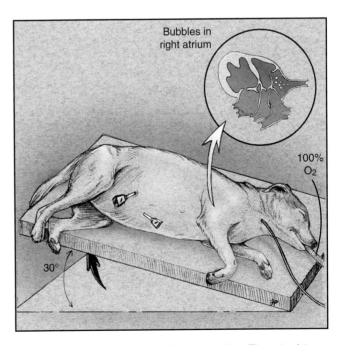

Fig. 6-12   Acute management of gas embolism. The animal is placed in left lateral recumbency with the head down. The pneumoperitoneum is released.

common bile duct that were not readily discernible with an endoscope. By highlighting the potential for these injuries at national meetings and in resident training programs, credentialing requirements, and peer reviews, the general surgeons were able to reduce the incidence of common bile duct injury to an acceptable level. For similar reasons, the early use in humans of vascular staplers in laparoscopic-assisted vaginal hysterectomies was associated with increased risk of ureteral injury. Just as the general surgeons did, gynecologists stressed the importance of intraoperative identification and avoidance of troublesome structures, subsequently reducing the risks.

TECHNICAL LIMITATIONS

Technical limitations of the two-dimensional view on video monitors, lack of tactile feedback, restricted range of motion, and unfamiliarity with new equipment may lead to complications in minimally invasive surgery. The two-dimensional view results in loss of depth perception. An instrument may be inserted more deeply or more aggressively than the surgeon intends. With little tactile feedback, the surgeon may grasp, pull, or manipulate tissue much more forcefully than he or she realizes. Motions are limited by the cannula and its point of insertion at the body wall. Unfamiliarity with equipment can also lead to problems. For example, trying to staple across the site of a previous clip application can lead to instrument breakage. Inability to obtain a clear view of the operative site can be caused by equipment malfunction and is a reason for conversion to an open procedure.

ELECTROSURGICAL INJURIES

Electrosurgical burns occur when an electrosurgical device is activated outside the field of view and contacts tissue. They can also occur from direct coupling of an activated instrument to another metal instrument in the field. Damaged insulation on the shaft of an electrosurgical device may allow stray current to travel to tissue in contact with the shaft of the instrument. Using metal trocars with plastic stability threads creates a condition known as *capacitive coupling*, in which the energy that would have been dispersed to the body wall travels to tissue in contact with the cannula (see Fig. 4-9). Each of these modes of tissue damage can be avoided if careful attention is paid to the principles of electrosurgery.

PERIPHERAL NERVE INJURY

Peripheral nerve damage can occur, but it is difficult to diagnose in animals. As with any surgical procedure, attention should be paid to providing adequate padding and proper positioning. Stapling mesh to the body wall in laparoscopic inguinal hernia repair in humans has been associated with a peripheral neuropathy caused by en-

trapment of the lateral cutaneous femoral nerve. The neuropathy is resolved when the staples are removed. Intercostal neuropathy after entrapment of an intercostal bundle between the trocar cannula and a rib has been reported in humans. This complication is minimized by proper port placement and use of flexible cannulas.

INCISIONAL HERNIA

Hernias containing omentum have developed through 5-mm laparoscopic ports in dogs.[20] Incisional hernias may be more likely in thin body walls when the openings in the peritoneum, fascia, and subcutaneous tissues are more nearly aligned.[21] The hernia can occur during trocar removal when abdominal contents are drawn up into the port tract, or following surgery (Fig. 6-13). An incisional hernia can occur despite fascial closure if sutures are placed too far apart. To prevent incisional hernias, remove the ports under direct endoscopic inspection, elevate the body wall during port removal, use sutures to elevate the rectus fascia during suturing, and close each fascial defect under direct vision.

TUMOR IMPLANTATION AT TROCAR SITES

Laparoscopic surgery has presented a new potential cause for alarm. Metastasis of abdominal and thoracic malignancies to trocar sites has been reported. Trocar-

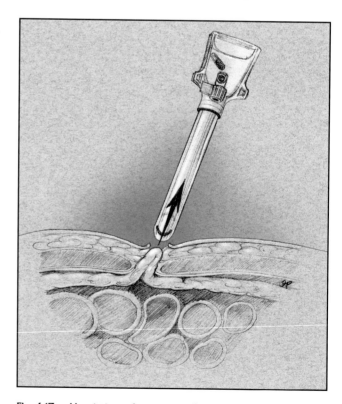

Fig. 6-13 Herniation of omentum through abdominal port sites. The condition may occur more often with a thin body wall. Closure of all 5-mm or larger port sites is recommended.

site implantation has been documented after laparoscopic resection or biopsy of cancers of the liver, gallbladder, stomach, appendix, lung, and ovary.[1] Metastases to abdominal incisions, drain sites, and fine-needle biopsy sites were documented.[22] Although it is unknown whether the incidence of abdominal wall metastasis is higher with laparoscopy than would have occurred with an open laparotomy, potential mechanisms of port site implantation are being explored.[23]

Trocar placement creates a zone of tissue trauma and disrupts the peritoneum, providing a site for tumor cells to implant and grow.[24] Surgeons performing laparoscopic surgery may use instruments to palpate a tumor, inadvertently incise a tumor, or accidentally open the lumen of an organ containing a tumor.[25] Neoplastic cells can be transferred to the port site during specimen removal, by contaminated instruments, or by making an aerosol of tumor cells. Insufflating the abdominal cavity of hamsters inoculated with colon cancer cells resulted in a threefold increase in the implantation of cancer cells at port sites.[26] A high-pressure CO_2 environment did not create an aerosol of viable tumor cells from solid tumors or liquids containing tumor cells, suggesting that an aerosol is not the means for transferring cells to the port sites.[27] Rapid desufflation through the trocar cannula may allow tumor cells in fluids to be transported to the port site. Tumor cells have been demonstrated experimentally on laparoscopic instruments, trocar cannulas, and stability threads and wound margins around the port site.[28] The ports used by the surgeon had higher numbers of tumor cells than those used by the assistant or the camera operator.[26]

To reduce the likelihood of port site metastasis, the surgeon should take steps to minimize handling a tumor. After the tumor is located, it can be identified with clips on the organ serosa. Handling and resection of neoplastic intestine should be performed at a distance from the tumor site. The vascular supply should be ligated so the intestine containing the tumor is isolated. Because it appears that rapid desufflation may be a means of transporting cells to a port site, surgeons should try to prevent a sudden loss of pneumoperitoneum. The cannulas should be secured to the body wall, reducer caps should be used, and the number of instrument exchanges should be minimized. To prevent direct contact of the tumor with the port site, a plastic disposable specimen retrieval bag and a wound protective device may be used.

At the end of the procedure, aspirating the CO_2 from the abdominal cavity is indicated.[1] Irrigation of port sites with solutions, such as povidone-iodine, chlorhexidine-cetrimide, or sodium hypochlorite, may be of value in killing tumor cells.[1] Intraperitoneal, systemic, or local chemotherapy may also be indicated in selected cases.[23]

Conclusion

As with open procedures, in minimally invasive surgery veterinary surgeons must anticipate potential complications and discuss these with the client or owner. The possibility, feasibility, and ease of conversion to an open procedure must be considered. Preparing the patient by established protocols that include monitoring, positioning, padding, wide surgical preparation, orogastric tubes, and urinary catheters will reduce the risk of complications. Taking a standardized approach to insufflation and trocar placement, monitoring the insertion of instruments and trocars, inspecting for injury, using energy precisely, evaluating port sites for bleeding, and closing port sites will further reduce the risk of complications. An experienced assistant, camera operator, and scrub nurse are invaluable resources in anticipating, preventing, and addressing complications of minimally invasive surgery.

REFERENCES

1. Nord HJ: Complications of laparoscopy. *Endoscopy* 24:693-700, 1992.
2. Phillips JM: Complications in laparoscopy. *Int J Gynaecol Obstet* 15:157-162, 1977.
3. Phillips J et al: Laparoscopic procedures: a national survey for 1975. *J Reprod Med* 18:219-226, 1977.
4. Phillips JR, Hulka JF, Peterson HB: American Association of Gynecologic Laparoscopists' 1982 membership survey. *J Reprod Med* 29:592-594, 1984.
5. Peterson HB, Hulka J, Phillips JM: American Association of Gynecologic Laparoscopists' 1988 membership survey. *J Reprod Med* 35:587-589, 1990.
6. Bailey RW: General considerations. In Bailey RW, Flowers JF, editors: Complications of laparoscopic surgery. St. Louis, 1995, Quality Medical Publishing.
7. Spitzer M et al: Repair of laparoscopic injury to abdominal wall arteries complicated by cutaneous necrosis. *J Am Assoc Gynecol Laparosc* 3:449-452, 1996.
8. Quint EH, Wang RL, Hurd WW: Laparoscopic transillumination for the location of anterior abdominal wall blood vessels. *J Laparoendosc Surg* 6:167-169, 1996.
9. Yuzpe AA: Pneumoperitoneum needle and trocar injuries in laparoscopy: a survey of possible contributing factors and prevention. *J Reprod Med* 35:485-490, 1990.
10. Freeman LJ: Unpublished data. 1991.
11. Rudston-Brown Blair CD et al: Effect of subcutaneous carbon dioxide insufflation on arterial pCO_2. *Am J Surg* 171:460-463, 1996.
12. Andrus CH, Wittgen CM, Naunheim KS: Anesthetic and physiological changes during laparoscopy and thoracoscopy: the surgeon's view. *Semin Laparosc Surg* 1:228-240, 1994.
13. Thompson SE: Unpublished data. 1992.
14. Potter L et al: Unpublished data. 1992.
15. Watson DI et al: Pneumothorax during laparoscopic dissection of the diaphragmatic hiatus. *Br J Surg* 80:1353-1354, 1993 (letter).
16. Marcus DR, Lau WM, Swanstrom LL: Carbon dioxide pneumothorax in laparoscopic surgery. *Am J Surg* 171:464-466, 1996.
17. Gilroy BA, Anson LW: Fatal air embolism during anesthesia for laparoscopy in a dog. *J Am Vet Med Assoc* 190:552-554, 1987.

18. Chan S: Anesthesia and thoracoscopic surgery. *Semin Laparosc Surg* 1:211-214, 1994.

19. Yacoub OF et al: Carbon dioxide embolization during laparoscopy. *Anesthesiology* 57:533-535, 1982.

20. Freeman LJ: Unpublished data. 1992.

21. Wound healing. In Hulka JF, Reich H, editors: Textbook of laparoscopy, ed 2, Philadelphia, 1994, WB Saunders.

22. Mouiel J et al: Port-site recurrence of cancer associated with laparoscopic diagnosis and resection: the European experience. *Semin Laparosc Surg* 2:167-175, 1995.

23. Mathew G et al: Wound metastasis following laparoscopic and open surgery for abdominal cancer in the rat model. *Br J Surg* 83:1087-1090, 1996.

24. Greene FL: Principles of cancer biology in relation to minimal access surgical techniques. *Semin Laparosc Surg* 2:155-157, 1995.

25. Treat MR, Bessler M, Whelan R: Mechanisms to reduce incidence of tumor implantation during minimal access procedures for colon cancer. *Semin Laparosc Surg* 2:176-178, 1995.

26. Jones DB et al: Impact of pneumoperitoneum on trocar site implantation of colon cancer in hamster model. *Dis Colon Rectum* 38:1182-1188, 1995.

27. Whelan RL et al: Trocar site recurrence is unlikely to result from aerosolization of tumor cells. *Dis Colon Rectum* 39:S7-S13, 1996.

28. Allardyce R, Morreau P, Bagshaw P: Tumor cell distribution following laparoscopic colectomy in a porcine model. *Dis Colon Rectum* 39:S47-S52, 1996.

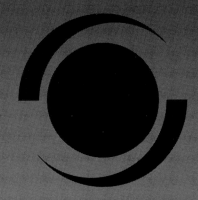

PART TWO

APPLICATIONS

OF

ENDOSURGERY

CHAPTER 7

MINIMALLY INVASIVE HERNIA REPAIR

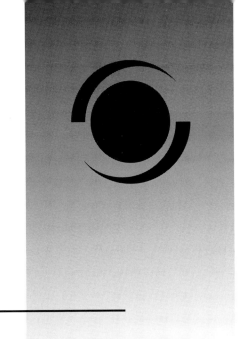

Suzanne E. Thompson, Dean A. Hendrickson

Hernia Repair

SUZANNE E. THOMPSON

Hernias are either congenital or acquired, secondary to trauma or incisional dehiscence. In humans, abdominal hernias are repaired laparoscopically with stapled polypropylene mesh prostheses.[1] The reported benefits include elimination of tension on the tissues and faster recovery to normal activities. Laparoscopic inguinal hernioplasty is reported in foals.[2] Dogs and pigs are used as animal models for surgical training, procedure development, and product testing for laparoscopic inguinal hernia surgery.

Laparoscopic hernioplasty may be considered in animals that have recurrence caused by excessive tissue tension. Large domestic animals or exotic species may benefit from a minimally invasive approach to hasten return to normal activities. Approaches for inguinal, femoral, diaphragmatic, and perineal hernias are described here. Veterinary surgeons must consider the benefits and risks of these approaches.

Inguinal and Femoral Hernias

Laparoscopic inguinal hernia repair has been described in dogs, pigs, and horses. With laparoscopy, the surgeon sees the entire abdominal cavity and both inguinal regions so bilateral hernias can be detected and repaired with minimal tissue trauma. Depending on the technique, there may be less chance of spermatic cord injury than with the open technique.

Laparoscopic inguinal hernia repair in humans is criticized for the risks associated with laparoscopy, such as general anesthesia and the potential for trocar injury. Some pediatric surgeons have expressed concern about using mesh implants because of the unknown interaction of mesh with growth in the inguinal area and because of the potential for reduced fertility and postoperative adhesions. Laparoscopic inguinal hernia repair is technically challenging and costs more than the open procedure, and the recurrence rates for animals are unknown.

ANATOMY

Inguinal hernias are classified as *indirect* if the contents pass through the internal, or deep, inguinal ring, or *direct* if the defect is adjacent to and distinct from the deep inguinal ring. *Femoral* hernias occur when abdominal contents pass into the femoral canal. Indirect, direct, and femoral hernias are difficult to differentiate by physical examination, and all may extend into the scrotum in males to produce a scrotal hernia.

In laparoscopy, the hernia is approached from the peritoneal instead of the external surface. That reverses the surgeon's perspective of the already distorted anatomy. Normal anatomy should be reviewed, with careful consideration of vital anatomic structures, before a laparoscopic approach is attempted (Fig. 7-1).

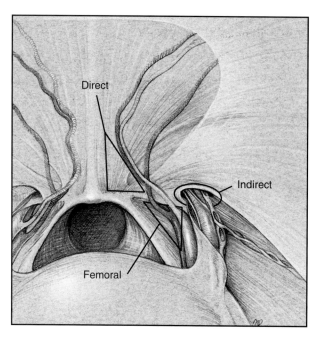

Fig. 7-1   Inguinal anatomy of the pig as seen laparoscopically. The locations of direct, indirect, and femoral hernias are outlined.

The internal inguinal ring is bordered by the inguinal ligament and the rectus abdominis and internal abdominal oblique muscles. In males, testicular vessels and the ductus deferens pass through the ring. They may be atrophied if the animal was castrated earlier. Cooper's ligament, the periosteum covering the brim of the pubis, is an important site for staple fixation in stapled mesh hernioplasty procedures in humans. The caudal epigastric vessels, which are branches of the external iliac vessels, are medial to the internal inguinal ring and enter the internal aspect of the rectus abdominis muscle. During laparoscopy, indirect hernias are seen lateral to the epigastric vessels, and direct hernias occur medial to these vessels.

INSTRUMENTATION
Box 7-1 lists the instrumentation necessary for most laparoscopic hernia repairs.

SURGICAL APPROACH
Position the animal in dorsal recumbency under general anesthesia. Pass a urinary catheter aseptically to drain the bladder. Establish pneumoperitoneum and insert the primary trocar cannula at the umbilicus by one of the techniques described in Chapter 3. Tilt the operating table with the animal's head downward (Trendelenburg position).

Inspect the hernia and abdominal viscera for adhesions or other abnormalities. Place secondary ports in each of the caudal abdominal quadrants (Fig. 7-2). Return any viscera remaining in the hernia to the abdomen with grasping forceps. Applying external pressure to the scro-

BOX 7-1

INSTRUMENTS REQUIRED FOR LAPAROSCOPIC HERNIA REPAIR

10/11 mm trocars (2)
5-mm trocar (1)
Grasping forceps
Dissecting forceps
Scissors with monopolar electrocautery
Electrosurgical generator
Prosthetic mesh material
10-mm introducer sleeve
Hernia stapler
Laparoscopic needle holders (optional)
Laparoscopic suture (optional)

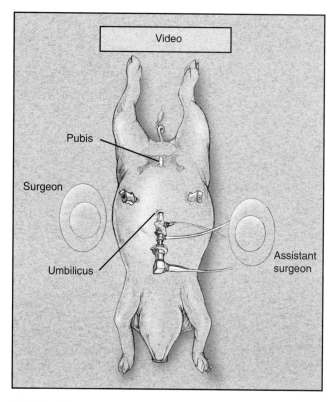

Fig. 7-2   Trocar port locations for laparoscopic inguinal hernia repair.

tum assists in reduction. Transect adhesions from the hernia contents to the inguinal ring with electrosurgical scissors.

Three techniques are used for minimally invasive herniorrhaphy.

Ligation of the Neck of the Hernia Sac
Small indirect hernias can be treated by ligating the neck of the hernia sac (Figs. 7-3 and 7-4). After the hernia has

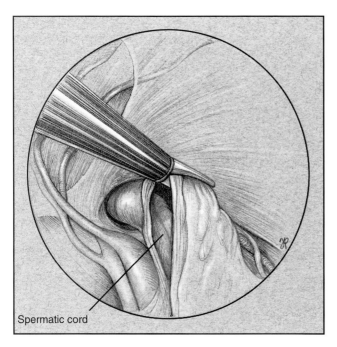

Fig. 7-3 The hernia sac is inverted and an incision is made to isolate the spermatic cord. The sac is ligated and amputated.

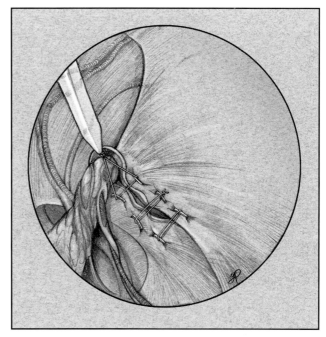

Fig. 7-4 The sac has been inverted, an incision made in the peritoneum, and borders of the defect identified. Staples have been placed circumferentially around the defect over a loop ligature. The ligature is then tightened.

been reduced, grasp the hernia sac and invert it into the abdominal cavity. Some species have a very long, delicate hernia sac that is difficult to invert without tearing the peritoneum. Torn peritoneum does not appear to be clinically significant. Open the sac by making a transperitoneal incision above the internal inguinal ring with scissors. Identify the structures of the spermatic cord. Amputate redundant sac with scissors. Close the neck of the sac with a loop ligature.

An alternative method of closing the neck of the hernia sac is to close the inguinal ring by fixing multiple loop ligatures to the structures surrounding the inguinal ring with endoscopic staples (see Fig. 7-4). Place a 5-mm trocar in each caudal abdominal quadrant. Reduce the hernia and make a transperitoneal incision above the internal inguinal ring. Dissect the hernia sac and ligate it. Insert a 5-mm laparoscope through the port opposite the defect. Introduce a loop ligature through the ipsilateral port and an endoscopic stapler through the umbilical port. Position the loop over the inguinal ring and fix it with staples in the transversalis fascia and muscle ventrally and in the iliopubic tract dorsally. Tighten the loop, drawing the edges of the inguinal ring together. Place three to six loops to close the defect, leaving approximately 5 mm between the spermatic cord and the closest suture. Close the peritoneal incision with staples. In a side-by-side comparison of the laparoscopic loop-staple closure with open repair in six pigs, external physical examination revealed no evidence of recurrence after

3 months. Enlargement of the internal inguinal ring was evident laparoscopically in one of the animals with the laparoscopic repair. There were no adhesions to the operative sites in either group of animals.[3]

Laparoscopic ligation of the neck of the hernia sac with special forceps and a handmade staple-applying instrument has been described.[4] Structures of the inguinal ring were approximated with the forceps, and the staples held the tissue in apposition. The initial animal studies were conducted in female beagle dogs with congenital inguinal hernias. Occlusion of the inguinal defects was satisfactory.

Prosthesis Onlay

An intraperitoneal onlay of a graft prosthesis is used if the peritoneum cannot be dissected from the tissues surrounding the hernia defect and the hernia is too large for simple ligation (Fig. 7-5). Graft materials include polypropylene mesh* and e-PTFE patch.[†] The ability to see anatomic structures through mesh allows precise placement of the graft over the defect. A mesh that results in the lowest rate of postoperative adhesions is desired, but the choice is still under investigation.[5-8] Attempts have been made to reduce adhesion formation

---

*Prolene, Ethicon, Inc., Somerville, NJ. 08876; Marlex, C.R. Bard, Inc., Billerica, Mass.; Surgipro, United States Surgical Corp., Norwalk, Conn. 06856.

†Goretex, W.L. Gore and Associates, Flagstaff, Ariz.

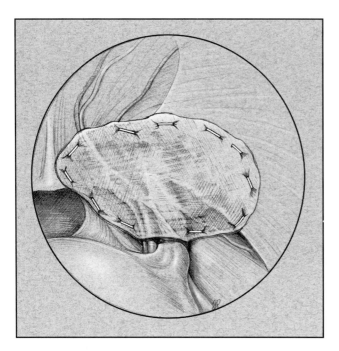

Fig. 7-5   A mesh patch is positioned over the defect and secured with staples.

by using an e-PTFE patch or combining mesh with agents such as oxidized regenerated cellulose (Interceed*) and poloxamer 407 (Pluronic F-127†).

To perform an intraperitoneal onlay of a mesh prosthesis, place two 5- or 10-mm trocars (depending on the stapler) and reduce the inguinal hernia as previously described. Identify the anatomic limits, including the abdominal midline medially, the external iliac artery and vein dorsally, and 1 to 2 cm lateral to the inguinal ring. Measure the width of the defect by spanning it with the open jaws of a 5-mm grasping forceps. Cut the mesh or patch to allow a generous overlap of the entire inguinal region. Roll the mesh or patch material and back load it into a 10-mm introducer sleeve for insertion into the abdominal cavity. Unroll and position the graft over the hernia. Staple the material to the inguinal ligament, the rectus abdominis muscle, and the internal abdominal oblique muscle. Do not place staples on or between the spermatic vessels and the ductus deferens to avoid injuring the underlying external iliac vessels (see Fig. 7-5). If possible, cover the mesh with omentum to minimize adhesions to vital structures.

This technique is technically the easiest to perform because no dissection is required and the peritoneum does not have to be closed. The tensile strength of mesh incorporation with the onlay repair technique was studied in

nine pigs.[7] The onlay technique resulted in weaker tensile strength than preperitoneal or extraperitoneal mesh placements. Laparoscopic intraperitoneal onlay hernia repair with three materials (Prolene, Marlex, and Goretex) and prototype hernia staplers was studied in 30 pigs.[9] Average operative times were 32 minutes for unilateral and 47 minutes for bilateral herniorrhaphy. During a 3-month postoperative period, complications included hernia recurrence and bowel obstruction attributed to inadequate staple fixation in three pigs. Adhesions to the mesh or staples occurred in two pigs. Testicular torsion and hydrocele formation, and erosion of the mesh into the urinary bladder each occurred in one pig. Gross and histologic evaluations revealed fibrous ingrowth of the prosthetic materials. Pigs with unilateral hernias were used to compare testicle sizes of the repaired side with the normal side. No differences were seen.

Fertility after laparoscopic inguinal herniorrhaphy with the mesh onlay technique in 21 swine was evaluated by examining the patency of the ductus deferens, measuring the size and weight of the testicles, and examining sperm.[10] There was no evidence of mesh erosion into the ductus deferens, and the ducts were patent. Testicular sizes and weights were within normal ranges. Three pigs had low sperm counts or abnormalities in sperm appearance or motility, but the authors attributed the abnormalities to factors other than the surgical repair.

Five types of mesh were implanted over the internal inguinal ring in 20 male pigs and evaluated 30 and 90 days after surgery for adhesions and effects on spermatic cord structures. Venous congestion of the spermatic vessels led to necrosis of the testis in two pigs. One occurred with Prolene mesh and one with Marlex mesh. Overall, the e-PTFE resulted in the fewest adhesions and the least inflammatory response.[11]

Preperitoneal Mesh Prosthesis
Preperitoneal mesh placement is advocated in large defects and bilateral repairs to reduce the potential for adhesions. The transabdominal approach uses laparoscopic techniques to place mesh in the preperitoneal space. The extraperitoneal approach does not enter the abdominal cavity.

TRANSABDOMINAL APPROACH
After insufflation and primary trocar placement, insert a 5- or 10-mm trocar in each caudal abdominal quadrant. Reduce the hernia and make a transperitoneal incision above the internal inguinal ring from the pubic tubercle laterally toward the abdominal wall (Fig. 7-6). Dissect the peritoneum from superficial structures around the defect to form pockets dorsally and ventrally in the preperitoneal space. Measure and cut the mesh to overlap the defect and place it in the preperitoneal space. Staple

---

*Interceed, Johnson and Johnson, New Brunswick, NJ.
†Pluronic F-127, BASF Corp., Parsippany, NJ.

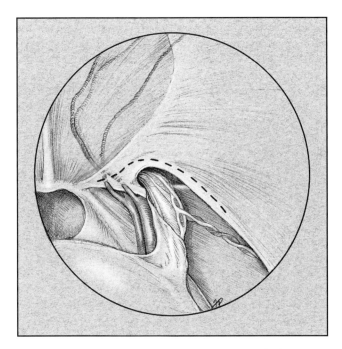

Fig. 7-6   A peritoneal incision is made cranial to the hernia defect. The peritoneum is dissected from the inguinal structures.

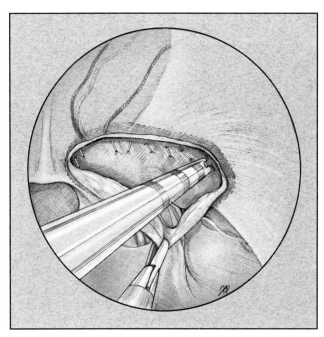

Fig. 7-7   The mesh is positioned over the defect and secured with staples. The peritoneum is reapposed with staples.

the mesh to the inguinal ligament, the rectus abdominis muscle, and the internal abdominal oblique muscle, as outlined previously (Fig. 7-7). Reduce the intraabdominal pressure to 5 to 7 mm Hg to make it easier to approximate the edges of the delicate peritoneum. Staple or suture the edges of the peritoneum together.

Laparoscopic mesh herniorrhaphy proved stronger than either open mesh repair of an inguinal hernia or normal inguinal regions in swine.[12] One month after surgery, the force required to disrupt the repair with a mechanical testing machine was two times higher with laparoscopic than with open mesh repair and three times higher than the normal inguinal canal.

Adhesions can occur with or without mesh. Adhesion rates after procedures with and without polypropylene mesh were compared in 21 pigs.[13] Adhesions developed where mesh was placed in 12 animals and on the side in 3 animals where no mesh was used. A further study compared laparoscopic preperitoneal herniorrhaphy with e-PTFE in 10 pigs with open repair in 31 pigs.[8] None of the pigs with the open repair had intraabdominal adhesions.

Adhesion to mesh placed in the preperitoneal space was compared with mesh placed intraperitoneally in three studies. When bilateral hernias were repaired in 30 pigs, adhesion rates were greater when the peritoneum was closed over the mesh covering the defect than when the mesh was left exposed.[14] In a study of 15 pigs, extraperitoneal mesh implantation resulted in two adhesions and intraperitoneal mesh placement

resulted in five adhesions.[15] Rates of adhesion formation in various placements of polypropylene mesh were compared in six dogs.[16] Intraperitoneal mesh onlay resulted in adhesions in all of the dogs. Transabdominal preperitoneal placement resulted in adhesions in two dogs.

EXTRAPERITONEAL APPROACH

Animals with a thick peritoneum and sufficient preperitoneal fat to facilitate easy separation of the peritoneum from the body wall are candidates for the extraperitoneal approach. All operating ports are inserted directly into the preperitoneal space so that the peritoneal cavity is not entered.

Use an open technique to place the initial port into the space between the muscle and the internal fascia of the rectus abdominis muscle (see Fig. 3-19). Make a skin incision 1 to 2 cm lateral to the midline on the side of the hernia. Continue the dissection through the subcutaneous tissue and external fascia of the rectus abdominis muscle, and bluntly dissect between the fibers of the rectus abdominis muscle. Do not enter the peritoneal cavity. Insert a balloon dissector toward the pubis between the rectus abdominis muscle and the internal fascia. Insert the laparoscope into the balloon dissector and fill the balloon with air or saline solution. Observe the progressive dissection through the wall of the balloon as the preperitoneal working space is created.

Alternatively, dissect the space with an operating laparoscope or with the end of the rigid telescope. Continue dissection until the optical cavity is large enough to accommodate ancillary ports. Remove the balloon dissector or the operating laparoscope, insert a trocar cannula, and insufflate the preperitoneal space with carbon dioxide (CO_2) at 12 to 14 mm Hg. Insert one 5-mm port just lateral to the midline, halfway between the umbilicus and the pubis, and another laterally at the same level. Complete the dissection of the hernia and inguinal region. Cut the mesh to cover the defect. Measure, cut, and introduce the mesh through one of the ports. Position the mesh over the hernia defect and staple it to Cooper's ligament, the transversalis fascia, and the internal abdominal oblique muscle. Do not place staples over the iliac artery and vein. Desufflate the preperitoneal space, remove the trocars, and close the port sites.

Because the extraperitoneal approach does not invade the abdominal cavity, adhesions are least likely to occur with this procedure. In the study of six dogs reported earlier, there were no adhesions with the extraperitoneal approach.[13]

Umbilical, Incisional, and Traumatic Hernias

Small umbilical, incisional, and traumatic hernias result from defects in the external abdominal wall that allow protrusion of abdominal contents.[17] They may be amenable to laparoscopic repair. If the defect is so large that skin resection is required or if there are significant adhesions to the skin and subcutaneous tissue, laparoscopic repair is not advised. Operating port placements depend on the location of the hernia.

Position the animal in dorsal or lateral recumbency. Insufflate the abdomen and insert at least three ports, with the camera port between the two instrument ports. Position the instrument ports to approach the hernia at 60° to 90° angles to each other (Fig. 7-8). Reduce the hernia. Make an incision in the peritoneum to expose the internal fascia of the tranversus or rectus abdominis muscle. Continue dissecting until a space large enough for insertion of the mesh is created. Insert the mesh and secure it to the internal fascia and underlying abdominal muscle with staples. Reduce the insufflation pressure and close the peritoneum over the mesh with staples.

The comparative strengths of mesh fixation with hernia staples and Prolene sutures were compared in a porcine abdominal wall defect model.[18] Mesh fixed with sutures had the greatest bursting strength. The sutures had the greatest depth of penetration and the strongest fixation. The bursting strength of the repair with mesh and hernia staples was 665 to 885 mm Hg, depending on the staple configuration. In animals, it is not known whether mesh repair with staples is strong enough to resist intraabdominal pressures associated with coughing, straining, or running, but mesh and staples appear to be

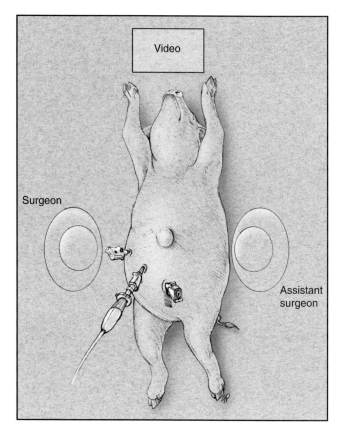

Fig. 7-8 Trocar port locations for a paracostal incisional hernia repair.

effective for repairing human abdominal wall hernias, where intraabdominal pressures reach 220 mm Hg.

Diaphragmatic Hernia

In both congenital and acquired diaphragmatic hernias, the peritoneal cavity communicates with the pleural cavity. Creation of pneumoperitoneum causes tension pneumothorax. Therefore, insufflation of the peritoneal cavity is contraindicated in any animal suspected of having a diaphragmatic defect. A gasless laparoscopic technique (see Chapter 3) or a video-assisted thoracic approach (see Chapter 9) should be used if minimally invasive repair of a diaphragmatic hernia is performed. Retracting the liver and stomach and releasing adhesions in the thorax may be more difficult than with an open approach. This procedure should be considered experimental, because no survival studies have been performed in animals.

Ancillary Procedures for Perineal Hernia

Perineal hernias result from disruption or weakening of the pelvic floor muscles, often secondary to chronic abdominal straining associated with rectal or prostatic dis-

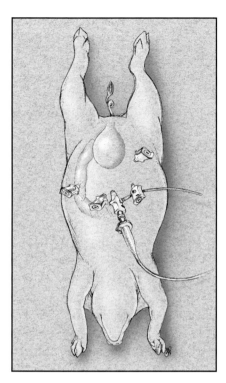

Fig. 7-9   Trocar port locations for a laparoscopic cystopexy, colopexy, and deferent duct fixation.

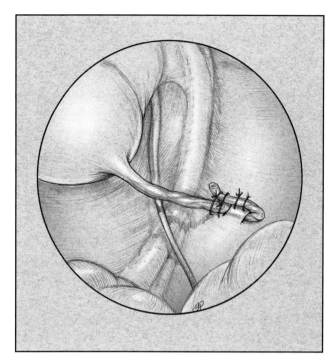

Fig. 7-10   Laparoscopically sutured deferent duct fixation.

ease.[19] Although the hernia itself should be repaired by conventional techniques, ancillary abdominal procedures, such as cryptorchid castration, cystopexy, colopexy, and deferent duct fixation, can be performed laparoscopically to reduce the recurrence of perineal hernia. Cryptorchid castration is described in Chapter 11.

LAPAROSCOPIC COLOPEXY AND CYSTOPEXY

Administer general anesthesia and position the animal in dorsal recumbency. Insert a urinary catheter aseptically. Create a pneumoperitoneum and insert the primary trocar cannula at the umbilicus by one of the techniques described in Chapter 3. Tilt the operating table with the animal's head in Trendelenburg position. Inspect the abdominal contents for adhesions or other abnormalities. Insert secondary ports in the caudal abdominal quadrants (Fig. 7-9).

Suture the descending colon or the urinary bladder, or both, to the abdominal wall with nonabsorbable sutures. Use laparoscopic suturing techniques to place sutures along the entire descending colon. Fixing the neck of the bladder allows the fundus to move as it is distended with urine. Do not penetrate the colonic or bladder mucosa.

LAPAROSCOPIC DEFERENT DUCT FIXATION

Laparoscopic fixation of the deferent ducts is performed to prevent herniation of the prostate.[20] Perform a pre-

scrotal or cryptorchid castration. Using a laparoscopic approach, identify the deferent ducts. Pull the deferent ducts from the inguinal canal into the abdominal cavity with grasping forceps. Mobilize the deferent ducts to the level of the prostate. Grasp the end of each duct and pass each one through an intermuscular tunnel created under the transversus abdominis muscle in the ipsilateral dorsolateral abdominal wall lateral to the colon. Suture each duct laparoscopically with nonabsorbable interrupted sutures (Fig. 7-10). Because it is important for the deferent ducts to be tight, use staples or vascular clips to stabilize the ducts in tension while placing the sutures.

To eliminate the need for laparoscopic suturing, a laparoscopically assisted technique can be used. Insert grasping forceps through the trocar ports on each side to grasp the ducts close to the prostate. Pull the prostate and urinary bladder forward by pulling the ducts into the trocar ports (Fig. 7-11). Remove the ports. Enlarge the skin incision and secure the ducts in the muscles of the abdominal wall with sutures.

This procedure has been performed in six dogs.[21] Four dogs had no clinical signs 8 months after the surgery. One dog had recurrence of straining at 6 months, and one was lost to follow-up. If the bladder and prostate are mobile, the chances of a successful outcome are considered to be better. Failure occurs if the ductus deferentia stretch or become detached when the animal exercises.

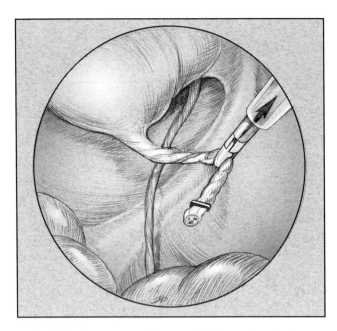

Fig. 7-11   Laparoscopically assisted deferent duct fixation.

Repairs of inguinal hernias with minimally invasive techniques should have results equivalent to those performed with open techniques while avoiding complications. The basic principle of tension-free defect closure must be followed. Although experimental studies in swine demonstrate the feasibility of laparoscopic inguinal herniorrhaphy, care should be used in extrapolating these results to all species.

REFERENCES

1. Arregui ME, Nagan RF, editors: Inguinal hernia: advances or controversies? New York, 1994, Radcliffe Medical Press.
2. Klohnen A, Wilson DG: Laparoscopic repair of scrotal hernia in two foals. *Vet Surg* 25:414-416, 1996.
3. Freeman LJ, Zelewski B: Unpublished data. 1993.
4. Ger R et al: Management of indirect inguinal hernias by laparoscopic closure of the neck of the sac. *Am J Surg* 159:370-373, 1990.
5. Beets GL, Go P, van Mameren H: Foreign body reactions to monofilament and braided polypropylene mesh used as preperitoneal implants in pigs. *Eur J Surg* 162:823-825, 1996.
6. Naim JO et al: Reduction of postoperative adhesions to Marlex mesh using experimental adhesion barriers in rats. *J Laparoendosc Surg* 3:187-189, 1993.
7. Rasim ZM et al: Comparison of adhesion formation and tensile strength after three laparoscopic herniorrhaphy techniques. *Surg Laparosc Endosc* 7:133-136, 1997.
8. Eller R et al: Intraperitoneal adhesions in laparoscopic and standard open herniorrhaphy: an experimental study. *Surg Endosc* 11:24-28, 1997.
9. Layman TS et al: Laparoscopic inguinal herniorrhaphy in a swine model. *Am Surg* 59:13-19, 1993.
10. Fitzgibbons RJ et al: A laparoscopic intraperitoneal onlay mesh technique for the repair of an indirect inguinal hernia. *Ann Surg* 219:144-156, 1994.
11. LeBlanc KA, Booth W, Whitaker JM: In vivo study of meshes implanted over the internal inguinal ring and external iliac vessels. *Surg Endosc* 11:174, 1997 (abstracts).
12. Horgan LF et al: Strengths and weaknesses of laparoscopic and open mesh inguinal hernia repair: a randomized controlled experimental study. *Br J Surg* 83:1463-1467, 1996.
13. Eller R et al: Abdominal adhesions in laparoscopic hernia repair: an experimental study. *Surg Endosc* 8:181-184, 1994.
14. Durstein-Decker C et al: Comparison of adhesion formation in transperitoneal laparoscopic herniorrhaphy techniques. *Am Surg* 60:157-159, 1994.
15. Attwood SEA et al: Adhesions after laparoscopic inguinal hernia repair: a comparison of extra versus intra peritoneal placement of a polypropylene mesh in an animal model. *Surg Endosc* 8:777-780, 1994.
16. Schlecter B et al: Intraabdominal mesh prosthesis in a canine model. *Surg Endosc* 8:127-129, 1994.
17. Smeak DD: Abdominal hernias. In Slatter DH, editor: Textbook of small animal surgery, ed 2, Philadelphia, 1993, WB Saunders.
18. Dion YM, Charara J, Guidoin R: Bursting strength evaluation: comparison of 0-Prolene sutures and endoscopic staples in an experimental prosthetic patch repair of abdominal wall defect. *Surg Endosc* 8:812-816, 1994.
19. Bellenger CR, Canfield RB: Perineal hernia. In Slatter DH, editor: Textbook of small animal surgery, ed 2, Philadelphia, 1993.
20. Bilbrey SA, Smeak DD, DeHoff W: Fixation of the deferent ducts for retrodisplacement of the urinary bladder and prostate in canine perineal hernia. *Vet Surg* 19:24-27, 1990.
21. Henderson RA: Unpublished data. 1991-1993.

Large Animal Inguinal Hernia Repair

DEAN A. HENDRICKSON

Laparoscopic repair of inguinal hernia has been reported in two Percheron foals and two stallions. All of the horses were positioned in dorsal recumbency. In the foals, the hernias were repaired with an automated stapling device designed for mesh implantation in humans.

In the stallions, the peritoneum over the internal inguinal ring was dissected and polypropylene mesh was secured to the inguinal region with an endoscopic stapler. The peritoneum was drawn over the mesh and closed with staples.

Surgical Preparation

Fast the horse for 24 to 48 hours to decrease the volume of intestinal contents and thereby improve visibility. Administer antibiotics and nonsteroidal antiinflammatory drugs following accepted principles governing their selection and use.

Anesthesia and Positioning

Induce general anesthesia and provide assisted ventilation because of the increased abdominal pressure caused by insufflation and dorsal recumbency, and the potential for peritoneal carbon dioxide (CO_2) absorption. Aseptically prepare the penis and prepuce and insert a stallion catheter to drain the bladder.

Aseptically prepare the abdomen. It may be helpful to tie the horse to the table to minimize slippage when the table is tilted. Drape the umbilicus, both folds of the flank, and the inguinal region for surgery. After the abdomen is insufflated and the primary trocar for the laparoscope has been inserted, tilt the table so that the horse's head is in Trendelenburg position. Position the video monitor caudal to the animal, or slightly to one side if the hind limbs are between the surgeon and the monitor. The surgeon and assistant stand on each side of the horse.

Procedure

INSUFFLATION
Use either of two techniques to gain access to and insufflate the abdomen.

Open Technique
Insert a trocar under direct observation through an incision in the linea alba at the level of the umbilicus and secure it with two sutures to the fascia. Insufflate the abdomen with CO_2 to a pressure of 15 to 20 mm Hg. Direct observation of the insertion helps avoid iatrogenic damage to the underlying viscera. However, if the incision is slightly large, CO_2 can escape around the cannula, making it difficult to maintain pneumoperitoneum.

Insufflation with a Veress Needle or Teat Cannula
Insert a Veress needle or a teat cannula into the peritoneal space through a small stab incision at the umbilicus. Connect the needle to a CO_2 insufflator to distend the abdomen to 15 to 20 mm Hg pressure. When the abdomen is distended, remove the Veress needle or teat cannula. Lengthen the skin incision to the size of the telescope cannula and place a trocar through the body wall with a slow, constant, twisting motion. Remove the obturator and connect the insufflation tubing, telescope, and video camera.

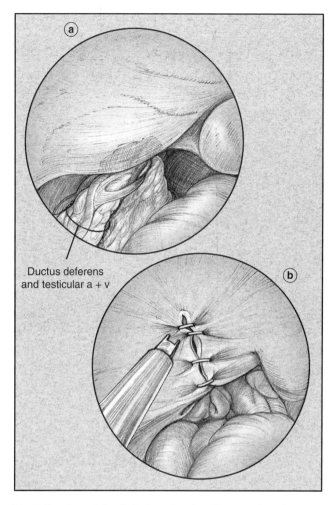

Ductus deferens
and testicular a + v

Fig. 7-12 Intraabdominal view of a dorsally recumbent horse during inguinal hernia repair with staples. Internal inguinal ring (*a*). Hernia staple applier with staples closing the vaginal ring (*b*).

PLACING SECONDARY PORTS
After an initial exploration, tilt the table so the horse's hind quarters are elevated (Trendelenburg position) to facilitate exploration and surgical manipulation in the caudal part of the abdomen. Place secondary ports under direct observation, using the same principles as described previously. Some surgeons prefer to preplace a spinal needle to determine the exact entry points of the additional cannulas. Place one secondary port on each side of the midline, approximately 10 cm cranial to the cranial aspect of the inguinal rings. Depending on the diameter of the endoscopic stapler used, ensure that at least one of the ports has a 12-mm cannula.

STAPLE TECHNIQUE[1]
If a loop of intestine is still within the ring, gently manipulate it back into the abdomen with atraumatic forceps. Externally massage the scrotum to assist in returning the bowel to the abdomen. After the hernia is reduced, ex-

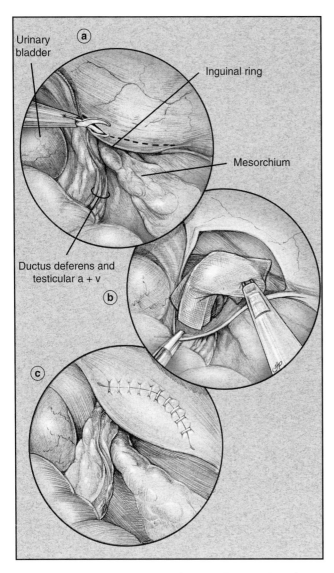

Fig. 7-13   Intraabdominal view of a dorsally recumbent horse during inguinal hernia repair with a nonabsorbable mesh and staples. Dissection of the peritoneum (*a*). Placement and attachment of mesh with stapler (*b*). Reattachment of the peritoneum (*c*).

amine the bowel for areas of devitalized tissue. Resect any devascularized segments through an open approach or by a closed, laparoscopic approach. Draw the testis into the abdomen and remove it as in cryptorchid castration, or leave it in place. Staple the peritoneum of the vaginal ring (Fig. 7-12, *a*) together with an endoscopic hernia stapler. Use as many staples as are necessary to close the entire ring (Fig. 7-12, *b*). Partially advance the staples to grasp one side of the vaginal ring. Move the end of the stapler to the opposite side of the vaginal ring and completely advance and close the staples. If the testis is left in situ, take care to avoid incorporating its vasculature or the ductus deferens in the closure. Both foals described in the

literature were castrated at the time of herniorrhaphy. Neither hernia had recurred 16 weeks after surgery.

STAPLE AND MESH TECHNIQUE[2]

Reduce the hernia as previously described. Using scissors, dissect the peritoneum from the ventral and cranial aspects of the internal inguinal ring to the caudal aspect of the inguinal ring. Dissect the caudal wall of the inguinal ring to create a free flap of peritoneum (Fig. 7-13, *a*). Control hemorrhage with electrocautery. If the testis is to be removed, draw it into the abdomen and amputate it as in cryptorchid castration. If the testis is to be salvaged, dissect the blood supply, mesoductus, and ductus deferens from the peritoneal flap. Introduce a 5-cm × 7-cm piece of nonabsorbable mesh into the abdomen through one of the cannulas. Unroll the mesh and position it across the inguinal ring. The mesh covers the ductus deferens and vascular supply. Staple the mesh in place with an endoscopic stapler (Fig. 7-13, *b*). Avoid stapling either the ductus deferens or the blood supply when attaching the mesh. Advance the peritoneum over the mesh and staple it in place (Fig. 7-13, *c*).

At the end of the procedure open the cannulas, release or actively aspirate the pneumoperitoneum, and remove the cannulas. Suture the incisions by using standard techniques. Allow the horse to exercise normally 30 days after surgery. In the published report, the testes were left in place in both stallions and on followup at year 2, there had been no recurrence of an inguinal hernia.

Complications

Potential complications of herniorrhaphy include breakdown of the herniorrhaphy site and stricture of the blood supply or ductus deferens if the testis is left in situ.

Conclusion

Inguinal herniorrhaphy can be performed successfully by using either the staple or the staple and mesh technique. The staple-only technique is less technically demanding and has been adequate when performed in foals. Concern has been expressed that the peritoneum may not be strong enough to prevent reherniation in an adult horse. Mesh can be implanted to reinforce the peritoneum and reduce the likelihood of dehiscence.

REFERENCES
1. Klohnen AAO, Wilson DG: Laparoscopic repair of scrotal hernia in two foals. *Vet Surg* 25:414-416, 1996.
2. Fischer AT, Vachon AM, Klein SR: Laparoscopic inguinal herniorrhaphy in two stallions. *J Am Vet Med Assoc* 207:1599-1601, 1995.

CHAPTER 8

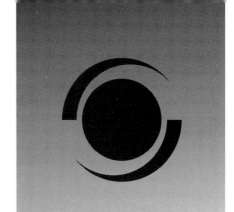

MINIMALLY INVASIVE SURGERY OF THE GASTROINTESTINAL SYSTEM

Lynetta J. Freeman, Ronald J. Kolata, Steven Trostle

Minimally Invasive Surgery of the Esophagus

LYNETTA J. FREEMAN

Conventional surgical approaches to the esophagus include a ventral midline approach to the cervical portion and a right intercostal thoracotomy to approach the thoracic portion cranial to the heart. If the animal has a persistent right aortic arch, a left thoracotomy is indicated.[1] Caudal to the heart, either a right or left thoracotomy can be used. The abdominal portion of the esophagus is approached from the abdomen.

The benefits of minimally invasive techniques to gain access to the cervical esophagus do not appear to outweigh the technical difficulty at this time. Although the optical cavity is relatively easy to establish with a balloon dissector, insufflating the cervical space above 12 mm Hg results in pneumomediastinum.[2] Therefore, very low pressure or a lift device without insufflation must be used. Both techniques result in a small optical cavity, and dissection in small spaces is difficult. Because morbidity with the conventional cervical approach is relatively low, minimally invasive procedures are not justified.

An endoscopic approach to the thoracic portion of the esophagus is justified because it makes thoracotomy unnecessary. Segmental blood supply, tension from head and neck movement, and motion from peristalsis may delay esophageal wound healing.[1] Difficulty in preventing or sealing esophageal leakage is attributed to lack of serosa or omentum. Gentle tissue handling, minimal contamination, minimal use of electrocautery, accurate tissue apposition, and proper selection of suture materials are necessary to avoid wound complications in both open and minimally invasive esophageal surgery.

Anatomy

The esophagus has cervical, thoracic, and abdominal portions.[3] The thoracic portion of the esophagus extends from the thoracic inlet to the esophageal hiatus of the diaphragm. Cranially, the esophagus lies to the left of the trachea. At the tracheal bifurcation, it crosses to the right and lies dorsal to the trachea. The azygos vein crosses over the esophagus on the right side (Fig. 8-1). Also at this level the aortic arch passes from the left of the esophagus to become dorsal to it (Fig. 8-2). Caudal to the base of the heart, the esophagus lies nearly in the median plane, ventral to the aorta. Dorsal branches of the right and left vagal nerves unite on the dorsal surface of the esophagus and pass through the dorsal part of the esophageal hiatus. The right and left ventral vagal nerves unite on the ventral surface of the esophagus and pass through the ventral port of the esophageal hiatus.

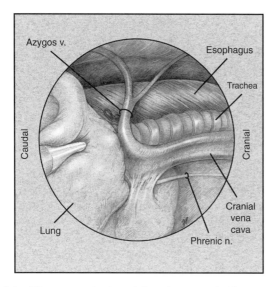

Fig. 8-1 Thoracoscopic view, right-side approach. The azygos vein is visible.

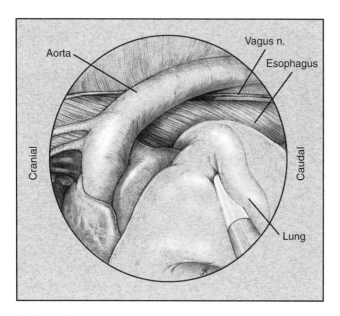

Fig. 8-2 Thoracoscopic view of the esophagus from the left side. The aortic arch is visible. Caudal to the heart, the esophagus is separate from the aorta. The vagus nerves are dorsal and ventral to the esophagus.

The esophagus has four layers: the *fibrous layer*, or *adventitia*; the *muscular layer*, consisting of two layers of striated muscle; the *submucosa*, loosely connected to the muscular coat; and the *mucosa*, lined with stratified squamous epithelium.[3] Blood supply to the cranial two thirds of the thoracic portion is provided by the broncho-esophageal artery, and the caudal one third is supplied by the esophageal branches of the aorta or the dorsal intercostal arteries, or both. The abdominal portion is supplied by the left gastric artery.

Indications

Because a conventional thoracotomy involves significant postoperative morbidity, performing this procedure thoracoscopically may improve the postoperative outcome. Retrieving an imbedded and penetrating fish hook that resists removal with an esophagoscope is one example. The barb can be cut off thoracoscopically and the rest of the hook retrieved with the endoscope. Closure of esophageal perforations, resection of esophageal diverticula, resection of vascular ring anomalies, biopsies of periesophageal masses, and esophagomyotomies are examples of procedures that may benefit from the use of minimally invasive techniques. Using thoracoscopy to access the esophagus and laparoscopy to mobilize a portion of omentum and bring it through the diaphragm could avoid simultaneous thoracotomy and laparotomy.

Surgeons must weigh the benefits of less tissue trauma and less postoperative pain against the risks of thoracoscopy. Animals with esophageal disease may have aspiration pneumonia, which could decrease the lung capacity and increase the anesthetic risk during one-lung ventilation. Thoracoscopic approaches may be associated with longer operative times. In any case, the surgeon must be prepared to convert to an open approach at any time.

Anesthesia

Preoperative preparation and anesthetic techniques for minimally invasive esophageal surgery are the same as for video-assisted thoracic surgery (VATS) (see Chapter 9). Special equipment needs are outlined in Box 8-1. Surgery that involves a nonperforated, nonleaking esophagus is considered clean contaminated and antibiotics are administered, following the accepted principles governing their selection and use.[1] The anesthetist should be prepared to pass an endoscope or orogastric tube if necessary during the procedure. A lateral thoracic radiograph is helpful for reference during the procedure.

Selected Procedures

THORACOSCOPIC APPROACH

The animal is positioned in lateral recumbency, and an intercostal approach is performed as described for VATS. Unless otherwise indicated, it is advisable to approach the esophagus from the right side. Vascular ring anomalies, such as persistent right aortic arch (PRAA), are approached from the left side. Disease involving the caudal portion of the thoracic esophagus can be approached from either side, according to the most likely site of disease and the surgeon's preference. Esophageal cardiomy-

BOX 8-1

EQUIPMENT FOR MINIMALLY INVASIVE ESOPHAGEAL SURGERY

Gastrointestinal endoscope
0° and 30° telescopes
Thoracic trocars
Grasping forceps
Dissecting forceps
Atraumatic lung clamps
Right-angled forceps
DeBakey forceps
Endoscopic Kittner (cherry, peanut) dissectors
Clip applier
Silk strands
Ultrasonic scalpel or microbipolar forceps
Needle holders
Irrigation/aspiration cannula

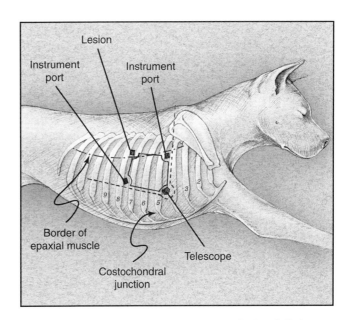

Fig. 8-3 Trocar site in thoracoscopy, using the baseball diamond plan. The telescope is inserted at home plate, looking toward the lesion at second base. Instrument ports are positioned at first base and third base.

otomy (Heller's myotomy) is usually performed from the left side.

Draping is done as widely as possible in case an open thoracotomy becomes necessary. The abdomen is prepared aseptically if omental harvest is anticipated. The omentum serves as a patch to seal defects in the esophagus. The camera port is placed after selective bronchial intubation and collapse of the superior (operative) lung.

To view the cranial portion of the thoracic part of the esophagus, place the camera port in the sixth or seventh intercostal space, midway between the costochondral junction and the ventral border of the epaxial muscles. To view the caudal portion, place the camera port in the fourth intercostal space at the same level. To plan port placement, think of a baseball diamond with the camera port as home plate and the primary surgery site as second base.[4] When the primary lesion is identified, insert two additional working ports at first base and third base (Fig. 8-3). In very small chests the ports may have to be moved farther from the surgical site to allow the instruments to open safely. If the surgeon is planning to use a large port for inserting a stapler or a 12-mm clip applier, consideration should be given to where the largest port can be used most effectively. Port placement varies with the surgical procedure, the size and location of the lesion, the size of the animal, and the surgeon's skill.

EXPLORATION

An exploratory procedure is performed to confirm a diagnosis, identify an extraluminal foreign body, assess the severity of perforating injuries, or assess the potential for esophageal resection and anastomosis.

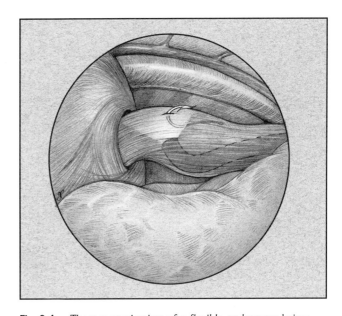

Fig. 8-4 Thoracoscopic view of a flexible endoscope being manipulated to identify the esophagus. A foreign body is identified and removed.

Unless thoracic radiographs or other diagnostic aids indicate disease confined to the left hemithorax, a right-side approach is used. The camera port is placed, and the esophagus is examined. Passing a lighted endoscope helps identify the esophagus and locate the lesion (Fig. 8-4). The tip of the endoscope is deflected to mark the site. Depending on the nature of the lesion, the surgeon may elect to obtain a biopsy specimen, resect a periesophageal mass, place additional ports, or convert to an open procedure. A bronchoesophageal fistula is an indication for thoracotomy. Although the esophagus could be repaired by using VATS techniques, lobectomy is usually required and a VATS lobectomy requires special instruments and advanced technical skills.

ESOPHAGOTOMY

Esophagotomy should be performed only by surgeons proficient in endoscopic suturing and intracorporeal knot tying. Esophagotomy is indicated to retrieve foreign bodies that cannot be dislodged by conventional methods, to relieve an intraluminal obstruction, or to resect an esophageal diverticulum. The esophagus proximal to a persistent obstruction is dilated and may contain fluid and particulate matter. Special care should be taken to minimize contamination of the thoracic cavity.

Beginning at the azygos vein, grasp the mediastinal pleura adjacent to the vein and elevate it. Snip the pleura with scissors and continue the pleural incision proximally and distally over the esophagus. Dissect the azygos vein from the esophagus and, if necessary, ligate the vein with sutures or clips and transect it. Dissect the esophagus circumferentially proximal to an obstruction and pass a silicone vascular tape around it. Use the tape for traction and mobilize the esophagus, ligating vascular branches from the aorta, if needed. To provide the best blood supply for the esophagus, minimize the number of vessels ligated. Pass a second tape around the esophagus distal to the lesion. If necessary, use the tapes to occlude the lumen of the esophagus to prevent spillage. Using grasping forceps to tent the periesophageal tissue, make a longitudinal esophagotomy with scissors (Fig. 8-5). The incision penetrates the muscle to the mucosa, which bulges out. Regrasp the muscle with grasping forceps and insert one tip of the scissors between the muscle and mucosa. Continue the myotomy for the appropriate length. Use an energy source, preferably microbipolar forceps or the ultrasonic scalpel, for hemostasis. Make a mucosal incision slightly shorter than the myotomy with scissors. Relieve the obstruction by delivering the foreign body through the incision. If possible, place the foreign body in a disposable specimen retrieval bag to reduce contamination during extraction.

Close the esophageal incision in two layers.[1] Suture the mucosa and submucosa with a simple continuous pattern of size 4/0 or 5/0 synthetic monofilament suture such as polydiaxanone. If possible, tie the knots in the lumen. Check for leakage and reinforce weak areas with simple interrupted sutures. Reappose the muscular layers with size 3/0 or 4/0 simple interrupted sutures of a synthetic monofilament suture (Fig. 8-6). Inspect and lavage the surgical site to reduce contamination.

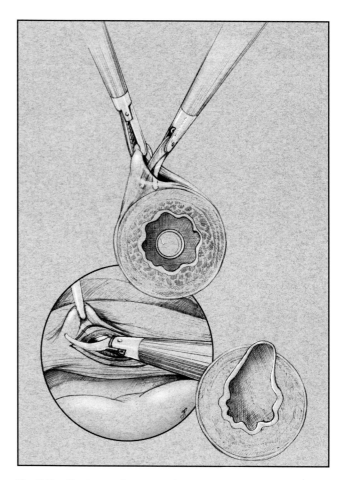

Fig. 8-5   Tenting and incising the muscles of the esophagus. *Inset,* cross-sectional view of esophagus with endoscope in esophageal lumen.

The surgeon may choose to reinforce the suture line with muscle, pericardium, or omentum.[1] It should be possible with thoracoscopy to harvest a pedicle graft of intercostal muscle, including the artery, vein, and nerve. In the caudal part of the thorax, a strip of diaphragm could be used. Strips of pericardium, 2 to 3 cm wide, can also be harvested by using techniques described for partial pericardectomy in Chapter 9.

OMENTAL PEDICLE PATCH

The usual technique for creating an omental pedicle involves a midline or paracostal laparotomy. Omental harvest can also be performed laparoscopically.[5] Three ports are used. Place the camera at the umbilicus and one additional port on each side of the umbilicus at the level of the greater curvature of the stomach. Ligate the gastroepiploic artery by developing a plane of dissection between the vessel and the greater curvature. For a pedicle based on the right gastroepiploic artery, the left gastroepiploic artery is ligated adjacent to the splenic branches. Continue dissection through the omental mesentery to

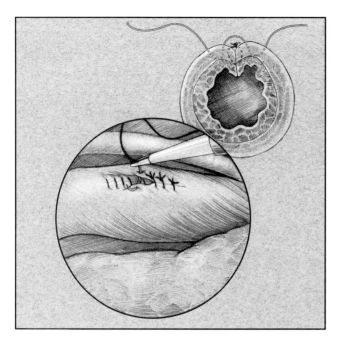

Fig. 8-6 Placing two rows of sutures in the esophagus.

free the omentum from the splenic mesentery. Ligate short branches between the gastroepiploic artery and the stomach with ligating clips or cauterize them with bipolar forceps and transect them with scissors, taking care to preserve the blood supply to the omentum (Fig. 8-7). Create a defect in the diaphragm to pass the omental pedicle into the thoracic cavity. The defect must be large enough to maintain the blood supply to the omentum and small enough to prevent a postoperative diaphragmatic hernia. Avoid excessive tension on the vascular pedicle that would impair the blood supply. The omentum can be sutured to the diaphragm. Within the thorax, bring the omentum to the surgical site to seal the incision. It may be possible to patch lesions in the caudal part of the thoracic portion of the esophagus by mobilizing the distal part of the omentum without ligating the short branches of the gastroepiploic artery to the greater curvature of the stomach.

DIVERTICULECTOMY

An esophageal diverticulum may involve only the mucosa, or it may involve all layers of the esophagus. If the diverticulum is single and relatively small, excision and two-layer closure of the esophagus are indicated. Resection of a small diverticulum requires approach, mobilization, and occlusion cranial and caudal to the lesion. The pouch is resected to reestablish a normal esophageal lumen diameter. The defect is closed as described for esophagotomy. If resection of a large diverticulum would not leave enough normal tissue for closure, esophageal resection and anastomosis are indicated.

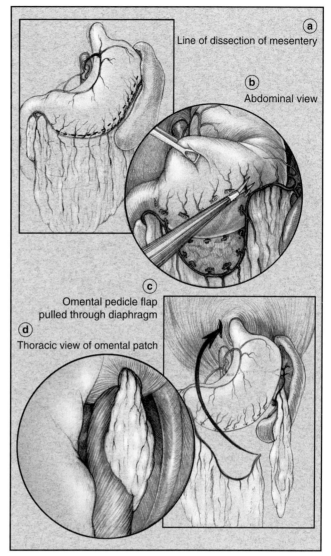

Fig. 8-7 Omental pedicle flap based on the right gastroepiploic vessels. A plane of dissection is developed between the gastroepiploic vessels and the greater curvature of the stomach (a). Short branches between the gastroepiploic artery and stomach are ligated with clips and transected to preserve the blood supply to the omentum (b). The left gastroepiploic vessels are ligated adjacent to the splenic branches, and the vascularized omentum is brought through a window in the diaphragm (c). Within the thorax, the omentum is brought to the surgical site to reinforce an esophageal suture line (d).

LIGATION OF VASCULAR RING ANOMALY

Persistent right aortic arch (PRAA) accounts for about 95% of the vascular ring anomalies in small animals.[4] The ductus arteriosus crosses from the pulmonary artery to the right aortic arch and compresses the esophagus, leading to cranial dilation of the esophagus. Surgical division of the ligamentum arteriosum is required to relieve the obstruction. Many animals with PRAA also have an aberrant subclavian artery that indents the esophagus cranial to the main stricture by the ligamentum arteriosum.[4] The aberrant subclavian artery rarely requires treatment. About 40% of the affected animals also have a persistent left cranial vena cava, which does not require treatment.[4]

The surgical approach for correcting PRAA is from the left side. Place the camera port in the sixth or seventh intercostal space at the midlateral aspect of the thorax. Place an additional port in the seventh intercostal space at the costochondral junction to allow a large organ retractor to be inserted. Additional working ports are placed in the fourth intercostal spaces, near the border of the epaxial muscles and near the costochondral junction.

Gently fold back the cranial lung lobe and hold it in place with the large organ retractor to expose the mediastinum. Incise and reflect the pleura over the descending aorta and ligamentum arteriosum. Bluntly dissect the ligament from the underlying esophagus with right-angle forceps and cherry dissectors. The goal is to encircle the ligament without exerting traction, which could tear the pulmonary artery. Take care not to injure the pulmonary artery or the recurrent laryngeal nerve that courses around the structure. Pass two size 0 silk sutures around the ligament and tie them, using an extracorporeal knotting technique (Fig. 8-8). Place one ligature next to the aorta and one next to the pulmonary artery. Transect the ligament between the ligatures. Perform additional dissection to release fibrotic bands without entering the esophagus.[1] Pass a Foley catheter by mouth past the site and inflate the balloon. Withdraw the Foley balloon to identify bands of fibrous tissue. When all tissue is released, inspect the cranial portion of the esophagus to determine if an aberrant subclavian artery is present. If necessary, perform an esophagotomy and remove any remaining material causing esophageal obstruction.

RESECTION AND ANASTOMOSIS

Thoracoscopic resection and anastomosis with surgical stapling devices has been attempted in several animal studies.[6] Results have been disappointing because of limited exposure, bleeding, incomplete lung collapse, and difficulty in obtaining a tension-free anastomosis, which is critical in esophageal surgery.[7] Minimally invasive esophageal resection and anastomosis are not recommended at this time.

ESOPHAGEAL CARDIOMYOTOMY (HELLER'S MYOTOMY)

Although Heller's myotomy is not endorsed as a primary tool for management of esophageal swallowing disorders, it could be a palliative treatment for animals with severe regurgitation.[4] The standard therapy for achalasia of the esophagus in humans is an esophageal myotomy. Camera and port placements are challenging in this procedure because at least one port usually has to work fac-

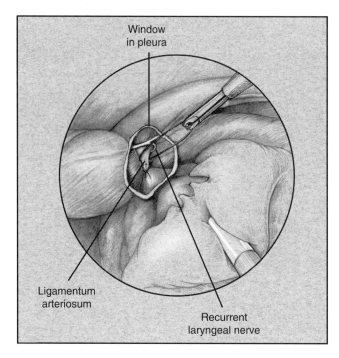

Fig. 8-8   Ligating the ligamentum arteriosum. The recurrent laryngeal nerve is identified and protected.

ing the scope, rather than being in line with it. The surgeon must adjust to paradoxical movement.

Position the animal in right lateral recumbency in head-down (Trendelenburg) position and collapse the superior (operative) lung. Insert the port for a 30° thoracoscope in the fourth intercostal space at the midlateral aspect of the thorax. Place two ports in the sixth intercostal space at the levels of the epaxial muscles and at the costochondral junction. Insert one port at the eighth or ninth intercostal space at the midlateral aspect of the thorax (Fig. 8-9). Advance a gastrointestinal endoscope into the esophagus to the level of dissection. Use the light from the endoscope to facilitate identification of the distal end of the esophagus through the thoracoscope.

With scissors, transect the pulmonary ligament from its attachment to the diaphragm and mediastinum cranially to the level of the pulmonary vein.[8] To provide appropriate countertraction, grasp the lung with the grasping forceps. Use scissors with cautery for the dissection. Incise and dissect the mediastinal pleura over the esophagus to expose and free the esophagus from the pulmonary vein to the esophageal hiatus.[9] As with the esophagotomy, begin the myotomy with scissors and deepen it to the level of the submucosa. Use scissors, electrocautery hook, or ultrasonic scalpel to divide the esophageal muscle. Do not penetrate the mucosa. To ensure that there is no leakage, instill saline in the thorax and withdraw the endoscope while insufflating air into the esophagus.[8] The lack of air bubbling indicates that the esophageal mucosa is intact. Irrigate and aspirate the

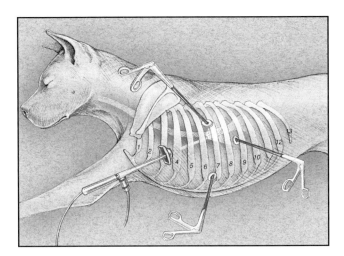

Fig. 8-9   Port placement for thoracoscopic Heller's myotomy.

surgical site and ensure absolute hemostasis. A chest tube is placed, the operative lung is inflated, the trocars are removed, and the skin is closed with sutures.

Postoperative Care

Although the incisions are small, thoracoscopic esophageal procedures are identical to procedures performed through a thoracotomy incision. Therefore, the standard postoperative treatment and analgesic regimens for animals undergoing thoracotomy are applied.

Complications

The most common complications of thoracoscopy are insufficient visibility, lung injury, and hemorrhage. Insufficient visibility occurs if the lung is not adequately collapsed, or if trocars are not placed properly. Lung injury occurs during trocar and instrument insertion and when traction is applied to a lung with grasping forceps. Safe trocar insertion techniques, monitoring instrument insertion and withdrawal, and gentle tissue handling reduce the risks of lung injury. Hemorrhage is avoided by careful dissection, proper identification of tissue planes, and judicious use of energy, clips, and sutures. The surgeon should always be ready to convert to an open procedure if hemorrhage cannot be controlled.

REFERENCES

1. Fingeroth JM: Surgical techniques for esophageal disease. In Slatter D, editor: Textbook of small animal surgery, ed 2, Philadelphia, 1993, WB Saunders.
2. Brunt LM et al: Videoendoscopic thyroidectomy in a canine model. *Minim Invasive Therapy* 4(suppl 1):47, 1995 (abstract).
3. The esophagus. In Evans HE: Miller's anatomy of the dog, ed 3, Philadelphia, 1993, WB Saunders.
4. Schropp KP: Basic thoracoscopy in children. In Lobe TE, Schropp KP, editors: Pediatric laparoscopy and thoracoscopy. Philadelphia, 1994, WB Saunders.
5. Pennino R, Freeman L: Laparoscopic harvesting of omentum for reconstructive purposes. International Symposium on Plastic Surgery, 1994 (abstract).
6. Tung P: Unpublished data. 1996.
7. Gossot D et al: Thoracoscopic dissection of the esophagus: an experimental study. *Surg Endosc* 6:59-61, 1992.
8. Heller myotomy. In Lobe TE, Schropp KP, editors: Pediatric laparoscopy and thoracoscopy. Philadelphia, 1994, WB Saunders.
9. Cheadle WG: Thoracoscopic esophageal myotomy. In Vitale GC, Sanfilippo JS, Perissat J, editors: Laparoscopic surgery: an atlas for general surgeons. Philadelphia, 1995, JB Lippincott.

Minimally Invasive Gastric Surgery

LYNETTA J. FREEMAN

Laparoscopic stapling devices allow difficult procedures to be completed through small incisions. Gastric resections and anastomosis have been completed using minimally invasive techniques in humans. Laparoscopic suturing techniques can be used for gastric surgery, but patience, persistence, and skill are required. As veterinary surgeons gain proficiency in minimally invasive surgery, gastric procedures will be commonly performed.

Anatomy

The stomach has four regions: the fundus, body, pyloric antrum, and pylorus. The esophagus enters at the cardiac ostium. The fundus is the portion of the stomach dorsal to the cardia. The angular incisure identifies the transition from the body to the pyloric antrum. The pylorus joins the antrum to the duodenum. From exterior to interior, the layers of the stomach are serosa, outer longitudinal and inner circular muscular layers, oblique fibers, submucosa, and mucosa. Vascular supply is by the left and right gastric arteries to the lesser curvature and the left and right gastroepiploic arteries to the greater curvature. The splenic artery also supplies branches to the greater curvature. Parasympathetic innervation is from the vagus nerve; sympathetic fibers are from the celiac plexus.

BOX 8-2

INSTRUMENTS REQUIRED FOR MINIMALLY INVASIVE GASTRIC PROCEDURES

Pyloromyotomy / Pyloroplasty

Gastrotomy / Gastrectomy

3 trocars
Grasping forceps
Dissecting forceps
Scissors
Needle holders
Energy source
Optional: Endoscopic stapler

Percutaneous Endoscopic Gastrostomy (PEG) Tube

Gastrointestinal endoscope
PEG tube kit

Laparoscopic Gastrostomy

2 5-mm trocars
PEG tube kit containing:
    T-bar anchors
    J wire

Dilators
Peelaway sheath
Gastrostomy tube
Optional: Endoscopic linear cutter
12-mm trocar
Babcock forceps

Pylorectomy and Enterostomy

Gastropexy

5 trocars
Grasping forceps
Dissecting forceps
Scissors
Needle holders
Energy source
Endoscopic linear cutter
Clip applier
Babcock forceps

Nissen Fundoplication

5 trocars
Babcock forceps
Grasping forceps
Dissecting forceps
Scissors
Needle holders
Knot pusher
Energy source
Large-organ retractor

Transgastric Approach to the Stomach

T-bar anchors
Gastrointestinal endoscope
Trocars

Indications

Minimally invasive gastric procedures are used when equivalent results can be obtained with smaller wounds. Typical applications include pyloromyotomy, feeding tube placement, and exploratory laparoscopy. More difficult techniques should be performed only by surgeons with advanced dissection and laparoscopic suturing skills.

Anesthesia

Anesthetic techniques are the same for closed surgery as for open surgery. If mask inhalation is used and the stomach is distended with gas, an orogastric tube is passed before a Veress needle or the first trocar is inserted to prevent inadvertent gastric injury.

Required Instrumentation

Standard laparoscopic instruments, including Babcock forceps, grasping forceps, scissors, needle holders, clip appliers, and endoscopic linear cutters are used for gastric procedures. Energy sources, such as electrocautery, laser, or ultrasonic energy, are essential for hemostasis. Instrumentation for minimally invasive surgery is listed by procedure in Box 8-2.

Selected Procedures

PYLOROMYOTOMY (FREDET-RAMSTEDT)

Pyloromyotomy is the least invasive of the procedures designed to relieve pyloric outflow obstruction and is recommended for minor pyloric obstruction not requiring tissue resection.[1] A longitudinal incision is made in the pyloric muscles to, but not through, the mucosa. The mucosa bulges through the incision. Laparoscopic pyloromyotomy is used to treat children with idiopathic hypertrophic pyloric stenosis.[2,3]

Position the animal in dorsal recumbency in head-up (reverse Trendelenburg) position. Establish pneumoperitoneum and insert the primary port as described in Chapter 3. Place a 5-mm port on each side of the umbilicus at the lateral edge of the rectus abdominis muscle (Fig. 8-10). Temporarily anchor the pylorus to the abdominal wall with two sutures passed through the skin and body wall, around the pylorus, and back through the body wall and skin. Make a serosal incision in a relatively avascular area over the pylorus with an ultrasonic scalpel, scissors, laser fiber, or endoscopic scalpel (Fig. 8-11). Use dissecting forceps to spread the muscle without penetrating the mucosa (Fig. 8-12). If unsure whether the mucosa has been penetrated, instill methylene blue into the stomach to identify a leak.[4] If a defect is found, repair it and perform a myotomy at another site, or su-

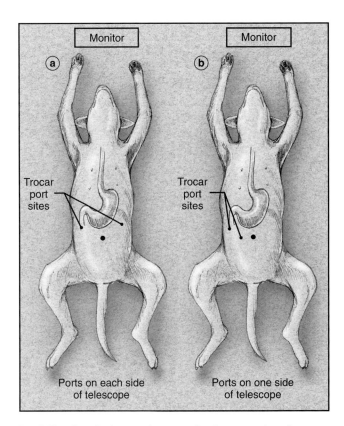

Fig. 8-10 Standard port placement for laparoscopic pyloroplasty and pyloromyotomy procedures. The camera is placed at the umbilicus. Having ports on the left and right sides of the animal requires that the surgeon "straddle" the camera port, which can become uncomfortable in long procedures (*a*). When both ports are on the animal's right side, they are not able to be placed at 30° to 60° angles to each other (*b*).

ture the mucosa and consider using an omental patch.[5] As an alternative, the pyloromyotomy can be converted to a pyloroplasty.[1]

PYLOROPLASTY (HEINEKE-MIKULICZ)

To perform a Heineke-Mikulicz pyloroplasty, establish pneumoperitoneum and place the laparoscopic ports as described for pyloromyotomy (see Fig. 8-10). Place two stay sutures, one on each side of the proposed incision, approximately 2 cm from the site. An assistant uses the stay sutures to stabilize the pylorus during the incision. Make a longitudinal incision through all layers of the pylorus with an ultrasonic scalpel, endoscopic scissors, or laser fiber. Avoid making the incision more than about 2 cm long; otherwise, it is difficult to close. Control bleeding with an energy source. The assistant holds the upper stay suture upward, toward the abdominal wall. Apply traction to the lower stay suture to convert the longitudinal incision into a transverse one. Beginning at the middle of the incision, pass one suture through the serosa, muscular layer, and mucosa, and out through the

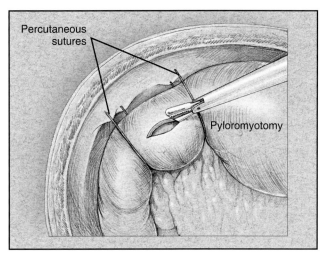

Fig. 8-11 Two sutures secure the pylorus to the abdominal wall. An incision through the pyloric muscle is made with an ultrasonic scalpel.

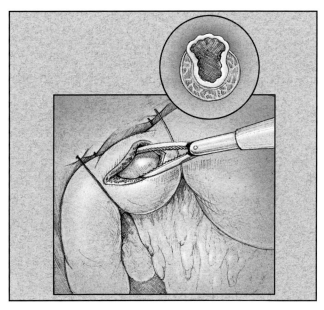

Fig. 8-12 Dissecting forceps are used to spread the muscle and allow the mucosa to bulge out of the incision.

opposite side to appose the middle portion of the incision (Fig. 8-13). Place several simple interrupted sutures with size 2-0 or 3-0 synthetic monofilament suture to close the incision. Closure can also be accomplished with Lapra-Ty* suture clips and size 3-0 polyglactin 910 suture (Fig. 8-14).[6] Apply a Lapra-Ty clip to a strand of suture approximately 3 mm from the suture tail. Pass the needle through tissue and draw the tissue into apposition. Instead of tying a knot, apply a second suture clip adjacent to the tissue. This procedure was performed

---

*Ethicon, Inc., Somerville, NJ. 08876.

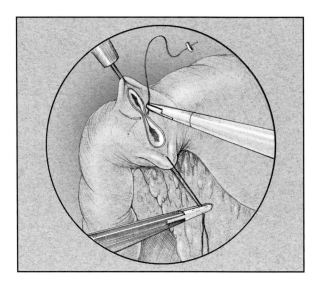

Fig. 8-13 A single suture is placed at the midpoint to appose the tissue edges. The clips are placed with the tissue under tension.

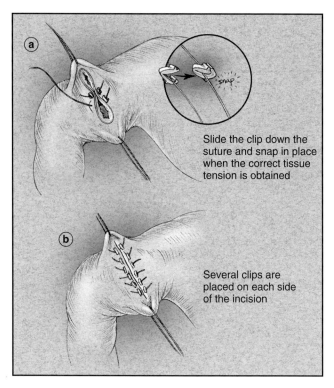

Slide the clip down the suture and snap in place when the correct tissue tension is obtained

Several clips are placed on each side of the incision

Fig. 8-14 Suture clips used to perform a pyloroplasty procedure in beagle dogs.

successfully in four beagle dogs. Mucosal ulcers from electrocautery-induced thermal injury were observed near the incision 2 weeks after surgery.[6]

GASTROTOMY CLOSURE

Gastrotomy is performed to confirm a diagnosis, retrieve a foreign body, or as part of another gastric surgical procedure. Laparoscopic gastrotomy may be indicated if the surgeon wishes to minimize the length of a laparotomy incision. To prevent contamination, thoroughly rinse and aspirate the stomach via an orogastric tube before surgery. Pass an indwelling orogastric tube. Establish pneumoperitoneum and place the laparoscopic ports as described for pyloromyotomy (see Fig. 8-10). Using laparoscopic suturing techniques, place two stay sutures at the ends of the proposed incision to stabilize the stomach and prevent excessive handling of the stomach with grasping forceps. Make an incision on the ventral aspect of the stomach, midway between the greater and lesser curvatures, with a laser fiber, endoscopic scissors, or an ultrasonic scalpel. Incise the serosa and the muscular layers. Grasp and elevate the mucosa and make a small incision through the mucosa. Lengthen the mucosal incision. Control bleeding that usually occurs between the mucosa and the muscularis with an energy source.

After the diagnostic or therapeutic procedures have been completed, close the gastric incision with a stapling device or sutures. Because it may be difficult to obtain ideal needle placement laparoscopically, a two-layer closure is recommended when suturing. Place a simple continuous suture through all layers to appose the wound edges. The ends of the suture may be secured with intra- or extracorporeal knots or suture clips. For the second

row, use a simple continuous Lembert suture that penetrates only the serosa and muscularis (Fig. 8-15). This technique was used successfully in four beagle dogs.[7] Two weeks after surgery, the incisions were healing uneventfully.

Depending on the length of the incision, a 60-mm endoscopic linear stapler can be used to close a gastrotomy incision. The wound edges are everted and held with two Babcock forceps. The stapler is applied proximal to the forceps. The instrument fires four rows of staples and cuts between the middle rows. The Babcock forceps containing the excised tissue are removed. The stapler is efficient and reliable; however, it requires a large port.

GASTROSTOMY

Gastrostomy provides enteral feeding for animals with anorexia and those that cannot swallow because of neurologic dysfunction, cranial trauma, or oropharyngeal cancer. A percutaneous endoscopic gastrostomy (PEG) tube is passed with the aid of a flexible endoscope. The surgeon may elect to perform a laparoscopically assisted PEG tube placement in animals with a perforated esophagus, failed PEG, or oropharyneal or esophageal obstruction; in animals with gastropexy for gastric volvulus; or under conditions in which the anatomy is unsure. A permanent gastrostomy is performed if the animal's temperament will not allow a tube to be kept in place.

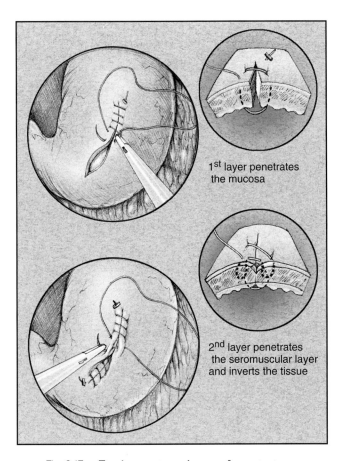

1st layer penetrates the mucosa

2nd layer penetrates the seromuscular layer and inverts the tissue

Fig. 8-15   Two-layer suture closure of a gastrotomy.

Percutaneous Endoscopic Gastrostomy (PEG) Tube[8,9]

Sedate the animal and pass a flexible endoscope into the stomach. Inflate the stomach with air through the endoscope and observe the interior of the stomach on the monitor. The inflated stomach moves closer to the abdominal wall. Prepare the surgical site aseptically.

Transilluminate the abdominal wall with the light from the endoscope. Depress the abdomen with a finger tip and observe it on the video monitor. Pass a snare through the endoscope and position the loop over the indentation in the stomach. Through a small skin incision, pass an intravenous catheter through the abdominal and gastric walls to land inside the loop of the snare inside the stomach. Tighten the loop and remove the catheter stylet. Pass a lubricated wire through the catheter and reposition the snare to grasp the wire. Pull the scope and wire up the esophagus and out of the animal's mouth. Tie the wire to the end of the gastrostomy tube. Pull the other end of the wire to pull the tube down the animal's esophagus and into the stomach. An assistant monitors the progress with the endoscope. Continued traction on the wire finally pulls the tapered end of the tube out of the stomach and through the abdominal wall, following the path of the catheter. Pull the tube out of the stomach and abdominal

wall until the mushroom tip lightly touches the gastric mucosa. Apply a crossbar over the outside of the gastrostomy tube and position it at skin level outside the body. Fix the bar to the skin with sutures.

Laparoscopic Gastrostomy

Anesthetize the animal and place it in head-up dorsal recumbency. Prepare the abdomen aseptically. Place a 5-mm port at the umbilicus for the laparoscope and a second 5-mm port in the left caudal portion of the abdomen (Fig. 8-16, *A*). Grasp the stomach with 5-mm grasping forceps and bring the middle portion of the body to the abdominal wall. Through a skin incision, insert a 5- to 7-cm needle through the skin and into the stomach under laparoscopic guidance. Secure the stomach to the abdominal wall with three or four T-bar anchors* (Fig. 8-16, *B*). Thread a J-wire through the needle and into the stomach. Pass progressively larger dilators over the guide wire until a 17 French peelaway sheath can be inserted into the stomach (Fig. 8-16, *C*). Slide a balloon catheter through the sheath into the stomach and inflate the balloon. Remove the peelaway sheath and secure the catheter in place by pulling the stomach up to the abdominal wall. Begin feeding the next day.

Permanent (Janeway) Gastrostomy

A permanent (Janeway) gastrostomy is created by using a stapling device to form a gastric tube.[10] After insufflation and primary port placement, insert two 5-mm ports lateral to the umbilicus at the lateral edge of the rectus abdominis muscle. Identify the site for the gastrostomy in the left cranial portion of the abdomen. Insert a 12-mm port at the proposed site. Pass the linear cutter and close it around a fold of the ventral surface of the stomach near the greater curvature. Firing the linear cutter creates a closed gastric tube (Fig. 8-17). Two firings may be needed, depending on the desired length of the tube. Place a reinforcing suture at the crotch of the staple line. Pass Babcock forceps through the 12-mm port and grasp the gastric tube. Remove the cannula and Babcock forceps, pulling the gastric tube out to the skin. Release the pneumoperitoneum to allow the stomach to come into apposition with the body wall. Cut off approximately 1 cm at the tip of the gastric tube and suture the gastric mucosa to the skin. Place a gastrostomy tube through the newly created stoma into the stomach during the immediate postoperative period.

PARTIAL GASTRECTOMY

Partial gastrectomy is usually performed to resect ischemic regions of the stomach after gastric dilation and volvulus in large breeds of dogs. Gastrectomy could be used to resect portions of the stomach to treat gastric

---

*Cope Suture Anchor, Cook Urological, Inc., Spencer, Ind. 47460.

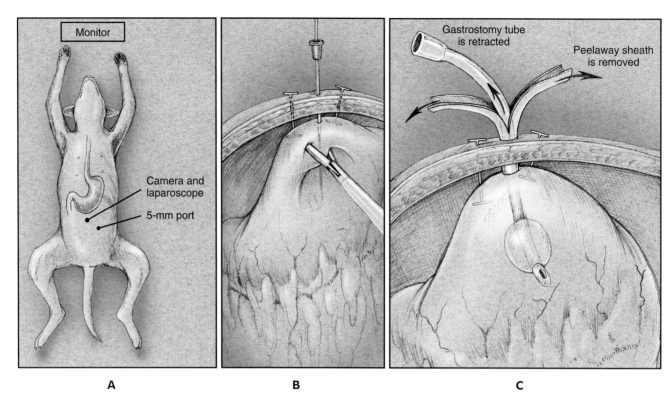

Fig. 8-16   **A,** Port placement for laparoscopic gastrostomy tube placement. **B,** T-bar anchors are placed through the skin and into the stomach under direct vision. The needle is passed transcutaneously into the stomach, and a J-wire is placed through the needle. **C,** The needle is removed, and a peelaway catheter and dilator are passed into the stomach over the guide wire. The dilator is removed and the gastrostomy tube is passed through the peelaway catheter. The balloon is inflated, and the sheath is removed. The stomach is pulled up to the abdominal wall.

ulcers or neoplasia. After a laparoscopic approach, use several firings of a mechanical stapler to resect the diseased tissue. The stapler staples and transects the tissue in a single step and thereby minimizes contamination of the surgical site. Invert the staple line by placing a continuous row of Lembert sutures to reinforce the staple line. The safety and efficacy of performing laparoscopy in animals with acute gastric dilation and volvulus has not been evaluated. Laparoscopy in dogs with gastric dilation and volvulus is not recommended at this time.

GASTROPEXY
Results of several studies have documented the feasibility of performing laparoscopic gastropexy in dogs. The strength of the adhesions in each of the studies was equivalent to the adhesions in the controls of the open circumcostal, incisional, and belt-loop gastropexy controls.[11-13] Laparoscopic and laparoscopically assisted gastropexies will be described.

Position the animal in dorsal recumbency under general anesthesia. Create the pneumoperitoneum and place the primary trocar cannula at the umbilicus by the open technique described in Chapter 3. Tilt the operating table with the animal's head up (reverse Trendelenburg position). It may be necessary to resect segments of the falciform ligament if that was not done during the initial port placement.

Laparoscopic Gastropexy
Use an endoscopic linear cutter to create a stapled incisional gastropexy. Place secondary ports (Fig. 8-18, *A*). To prevent excessive subcutaneous emphysema, insufflation gas pressures should not exceed 10 mm Hg.

Grasp the gastric wall with Babcock forceps at the junction of the fundus and pyloric antrum. Using scissors, create a seromuscular incision in the wall of the stomach at the junction of the fundus and the pyloric antrum. Use blunt dissection to create a 4- to 6-cm tunnel between the muscularis and the mucosa toward the pylorus. Take care to avoid penetrating the mucosa. Make an incision in the peritoneum and transverse abdominal muscle on the right side, 3 cm caudal to the eleventh rib and approximately 10 cm lateral to the ventral midline. Develop a tunnel by bluntly dissecting the intermuscular space. Position the endoscopic linear cutter with one fork in the subseromuscular gastric tunnel

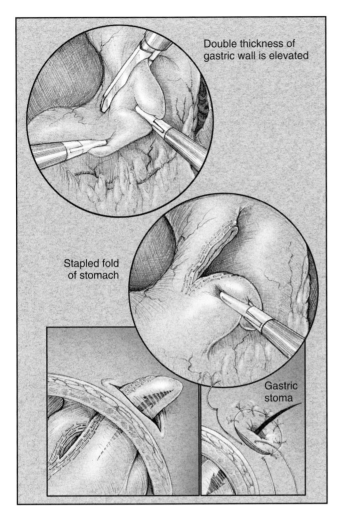

Fig. 8-17 The stapler is positioned across a fold of stomach and fired to create a stapled tube. The gastric diverticulum is brought out through a 12-mm port, opened, and sutured to the skin.

and the other fork in the intermuscular abdominal wall tunnel (see Fig. 8-18, *B*). Close, fire, and release the linear cutter, creating a stapled incisional gastropexy. Because mucosal perforations may be difficult to detect, pass an orogastric tube and inflate the stomach. If a perforation exists, the stomach will not inflate well because the gas passes into the abdominal cavity. Close any perforations of the mucosa with sutures. Close the remaining defect with endoscopic staples or sutures. Some gas will insufflate the intermuscular space, causing transient postoperative subcutaneous and intermuscular emphysema.

Laparoscopically Assisted Gastropexy

For laparoscopically assisted gastropexy, place trocar ports as illustrated in Fig. 8-19. Using scissors and grasping forceps, create a 3 cm wide by 5 cm long seromuscular flap approximately 4 cm proximal to the pylorus. Center the flap over a branch of the gastroepiploic ves-

sels. Remove the right subcostal port and extend the incision 3 cm cranially. Pull the gastric flap into the incision, tunneling it between the internal and external abdominal oblique muscles, and suture it to the external rectus fascia with absorbable interrupted sutures. Close the remaining incisions.

GASTRIC ANTRECTOMY AND ENTEROSTOMY

If a full-thickness defect of the antral portion of the stomach wall or pylorus is present, resection is required. If the disease process involves the duodenum, jejunostomy is required. The feasibility of performing these procedures laparoscopically has been proven; however, advanced laparoscopic skills and mechanical stapling devices are required.[14-16]

Gastric antrectomy and gastrojejunostomy (Billroth II) was performed laparoscopically in six mongrel dogs.[14] Each animal was anesthetized, positioned in dorsal recumbency, and prepared for aseptic surgery. An orogastric tube was passed to decompress the stomach. The abdomen was insufflated, and the primary camera port was placed caudal to the umbilicus. Five additional ports were used (Fig. 8-20). The angular incisure, representing the junction between the antrum and the body of the stomach, was identified by the "crow's feet" distribution of the vagus nerves on the lesser curvature. The gastroepiploic vessels along the greater curvature were ligated from the proposed line of resection to the pylorus. Vessels on the lesser curvature were dissected and ligated from the pylorus to the angular incisure. The common bile duct was identified and avoided. After the proposed site of resection was completely devascularized, the duodenum was transected between the pylorus and the common bile duct with a linear stapler. The antrum of the stomach was resected by using multiple applications of the linear stapler (Fig. 8-21). The resected tissue was placed over the liver for later removal. A loop of jejunum was identified and brought up to the ventral aspect of the stomach. A small incision was made in the jejunum and in the stomach approximately 1 cm proximal to the staple line, midway between the greater and lesser curvature on the ventral aspect of the stomach. A 60-mm linear stapler was introduced, with one fork in the stomach and the other in the jejunum, and fired to perform a side-to-side stapled anastomosis (Fig. 8-22). The common opening of the stomach and intestine was closed with another firing of the 60-mm stapler, taking care not to narrow the lumen of the jejunum. The anastomosis was inspected, irrigated, and aspirated. The specimen was removed through one of the trocar sites. Operative time averaged under 3 hours. One dog had diarrhea and lost weight because the stomach was erroneously anastomosed to the distal end of the ileum, rather than to the proximal end of the jejunum. There was no evidence of

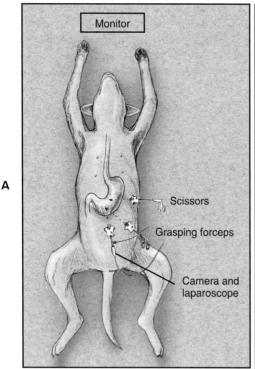

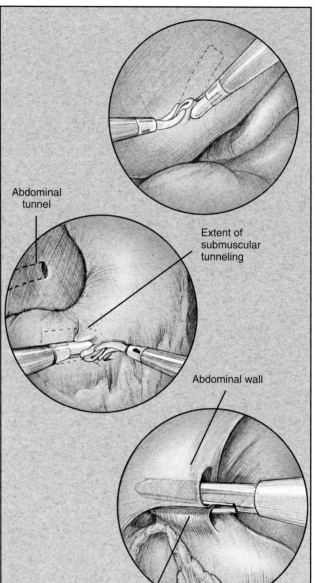

Fig. 8-18   A, Standard operative port placement for the laparoscopic stapled incisional gastropexy. **B,** The endoscopic linear cutter is positioned in the subseromuscular and intermuscular tunnels and fired to create an incisional gastropexy.

leakage, obstruction, or peritonitis and all other dogs maintained their preoperative weights. The average luminal diameter was 2 cm.

Laparoscopic antrectomy and gastroduodenal anastomosis (Billroth I) are performed in the same manner as Billroth II gastrojejunostomy to the point of the anastomosis. A gastroduodenostomy is accomplished with a circular stapling device inserted through a 33-mm port. After the duodenum has been transected near the pylorus, the distal staple line is removed and a purse-string suture is sewn around the duodenum. The anvil of the circular stapler is inserted into the proximal segment of duodenum, and the purse string is tied (Fig. 8-23).

A 2-cm gastrotomy incision is made on the ventral surface of the stomach to allow the shaft of the circular stapler to be inserted. The trocar of the circular stapler is extended adjacent to the staple line at the greater curvature of the stomach. The anvil is placed on the shaft of the stapler, and the stapler is closed and fired to unite the stomach and duodenum (Fig. 8-24). The circular stapler is removed, and the gastrotomy incision is closed with sutures or staples.

NISSEN FUNDOPLICATION

Antireflux surgery is performed when animals with esophageal reflux fail to respond to medical therapy. The

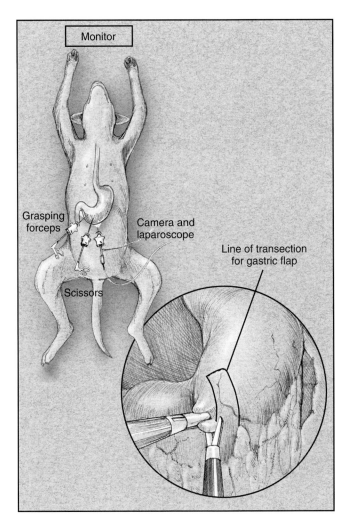

Fig. 8-19   Standard operative port placement for laparoscopically assisted gastropexy. Grasping forceps are introduced from the lateral port. Scissors are brought in from the medial port, directly in line with the line of transection for the gastric flap.

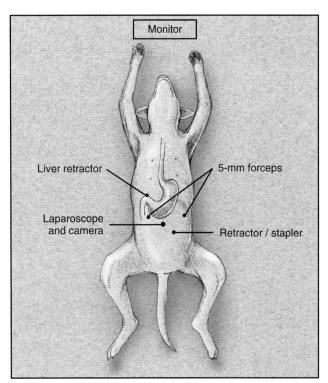

Fig. 8-20   Port placement for laparoscopic gastroenterostomy procedure.

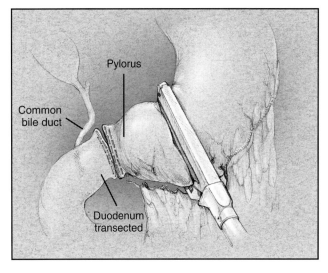

Fig. 8-21   Gastric resection using multiple firings of an endoscopic linear cutter.

Nissen fundoplication is one antireflux surgical technique. The laparoscopic approach is used to reduce the risk of atelectasis and pneumonia in children with impaired pulmonary function and because it may reduce wound adhesions.[17] In adults, the laparoscopic approach is becoming widely adopted for patients who are refractory to medical therapy and in those wishing to discontinue lifelong medical therapy. A successful outcome increases the length of the intraabdominal segment of the esophagus, increases the angle of His, and creates a valve at the gastroesophageal junction. The feasibility of this procedure in animals was demonstrated in a survival study in pigs.[18]

The animal is anesthetized, placed in head-up position, and prepared for aseptic surgery. An orogastric tube is passed to empty the stomach. Pneumoperitoneum is established with carbon dioxide (CO_2), and the laparo-

scope is placed through an umbilical cannula as described in Chapter 3. Four additional 5- or 10-mm ports are placed (Fig. 8-25). A liver retractor is placed through the right caudal port. The stomach is grasped along the greater curvature with Babcock forceps inserted through the left caudal port. If necessary to achieve adequate mo-

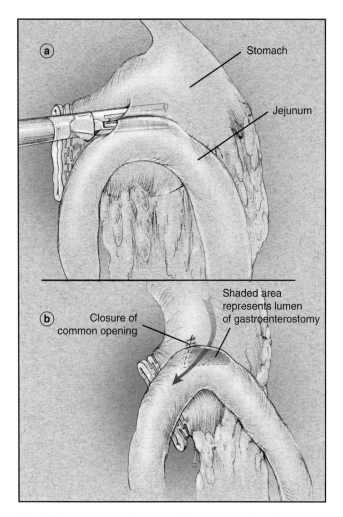

Fig. 8-22   A side-to-side gastrojejunostomy with a linear cutter. The jejunum is positioned adjacent to the ventral aspect of the stomach, midway between the greater and lesser curvatures. The forks of the stapler are introduced through openings in the stomach and intestine and a stapled gastrojejunostomy is created (*a*). The opening remaining from introduction of the stapler (common opening) is closed with sutures or staples (*b*).

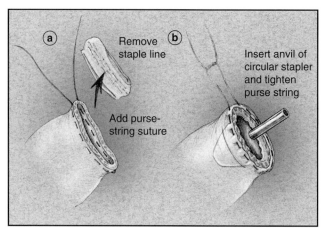

Fig. 8-23   A purse-string suture is sewn around the proximal portion of the duodenum. The anvil of the circular stapler is inserted into the proximal duodenum, and the purse-string suture is tied.

bility, the short gastric vessels are occluded with bipolar forceps, ultrasonic forceps, or clips and divided along the proximal portion of the greater curvature of the stomach. The peritoneum over the esophageal hiatus is grasped and elevated. Dissection of the peritoneum and tissue overlying the lesser curvature of the stomach is continued toward the esophagus, being careful to preserve the vagus nerve (Fig. 8-26, *a*). The phrenoesophageal membrane is incised just below the hiatus. The esophagus is dissected free by creating a window in the retroesophageal space. Pneumothorax may be created with this step. Management of tension pneumothorax is discussed in Chapters 2 and 6.

Once the esophagus is freed, umbilical tape can be passed behind the esophagus and traction exerted to expose the left and right diaphragmatic crura (see Fig. 8-26, *b*). The hiatal hernia, if present, is reduced. The crura are apposed with simple interrupted sutures (see Fig. 8-26, *c*). Extracorporeal knotting techniques provide the best tissue apposition. The cranial wall of the fundus is passed behind the esophagus (Fig. 8-26, *d*). Babcock forceps are inserted behind the esophagus to grasp the fundus and bring it to the right side of the esophagus. The gastric wrap should be tension-free and not too tight. Approximately four seromuscular sutures are used to secure the wrap (Fig. 8-26, *e*). The sutures pass through the fundus, esophagus, and gastric wrap and are tied with extracorporeal knots. Aftercare and complications are similar to an open fundoplication.

TRANSGASTRIC APPROACH TO THE STOMACH

An unusual approach that provides an excellent view of the gastric mucosa and cardia is the transgastric procedure. The technique was developed by investigators searching for a better way to perform antireflux procedures in humans.[19] The animal is anesthetized and placed in dorsal recumbency with the head up. A gastroscope is passed into the stomach and angled toward the body wall to transilluminate the abdominal wall and identify the site for trocar insertion. The stomach is insufflated with air to 15 cm H_2O pressure, and nylon T-bar fixation devices (4-inch nylon clothes tags) are inserted into the stomach (Fig. 8-27). A 14-gauge needle is passed into the lumen of the stomach under endoscopic guidance. The T-bar is inserted into the needle

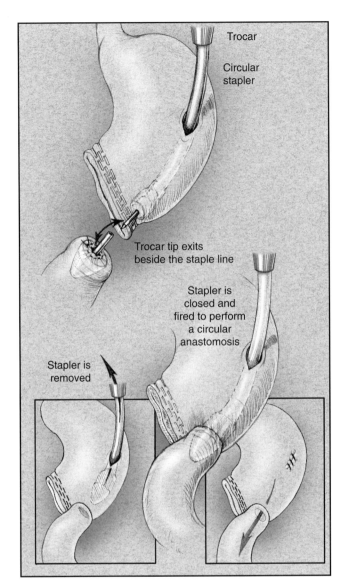

Fig. 8-24 The trocar shaft of the circular stapler is extended adjacent to the staple line from the gastric resection. The trocar is joined to the anvil shaft, and the instrument is closed and fired to perform the anastomosis. The gastrotomy incision is closed with sutures or staples.

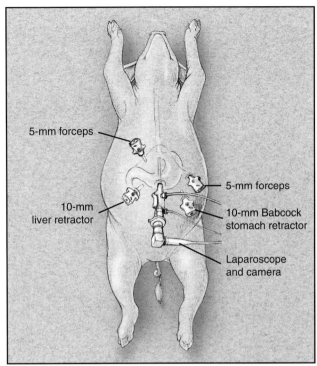

Fig. 8-25 Port placement for laparoscopic Nissen fundoplication.

and pushed out to deploy the crossbar when it exits the needle. The needle is removed and used again to place another T-bar. The external ends of the T-bars are clamped outside the abdominal wall with forceps to secure the stomach to the abdominal wall. One 10-mm port is passed through the abdominal wall into the stomach. The laparoscope is inserted to view the stomach interior (Fig. 8-28). Additional ports are placed as necessary to perform an operative procedure. The transgastric approach has been used experimentally to provide access for creating a nipple valve at the distal end of the esophagus to prevent gastroesophageal reflux.[18a] This ap-

proach provides access to suture bleeding gastric ulcers.[20] After removing the trocar cannulas, the gastrotomy sites are closed laparoscopically. The abdominal wall is closed with sutures.

Closure

After the procedure is completed, the surgical site is inspected, lavaged, aspirated, and observed to ensure hemostasis. The cannulas are removed, and the port sites are closed in two layers.

Complications

Complications of a laparoscopic approach to the stomach are the same as for open gastric procedures. Leakage may occur if there is disruption of the wound or of the staple line. Leakage and stricture can be avoided by ensuring adequate blood supply and a tension-free closure. Staple lines are inspected and evaluated for leakage before closure. If uncontrollable hemorrhage occurs during dissection, the surgeon should convert to a laparotomy. Adhesions are minimized by lavage and aspiration before closure. Placing omentum over staple lines may prevent adhesions to other structures. Occasionally the gastric wrap in the fundoplication procedure is wrapped too tightly, resulting in dysphagia.

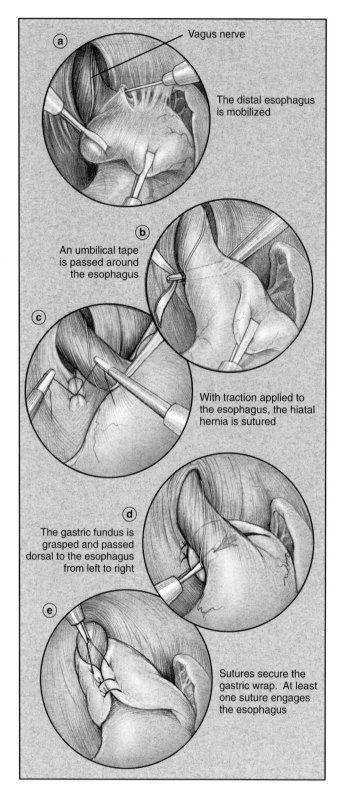

Vagus nerve

The distal esophagus is mobilized

(b) An umbilical tape is passed around the esophagus

(c)

With traction applied to the esophagus, the hiatal hernia is sutured

(d) The gastric fundus is grasped and passed dorsal to the esophagus from left to right

(e)

Sutures secure the gastric wrap. At least one suture engages the esophagus

Fig. 8-26   Laparoscopic Nissen fundoplication. An energy source is used to mobilize the distal portion of the esophagus (a). Umbilical tape is passed dorsal to the esophagus to provide distal traction (b). Simple interrupted sutures are used to close the crural defect (c). Babcock forceps grasp the fundus and bring it dorsal to the esophagus (d). The gastric wrap is secured with sutures (e).

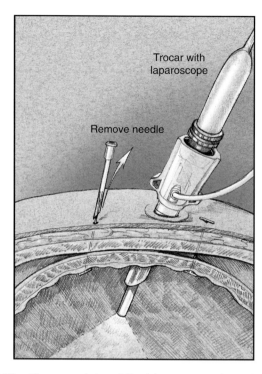

Trocar with laparoscope

Remove needle

Fig. 8-27   The stomach is stabilized by passing nylon T-bars through the abdominal wall and into the stomach. The trocar is inserted directly into the stomach.

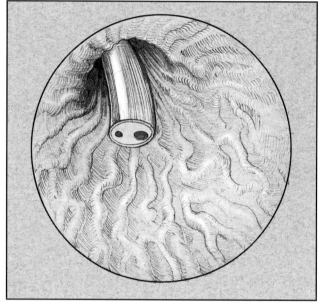

Fig. 8-28   The lumen of the stomach viewed through a laparoscope. The gastrointestinal endoscope is visible in the esophagus.

REFERENCES

1. Matthiesen DT: Stomach. In Slatter DH, editor: Textbook of small animal surgery, ed 2, Philadelphia, 1993, WB Saunders.
2. Najmaldin A, Tan HL: Early experience with laparoscopic pyloromyotomy for infantile hypertrophic pyloric stenosis. *J Pediatr Surg* 30:37-38, 1995.
3. Greason KL et al: Laparoscopic pyloromyotomy for infantile hypertrophic pyloric stenosis: report of 11 cases. *J Pediatr Surg* 30:1571-1574, 1995.
4. Pyloromyotomy. In Lobe TE, Schropp KP, editors: Pediatric laparoscopy and thoracoscopy, Philadelphia, 1994, WB Saunders.
5. Royal RE et al: Repair of mucosal perforation during pyloromyotomy: surgeon's choice. *J Pediatr Surg* 30:1430-1432, 1995.
6. Freeman LJ: Unpublished data. 1991.
7. Freeman LJ: Unpublished data. 1991.
8. Percutaneous endoscopic gastrostomy. In Ponsky JL, editor: Atlas of surgical endoscopy. St. Louis, 1992, Mosby.
9. Abood SK et al: Nutritional support of hospitalized patients. In Slatter DH, editor: Textbook of small animal surgery, ed 2, Philadelphia, 1993, WB Saunders.
10. Sangster W, Hunter JG: Surgical access for enteral nutrition. In Hunter JG, Sackier JM, editors: Minimally invasive surgery. New York, 1993, McGraw-Hill.
11. Thompson SE et al: Laparoscopic stapled incisional gastropexy. Proceedings ACVS Veterinary Symposium, Miami, Fla., 1992 (abstract).
12. Hardie RJ, Flanders JA, Short CE: Laparoscopic stapled gastropexy. Proceedings ACVS Veterinary Symposium 29, Washington, D.C., 1994 (abstract).
13. Wilson ER et al: A comparison of laparoscopic and belt-loop gastropexy in dogs. *Vet Surg* 25:221-227, 1996.
14. Soper NJ et al: Laparoscopic Billroth II gastrectomy in the canine model. *Surg Endosc* 8:1395-1398, 1994.
15. Frantzides CT, Carlson MA, Schulte WJ: Laparoscopic gastric bypass in a porcine model. *J Laparoendosc Surg* 5:97-100, 1995.
16. Nagai Y et al: Laparoscope-assisted Billroth I gastrectomy. *Surg Laparosc Endosc* 5:281-287, 1995.
17. Fundoplication. In Lobe TE, Schropp KP, editors: Pediatric laparoscopy and thoracoscopy, Philadelphia, 1994, WB Saunders.
18. Thompson SE: Unpublished data. 1997.
18a. Mason RJ et al: A new intraluminal antigastroesophageal reflux procedure in baboons. *Gastrointest Endosc* 45:283-290, 1997.
19. Jennings RW et al: A novel endoscopic transgastric fundoplication procedure for gastroesophageal reflux: an initial animal evaluation. *J Laparoendosc Surg* 2:207-213, 1992.
20. Potvin M, Gagner J, Pomp A: Laparoscopic transgastric suturing for bleeding peptic ulcers. *Surg Endosc* 10:400-402, 1996.

Minimally Invasive Small Intestinal Surgery

LYNETTA J. FREEMAN

Minimally invasive surgery of the small intestine must adhere to the principles established for open surgery. Bacterial contamination of the peritoneal cavity must be minimized. Tissue must be handled gently. Blood supply to anastomotic sites must be maintained. Sutures or staples should incorporate the submucosa as the holding layer. The anastomosis should be water tight. To reduce postoperative peritoneal adhesions, tissue eversion should be minimized. A patent lumen, large enough to prevent postoperative obstruction or stricture, must be provided.

Indications

Indications for laparoscopy are the same as for open surgery, except when distended loops of bowel make trocar insertion unsafe. Although the feasibility of performing laparoscopic hand-sewn colonic anastomoses[1] and Nissen fundoplication[2] in rats has been demonstrated, if the body cavity is too small to accommodate a surgical stapler, it is probably also too small for a hand-sewn anastomosis. Significant adhesions, which may be likely after previous abdominal surgery, can be a contraindication to the laparoscopic approach.

Conditions that require less complex laparoscopic skills may be the most amenable to a definitive laparoscopic procedure. Simple adhesiolysis, intestinal biopsy, laparoscopically assisted small bowel anastomosis, and feeding tube jejunostomy are the least complex. As the surgeon's laparoscopic skills improve, more complex procedures can be attempted. Extensive adhesiolysis, enterotomy closure, and stapled intracorporeal anastomosis require more skill. Hand-sewn intracorporeal anastomosis requires the most skill.

Equipment

Handheld instrumentation depends on the procedure being performed. Typical instruments used for laparoscopic intestinal surgery are listed in Box 8-3.

BOX 8-3

LAPAROSCOPIC INSTRUMENTATION FOR SURGERY OF THE SMALL INTESTINE

---

3 to 5 trocars, depending on the procedure
Grasping forceps
Dissecting forceps
Scissors
Energy source
Irrigation/aspiration
2 needle holders
Babcock forceps (optional)
Endoscopic linear cutter (optional)
Endoscopic stapler (optional)

Preoperative Treatment

Preoperative treatment of an animal for the laparoscopic approach is similar to that for open intestinal surgery. The cardiovascular status of the patient is assessed and corrected. An orogastric tube is used to decompress the stomach.

Positioning and Port Placement

The animal is anesthetized and placed in dorsal recumbency. Preoperative preparation and laparoscopic access are accomplished as described in Chapter 3. The primary trocar is inserted at the umbilicus after the falciform ligament has been excised. Secondary port placement depends on the procedure being performed. Two, three, or four additional ports are placed. Usually one port is placed in each of the abdominal quadrants. Two ports are used by the surgeon and two by the assistant (Fig. 8-29). The table is tilted to provide access to the area of interest.

Laparoscopic Anatomy

The intestines are covered by the omentum, a thick, fat-streaked, double layer of peritoneum. The omentum is reflected by grasping it in the right caudal abdominal quadrant and moving it cranially. Two grasping forceps are necessary to perform this procedure efficiently. When the omentum is fully retracted, it rests on the ventral surface of the stomach. The duodenum runs caudally from the pylorus on the right side of the abdomen until it makes a U-shaped turn to pass cranially and to the left under loops of jejunum. The U-shaped turn is anchored by a ligament that connects the duodenum to the colon. It is practically impossible to retract the jejunal loops sufficiently to continue tracing the ascending portion of the duodenum to the duodenojejunal flexure.

Multiple jejunal loops with attached mesentery are located beneath the umbilicus. The jejunum begins at the jejunoduodenal flexure in the left cranial abdominal quadrant and terminates at the ileum in the right cranial abdominal quadrant. The ileum is attached to the cecum by the ileocecal fold.

Exploratory Laparoscopy

Before performing a surgical procedure, the abdominal cavity is surveyed to identify potential problems. Reddened peritoneal surfaces and fluid in the abdomen indicate peritonitis. Cyanosis, hematomas, adhesions, or the presence of intestinal contents warrant further examination. Because magnification allows closer examination of intestinal color, mesenteric arterial pulsation, and peri-

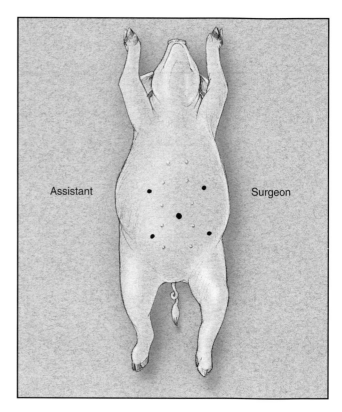

Fig. 8-29 Typical port placement for laparoscopic intestinal surgery. Two ports are used by the surgeon and two by the assistant surgeon.

stalsis, assessment of intestinal viability may be enhanced by laparoscopy. To aid in identifying ischemic intestinal segments, fluorescein dye may be given intravenously and the intestine examined with an argon laser with a quartz fiber.[3] Ischemia is usually apparent. Once the lesion or disease process is identified, a decision is made to insert a feeding tube; perform an enterotomy, an intestinal biopsy, a laparoscopic or laparoscopically assisted resection, or convert to open laparotomy.

Feeding Tube Jejunostomy

A feeding tube provides nutritional support to animals when the stomach must be bypassed. Animals with chronic vomiting and pancreatitis are considered ideal candidates for this procedure. The technique may be performed in a heavily sedated animal with local anesthesia. Several techniques are mentioned in the literature, and all are considered experimental at this time.

Percutaneous Technique[4]

With the animal in dorsal recumbency, the camera port is placed at the umbilicus. The site for tube insertion is identified in the distal portion of the duodenum or proximal portion of the jejunum. To select the site for the jejunostomy tube exit, indent the abdominal wall externally while observing the site with the laparoscope. Insert a 10-mm trocar at the site. Using racheting grasping forceps through the 10-mm working port, grasp the antimesenteric border of the jejunum and withdraw the forceps and the jejunum until the intestine contacts the cannula. Continue withdrawal of the cannula and forceps until the jejunum protrudes through the abdominal puncture. To secure the intestine, place four absorbable sutures from the intestine to the muscles of the abdominal wall. Sew a purse-string suture in the intestine at the proposed tube insertion site and make a small incision in the center of the purse string. Insert a 5 French, 36-inch infant feeding tube* and feed it into the lumen of the intestine (Fig. 8-30). Ideally, the tube should be directed aborally; however, the direction may be difficult to determine. The clinical significance of a misdirected tube has not been determined. Tie the purse-string suture and anchor the tube to the abdominal wall with sutures. Flush the tube with sterile water and observe the tube with the laparoscope to ensure that there is no leakage. The tube should be kept in place for at least 1 week before removal. Refer to other sources for management of jejunostomy feeding tubes.[5]

Laparoscopic Technique

Position the animal in dorsal recumbency and place the camera port at the umbilicus. Identify the proximal portion of the jejunum and locate the abdominal wall exit site. Secure the jejunum to the body wall inside the abdominal cavity with two sutures. Pass a Keith needle and suture percutaneously through the body wall, through the antimesenteric border of the jejunum, and back through the body wall.[6] Tie the sutures externally. Alternatively, use four T-fasteners (nylon clothing tags) by passing the fastener through the body wall and into the lumen of the intestine.[7] Deploy the fastener and apply external traction to secure the intestine to the body wall.[8] Box-shaped hernia staples and intracorporeally placed sutures have also been used to anchor the intestine to the inside surface of the body wall.[9]

After the intestine is anchored to the body wall, insert the jejunostomy tube (see Fig. 8-30). Human jejunostomy kits contain a needle, guide wire, dilators, and tubes with peelaway sheaths. If these devices are used to progressively enlarge the opening, a purse-string suture may not be required. Some advocate placing a purse-string suture at the antimesenteric border of the jejunum and securing the suture around the tube. To overcome potential problems with leakage at the tube insertion

---

* Argyle Infant Feeding Tube, Argyle Quest, St. Louis, Mo. 63103.

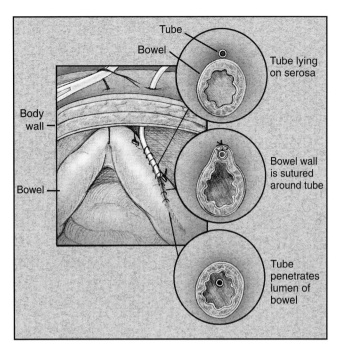

Fig. 8-30   Laparoscopic jejunostomy tube placement and creation of a Witzel tunnel with intracorporeal suturing and suture clips.

site, suture a Witzel tunnel laparoscopically and secure the sutures with Lapra-Ty suture clips.[10] All of these techniques were developed in animals and used in humans. A survival study of laparoscopic jejunostomy tube placement in eight beagle dogs confirmed that an intracorporeal purse-string suture and Witzel tunnel could be placed successfully without reducing the jejunal lumen diameter.[11]

Potential complications of the percutaneous technique include small bowel obstruction if the intestinal lumen is reduced by the fixation method at the body wall. Bleeding, wound infection, passage of the needle through the back wall of the jejunum, tube obstruction, and leakage are potential complications of jejunostomy tubes.

Enterotomy

An enterotomy allows removal of foreign bodies of <1 cm and examination of the mucosal surface of the intestine. With the optical port at the umbilicus, place three additional ports. Isolate the intestinal loop and elevate it with atraumatic forceps. Use grasping forceps to free the isolated segment of ingesta. Using scissors, make a full-thickness incision in the intestine at the antimesenteric border. Avoid using monopolar electrocautery to make the incision because the thermally damaged tissue is weaker and may predispose the incision to dehiscence. Bleeding is usually minimal and can be controlled with pressure. Close the incision with sutures or staples. If necessary, close longitudinal incisions transversely to preserve lumen diameter.

Intestinal Biopsy

Simple intestinal biopsy is performed with three 5-mm ports. Place the primary port near the umbilicus. Use grasping forceps and scissors to obtain a full-thickness biopsy specimen by making a longitudinal incision on the antimesenteric border. Close the incision with simple interrupted sutures (Fig. 8-31). A modified 4-mm skin punch biopsy has been used experimentally to obtain a satisfactory specimen, but it was difficult to remove the specimen and control the depth of penetration.[12] Two to four sutures were required to close the wound.

Laparoscopically Assisted Small Intestinal Anastomosis

Laparoscopically assisted anastomosis allows a complete and thorough exploration to be made using only a minimal incision. Identify the lesion laparoscopically and determine the extent of the intended resection. Use scissors or an energy source to lyse adhesions that prevent mobilization of the mesentery. Introduce Babcock forceps through one of the trocars to grasp the intestine. Retract the intestine and the trocar and as they are removed, enlarge the umbilical incision to allow the intestine to be brought externally (Fig. 8-32). Perform the anastomosis using standard operative techniques and replace the intestine into the abdomen. Close the incision in the linea alba with sutures. If desired, insert the laparoscope and insufflate the abdomen again to inspect, irrigate, lavage, and aspirate the abdominal cavity.

Laparoendoscopy

Endoscopists try to identify occult bleeding by examining the mucosal surface of the stomach, intestine, and colon with a flexible endoscope. Although it may be necessary to examine the entire small intestine, the oral approach does not allow a complete evaluation. Two laparoscopic techniques have been described to facilitate endoscopic examination of the entire small intestine. The so-called laparoscopically assisted panenteroscopy is performed with the endoscope passed through the mouth.[13] Four trocars are placed in a semicircular fashion in the midabdomen, and Babcock forceps are inserted to advance the bowel over the shaft of the endoscope. Pulling the intestine slowly off the endoscope tip while insufflating with air from the endoscope provides an excellent view of the mucosa. In another technique, a segment of small intestine is exteriorized.[14] An enterotomy is per-

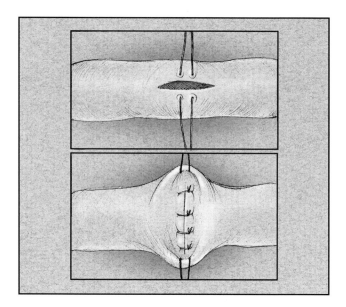

Fig. 8-31 Transverse closure of a longitudinal incision to obtain an intestinal biopsy.

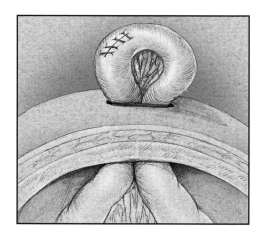

Fig. 8-32 The umbilical trocar site is enlarged to allow bowel to be brought externally. A biopsy or intestinal anastomosis may be performed.

formed, and a disinfected colonoscope is passed proximally and distally from the enterotomy site so that the entire small intestine can be inspected (Fig. 8-33). After examination, the enterotomy site is closed and the intestine is replaced in the abdomen.

Small Intestinal Anastomosis

Steps for performing laparoscopic small intestinal anastomoses are access, mobilization, devascularization, resection, anastomosis, inspection, and closure. Because laparoscopic suturing is difficult and time-consuming, many surgeons prefer to use automatic stapling devices

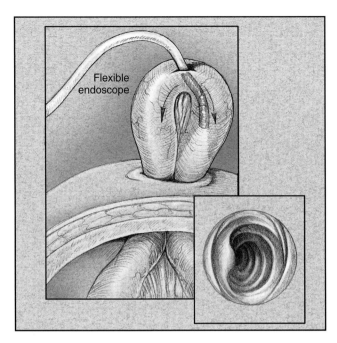

Fig. 8-33   An enterotomy allows access to all portions of the intestinal tract with an endoscope.

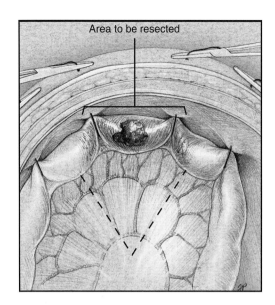

Fig. 8-34   The intestinal segment to be resected may be attached to the body wall with four to six sutures.

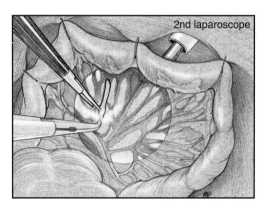

Fig. 8-35   Transillumination of intestinal mesentery is performed with another laparoscope and light source serving as a back light to help identify mesenteric blood vessels.

to perform the resection and anastomosis.[15] Suturing and stapling techniques are described on pp. 138 to 142.

ACCESS
Use the techniques described in Chapter 3 to place the primary port at the umbilicus. Place additional ports in each of the abdominal quadrants.

MOBILIZATION
After survey laparoscopy has been performed and the lesion identified, isolate and mobilize the small intestine to facilitate the resection. If the intestine is mobile and of sufficient thickness to hold sutures, hold it against the abdominal wall by passing a straight Keith needle swaged to 2-0 monofilament suture through the ventral abdominal wall, the antimesenteric portion of the jejunum, and then back out of the abdominal cavity.[16] Place four to six sutures to suspend the segment to be resected (Fig. 8-34). Draw the sutures up and clamp them externally with Kelly forceps to secure the segment. Alternatively, have the assistant surgeon use two grasping forceps or Babcock forceps to suspend the intestine. Resect a sufficient portion of intestine to ensure adequate margins in the case of neoplasia, or good blood supply in potentially devitalized tissue.

DEVASCULARIZATION AND RESECTION
To begin the resection, incise the visceral peritoneum over the mesentery in an avascular area. Use another laparoscope and light source to transilluminate the mesen-

tery and assist in identifying the vascular structures if the mesentery contains large amounts of adipose tissue (Fig. 8-35). Use dissecting forceps to dissect the adipose tissue around the vessels and ligating clips, sutures, staples, or an energy source to obtain hemostasis. Identify, ligate, and transect the major vascular pedicle and the arcuate vessels. Placing atraumatic occluding clamps or bands proximal and distal to the proposed resection site requires additional ports but helps prevent contamination. If the intestine is suspended, occlusion to prevent contamination is usually not necessary.

Use an endoscopic linear cutter that fires six rows of staples and cuts between the middle rows as the simplest way to resect tissue. The staples minimize spillage of intestinal contents or mucosal cells and help control bleeding from the wound edges in preparation for anastomosis. If an endoscopic stapler is not available, use scissors to transect the intestine. Control bleeding from the cut edge by applying pressure or using minimal amounts of bipolar electrocautery. Remove the resected tissue from the abdominal cavity through one of the ports.

ANASTOMOSIS

Because of the operative skill required, good teamwork is essential in performing laparoscopic intestinal anastomosis. These procedures should not be used to train a new camera operator or surgical assistant. Suturing techniques should be worked out and patience developed in an inanimate training box before attempting extensive laparoscopic suturing. Alternating between two surgeons experienced in laparoscopic suturing is helpful in providing relief from the stresses associated with intracorporeal suturing during the surgical procedure.

Hand-Sewn Anastomosis

Anastomoses are termed *inverting* if the tissue margins are turned inward, *everting* if the tissue margins are turned outward, and *approximating* if the tissue edges appose each other. Approximating anastomosis results in larger luminal diameter and more rapid mucosal regeneration. Approximating anastomoses are easier to apply, incite minimal adhesions, and provide good protection against leakage.[17] Needles, suture materials, and suture patterns are matters of the surgeon's preference. Short suture strands (~10 cm) and intracorporeal ties are used.

Suture and Needle Selection

Sutures are selected based on their tissue absorption profile, ease of passage through tissue, and ease of tying. Except for chromic gut and perhaps Monocryl (poliglecaprone 25), the commonly used absorbable sutures maintain their tensile strength through the period of intestinal wound healing. Selection becomes a choice between ease of suture passage and ease of tying. Generally, if a suture is easy to pass, it is hard to tie. Vicryl (polyglactin 910) or surgical silk is preferred by most surgeons. Intracorporeal sutures are more difficult to tie with polypropylene and polydiaxanone sutures because the suture ends are springy and the material has memory.

Straight, half-curved ("ski"), and curved needles have been used for laparoscopic suturing. Straight needles are easier to position in the needle holder and are relatively easy to pass through tissue; however, imprecise movement in positioning tissue on a straight needle can result in tearing through tissue. Ski needles offer an advantage in tying because the straight portion of the needle can be used to facilitate an intracorporeal tie, but the needle path created when the straight portion is pulled through tissue is larger than with a curved needle (Fig. 8-36). Curved needles are initially more difficult to load and orient correctly in the needle holder. Once the skill of

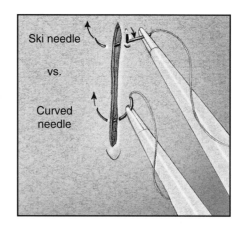

Fig. 8-36 Path of ski needle and curved needle through tissue.

loading the needle and supinating the hand and instrument during needle passage is mastered, curved needles are preferred. Curved needle passage is similar to open surgery, and the needle tip exit site is more predictable. We prefer the SH half-curved, taper-point needles, with suture sizes 2/0 and 3/0, and RB for sizes 4/0 and smaller.

Tissue Apposition

In open surgery, bowel edges are held in apposition by an assistant holding Doyen intestinal forceps parallel to each other. Suturing is begun at the mesenteric border and continued circumferentially. In laparoscopic surgery, occluding clamps must stay in one plane because the trocar cannulas are fixed at the abdominal wall. One group of surgeons showed that operating time was reduced when special parallel closing clamps* were used to hold the bowel in apposition during suturing.[18] Surgeons usually rely on stay sutures to hold tissue approximated during suturing. The stay sutures are tensed to align the tissue edges. If the assistant applies too much force, the stay sutures will tear out of the tissue.

Insert the first stay suture on the antimesenteric border because it is easiest. Take the suture bite from external to internal on one side and internal to external on the other side. Bring the tissue together and tie the suture. Leave the ends long and remove the needle. If a continuous suture is planned, leave the needle attached to the suture and lodge it in the abdominal wall to be used later in the procedure. For the second suture, on the mesenteric border, drive the needle in a "reverse" direction (Fig. 8-37). Tie the suture; leave the ends long to use for traction.

Suture Pattern

Simple interrupted and simple continuous patterns are used in intestinal surgery. Each of these patterns may be secured with intracorporeal knots or suture clips. The

---

*Endo-Gauge, United States Surgical Corp, Norwalk, Conn.

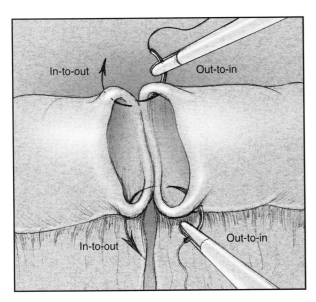

Fig. 8-37 Placing stay sutures for end-to-end hand-sewn intestinal anastomosis.

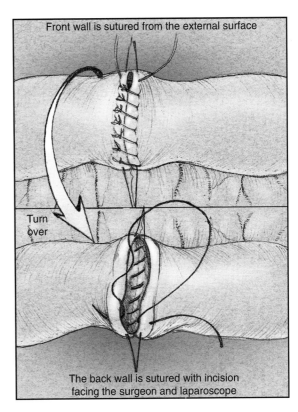

Fig. 8-38 The rotation technique for suturing intestinal anastomoses.

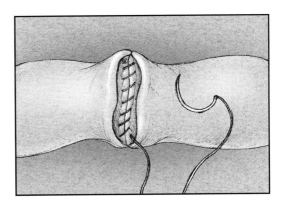

Fig. 8-39 If the back wall of the intestine is sutured from the inside, no rotation is required.

safety and efficacy of each of these techniques have been demonstrated by animal studies.[19] Simple interrupted sutures require approximately 20 minutes longer than a continuous suture secured with knots and 30 minutes longer than simple interrupted sutures secured with suture clips.[20] Simple interrupted sutures appeared to result in better alignment of the mucosa than did continuous sutures, resulting in fewer adhesions. One potential disadvantage of suture clips is that they can migrate through the bowel into the lumen if too much tension is applied. If the migration tract remains patent, leakage may occur.

With simple interrupted sutures, suture the front wall of the anastomosis from the external surface (Fig. 8-38). Rotate the intestine so the back wall faces the laparoscope and the surgeon. Suture the back wall from the external surface also. Use a similar technique for slightly faster continuous suturing. Start continuous sutures on the internal surface of the back wall and continue suturing to the external surface of the front wall without rotating the intestine (Fig. 8-39).[21]

Stapling Techniques

When properly applied, stapled anastomoses are tension-free and leak-free and heal by second intention. Automatic stapling devices have been used extensively in human surgery for approximately 20 years and were tested in animals before that. Three types of staplers are used. The linear cutter devices (GIA,* Proximate TLC†,

EndoGIA, Endopath ETS) apply four to six rows of staples and cut between the middle rows. The linear stapler devices (TA,* Proximate TX†) apply two or three rows of staples, and the tissue is cut by the surgeon. Disposable skin staplers or hernia staplers can be used to apply individual box-shaped staples.

---

*GIA, EndoGIA, TA United States Surgical Corp, Norwalk, Conn.
†Proximate TLC, Endopath ETS, Ethicon Endo-Surgery, Inc, Cincinnati, Ohio.

*TA, United States Surgical Corp, Norwalk, Conn.
†Proximate TX, Ethicon Endo-Surgery, Inc, Cincinnati, Ohio.

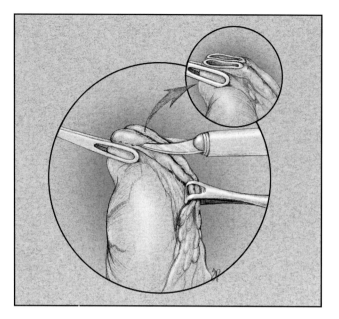

Fig. 8-40 After the linear cutter is applied, the antimesenteric corners of the two staple lines are resected. One fork of the stapler is inserted into each segment.

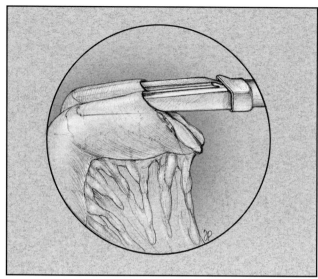

Fig. 8-4l A stapled side-to-side anastomosis is created when the stapler joins the bowel with six rows of staples and cuts between the middle rows.

Linear Cutters

Endoscopic linear cutters are used to perform a functional end-to-end anastomosis. The functional end-to-end anastomosis is, in reality, a side-to-side anastomosis because the antimesenteric borders of the intestine are positioned side by side during stapling. The function is equivalent to an end-to-end anastomosis. The feasibility of these techniques has been proved in pigs, dogs, and humans.[22-24]

Apply two firings of an endoscopic stapler to excise a segment of intestine and close the cut ends. Excise the antimesenteric corners of the two staple lines with scissors (Fig. 8-40). Insert the endoscopic stapler and one of the forks into the proximal portion of bowel through the enterotomy created by excising the corner of the staple line. Insert the other fork into the distal portion of bowel. Align the mesenteric attachments to ensure that the bowel is not twisted. Close and fire the stapler to perform a side-to-side anastomosis (Fig. 8-41). Open the stapler and remove it so that the staple line can be examined to ensure hemostasis. The 30- or 35-mm staplers do not create an adequate anastomotic lumen.[25] Reload the stapler with another cartridge and place it into the common enterotomy. Advance the intestine over the stapler while the forks are inserted into the limbs of the bowel (Fig. 8-42). Close and fire the stapler, crossing the previous staple line. Open and remove the stapler, and examine the staple line for bleeding.

Close the common opening on the antimesenteric border. Use grasping forceps to distract the staple lines,

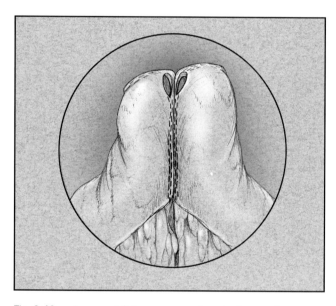

Fig. 8-42 A second firing ensures adequate lumen diameter when a 30-mm stapler is used.

thereby creating the greatest anastomotic lumen diameter. Position Babcock forceps to hold the everted tissue edges in apposition. Position the linear cutter below the Babcock forceps and close it. Fire the stapler to close the common opening and excise the everted tissue from the margins of the enterotomy (Fig. 8-43). Remove the excised tissue from the abdominal cavity. Evaluate the staple lines to ensure that they are intact. Use sutures if necessary to reinforce defects at the junction of the crossing

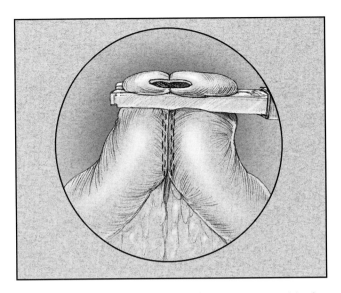

Fig. 8-43 Closure of the common opening is obtained by firing an endoscopic linear cutter.

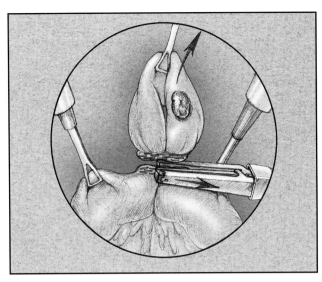

Fig. 8-45 To ensure correct mesenteric alignment, the endoscopic linear cutter can be used to appose the tissue and resect the specimen.

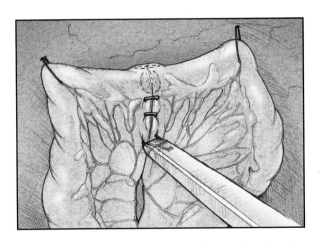

Fig. 8-44 The mesentery is closed with box-shaped staples.

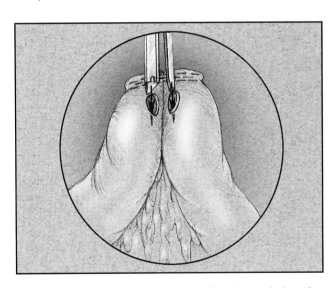

Fig. 8-46 An enterotomy is created below the staple lines for introduction of the forks of the linear cutter.

staple lines. Suture or staple the mesentery with box-shaped staples (Fig. 8-44).

An alternative technique for anastomosis ensures mesenteric alignment but may reduce the diameter of the lumen.[23] The mobilized segment is not transected first. Instead, the center of the bowel segment to be removed is grasped and elevated. The stapler is placed across the surviving limbs of bowel and the four walls are stapled together, maintaining the correct mesenteric alignment (Fig. 8-45). The excised bowel is removed from the abdomen. An enterotomy incision is made in the antimesenteric border of each limb. The stapler

is introduced and fired twice, as described previously (Fig. 8-46). The stapler is then placed across the bowel below the enterotomies and fired to amputate the tissue containing the enterotomies and complete the anastomosis (Fig. 8-47).

Linear Staplers

Use linear staplers, which apply staples but do not cut the tissue, to create end-to-end everting anastomoses. Transect the intestine with scissors. Hold the ends of the intestine in apposition with three stay sutures placed at 12 o'clock, 4 o'clock, and 8 o'clock. Separate the stay sutures to triangulate the bowel. Staple each side of the

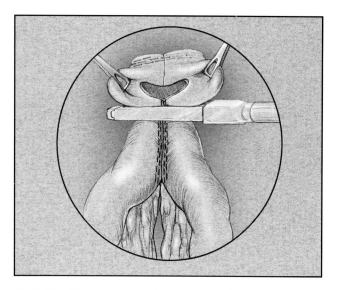

Fig. 8-47   The enterotomy sites are resected, and the common opening is closed.

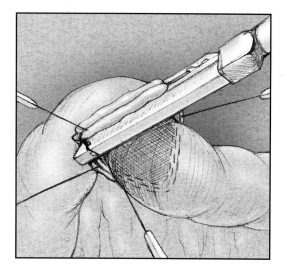

Fig. 8-48   Triangulated end-to-end intestinal anastomosis with a linear stapler.

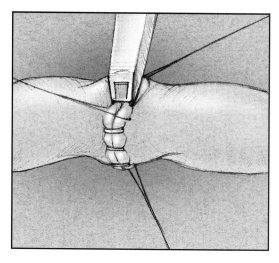

Fig. 8-49   Everted technique for end-to-end intestinal anastomosis with a hernia stapler.

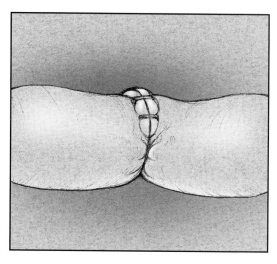

Fig. 8-50   Two-thirds inverted, one-third everted technique for end-to-end intestinal anastomosis with a hernia stapler.

triangle with the linear stapler and remove the stay sutures (Fig. 8-48). Everted stapled anastomoses provide larger lumen diameters than other end-to-end anastomosis techniques.[26]

Box-shaped Staples

Box-shaped staples are applied with laparoscopic hernia staplers. Individually applied metal staples resulted in primary intestinal wound healing in experimental studies in dogs and pigs.[27-30] Two laparoscopic methods of application were compared.[26] A wholly everted technique was performed by placing three stay sutures to triangulate the bowel ends. Staples were applied to the everted tissue edges approximately 2 mm apart (Fig. 8-49). The stay sutures were tied. In the other technique, staples were applied to inverted tissue for two thirds of the circumference of the bowel and everted tissue for the remaining one third (Fig. 8-50). Two weeks after surgery, some of the staples with both techniques had migrated into the lumen of the intestine. The wounds appeared to have healed by second intention but had acceptable clinical results in that there was no evidence of leakage or bowel obstruction. The burst pressures were comparable to sutured anastomoses.

INSPECTION AND CLOSURE

With sutured anastomoses, taking time to evaluate the anastomotic site for leakage may prevent postoperative complications. Occlude the bowel proximal and distal to

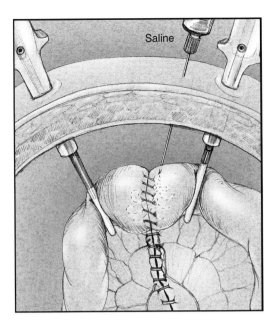

Fig. 8-51   Method to evaluate suture line leakage.

the anastomosis with endoscopic bowel clamps. Bring the intestinal segment near the abdominal wall and pass a spinal needle attached to a fluid-filled syringe through the wall and into the intestine. Inject fluid to distend the bowel (Fig. 8-51). Reinforce areas of leakage with additional laparoscopically placed sutures. Wash the anastomosis with saline and wrap it in omentum. Lavage and aspirate the abdomen and close the trocar sites.

Stapled anastomoses are usually not evaluated for leakage because the reliability of the mechanical devices is so high. The staple line is inspected, lavaged, and aspirated. If no defects are found, the abdomen is lavaged, aspirated, and closed.

Complications

Complications of laparoscopic surgery of the small intestine are the same as for open procedures and are managed similarly. The possibilities include obstruction, stricture, leakage, peritonitis, adhesion formation, and ileus.

REFERENCES

1. Berguer R, Gutt CN: Laparoscopic colon surgery in a rat model: a preliminary report. *Surg Endosc* 8:1195-1197, 1994.
2. Berguer R, Gutt C, Stiegmann GV: Laparoscopic surgery in the rat: description of a new technique. *Surg Endosc* 7:345-347, 1993.
3. Kam DM, Scheeres DE: Fluorescein-assisted laparoscopy in the identification of arterial mesenteric ischemia. *Surg Endosc* 7:75-78, 1993.
4. Twedt DC: Percutaneous laparoscopic jejunostomy tube placement (PLJ). Notes from Fourth International Course in Small Animal Rigid Endoscopy, Colorado State University, March 21-22, 1997.
5. Abood SK et al: Nutritional support of hospitalized patients. In Slatter DH, editor: Textbook of small animal surgery, ed 2, Philadelphia, 1993, WB Saunders.
6. Hotokezaka M et al: Laparoscopic percutaneous jejunostomy for long-term enteral access. *Surg Endosc* 10:1008-1011, 1996.
7. Duh QY et al: Prospective evaluation of the safety and efficacy of laparoscopic jejunostomy. *West J Med* 162:117-122, 1995.
8. Duh QY, Way LW: Laparoscopic jejunostomy using T-fasteners as retractors and anchors. *Arch Surg* 128:105-108, 1993.
9. Saiz AA et al: Laparoscopic feeding jejunostomy: a new technique. *J Laparoendosc Surg* 5:241-244, 1995.
10. Ellis LM et al: Laparoscopic feeding jejunostomy tube in oncology patients. *Surg Oncol* 1:245-249, 1992.
11. Clem MF et al: Laparoscopic feeding jejunostomy tube placement. SAGES abstract.
12. Freeman LJ: Unpublished data. 1996.
13. Bleau BL et al: Laparoscopically assisted panenteroscopy: a feasibility study in pigs. *Gastrointest Endosc* 41:154-156, 1995.
14. Phillips E, Hakim MH, Saxe A: Laparoendoscopy (laparoscopy assisted enteroscopy) and partial resection of small bowel. *Surg Endosc* 8:686-688, 1994.
15. Noel P et al: Resection anastomose de l'intestin grele par coelioscopie che le porc: etude experimentale comparative entre anastomose mecanique et manuelle. *Ann Chir* 48:921-929, 1994.
16. Staley CA et al: Laparoscopic intracorporeal harvest of jejunal tissue for autologous transplantation. *Surg Laparosc Endosc* 4:192-195, 1994.
17. Orsher RJ, Rosin E: Small intestine. In Slatter DH, editor: Textbook of small animal surgery, ed 2, Philadelphia, 1993, WB Saunders.
18. Schuder G et al: Technik und qualitat laparosckopisch handgenahter darmananstomosen im experiment. *Zentralbl Chir* 120:409-414, 1995.
19. Freeman LJ: Unpublished data. 1991-1993.
20. Waninger J et al: Comparison of laparoscopic handsewn suture techniques for experimental small-bowel anastomoses. *Surg Laparosc Endosc* 6:282-289, 1996.
21. Schuder G et al: Technik und qualitat laparosckopisch handgenahter darmananstomosen im experiment. *Zentralbl Chir* 120:409-414, 1995.
22. Soper NJ et al: Laparoscopic small bowel resection and anastomosis. *Surg Laparosc Endosc* 3:6-12, 1993.
23. Pietrafitta JJ et al: An experimental technique of laparoscopic bowel resection and reanastomosis. *Surg Laparosc Endosc* 2:205-211, 1992.
24. Thompson SE: Laparoscopic intestinal anastomosis. ACVS, 1992 (abstract).
25. Freeman LJ: Unpublished data. 1996.
26. Lange V et al: Different techniques of laparoscopic end-to-end small-bowel anastomoses. *Surg Endosc* 9:82-87, 1995.
27. Chung RS: Gastrointestinal anastomoses constructed with singly placed staples. *Am J Surg* 139:876-879, 1980.
28. Howell GP et al: Assessment of the use of disposable staplers in bowel anastomoses to reduce laparotomy time in penetrating ballistic injury to the abdomen. *Ann R Coll Surg Engl* 73:87-90, 1991.
29. Okudaira Y et al: Experimental study of singly placed staples for an everted intestinal anastomosis. *Am J Surg* 147:234-236, 1984.
30. Wetherall AP et al: Use of disposable skin staplers for bowel anastomosis to reduce laparotomy time in war. *Ann R Coll Surg Engl* 74:200-204, 1992.

Laparoscopic Colorectal Surgery

LYNETTA J. FREEMAN

Because of the high incidence of colon cancer in humans, extensive experiments have been conducted in animals to develop and refine techniques for laparoscopic colon surgery. Minimally invasive procedures in humans appear to result in shorter postoperative hospitalization, less pain, less ileus, and faster return to work or normal activity.[1] In rats, cell-mediated immune function was better after laparoscopic colon surgery than after open laparotomy.[2]

The feasibility of performing leak-free intracorporeal and laparoscopically assisted (extracorporeal) end-to-end anastomoses with circular staplers was demonstrated in dogs and pigs.[3,4] The surgical procedures required more time than an open procedure, but they resulted in equivalent burst pressures and histologic parameters.[5,6] Adhesions were minimal, gastrointestinal motility returned faster, and complete resection of mesenteric lymph nodes was possible.[7-9] Metastasis to trocar sites is being reported, but it is uncertain whether port site recurrence rates are higher than those observed with open surgery.[10-12]

Anatomy

In dogs, the blood supply to the descending colon is provided by the caudal mesenteric artery, which gives off the cranial rectal artery to supply the rectum (Fig. 8-52). The caudal mesenteric artery follows the border of the descending colon to join the middle colic artery at the middle portion of the descending colon. The left colic artery gives off numerous vasa recta to supply the colon. The vessels to the descending colon are contained in thin mesentery and are easily seen. Lymph nodes are located in the mesentery to the descending colon. The cranial mesenteric artery branches into the ileocolic artery, which forms the middle colic and right colic arteries and supplies the ascending and transverse colon. The mesentery to the ascending colon and the transverse colon is thick and consists of lymph nodes, fat, and blood vessels covered by peritoneum.

Indications

The ideal procedures for a laparoscopic approach in small animals are biopsy, colopexy or rectopexy, and defined lesions of the descending colon requiring minimal resection and anastomosis.

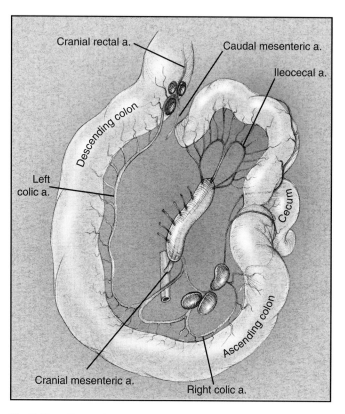

Fig. 8-52 Canine large intestine, illustrating blood supply, lymph nodes, cranial rectal artery, left colic artery, right colic artery, ileocecal artery, caudal mesenteric artery, and cranial mesenteric artery.

Contraindications

Animals with obstipation or obstruction are not candidates for a laparoscopic approach. Laparoscopic colon surgery requires advanced skills to mobilize, devascularize, and anastomose or suture the colon.[13] Procedures that require these skills should be performed only by experienced laparoscopists.

Bowel Preparation

Because spillage may be difficult to control, a laparoscopic approach should not be performed unless bowel preparation is thorough and the colon is clean and devoid of fluid and feces (Table 8-1). Administer antimicrobial prophylaxis according to established guidelines. To ensure adequacy of bowel preparation, perform

TABLE 8-1

Protocol for Preoperative Colorectal Cleansing

DRUG	HOURS BEFORE PROCEDURE	DOSE	ROUTE
Metoclopramide	18.25	0.3 mg/kg	Intramuscular (IM)
Magnesium citrate	18	20-35 mL/kg	Oral[†]
Metoclopramide	12.25	0.3 mg/kg	IM
Colon electrolyte lavage*	12	20-25 mL/kg	Oral[†]
Metoclopramide	4.25	0.3 mg/kg	IM
Colon electrolyte lavage*	4	20-25 mL/kg	Oral[†]
Optional:			
Metoclopramide	2.25	0.3 mg/kg	IM
Colon electrolyte lavage*	2	20-25 mL/kg	Oral[†]
Glycerin suppository	1		

*GoLytely-Peg 3350, Braintree Laboratories, Inc, Braintree, Mass 02184.
[†]Usually administered via an orogastric tube.

BOX 8-4

INSTRUMENTATION NEEDS FOR COLORECTAL SURGERY

Colotomy / Biopsy / Colopexy
3 trocars
Grasping forceps
Scissors
2 needle holders
Electrocautery

Rectopexy
3 trocars
Hernia stapler
Polypropylene mesh
Grasping forceps
Scissors

Typhlectomy
5 trocars
Grasping forceps

Typhlectomy, cont'd
Scissors
Clip applier
Endoscopic linear cutter
Electrocautery

Colonic Anastomosis
5 trocars
1 large trocar
2 Babcock forceps
Grasping forceps
Dissecting forceps
Scissors
Endoscopic linear stapler
Clip applier
Circular stapler
Loop ligature

---

colonoscopy after induction of anesthesia and mechanically remove any remaining fecal material by irrigating with a solution of 10% povidone-iodine in saline. Insert a urinary catheter to evacuate the bladder.

Equipment

Laparoscopic colorectal surgery requires a laparoscopic camera system, insufflator, irrigation-aspiration device, and a complete set of laparoscopic instruments, including staplers and clip appliers (Box 8-4).

Patient Positioning and Trocar Placement

Anesthetize the animal and position it in dorsal recumbency with the head down (Trendelenburg position). Position the video monitor, camera, and insufflator at the foot of the operating table. Make a 1-cm skin incision just caudal to the umbilicus to avoid the falciform ligament. Insert the primary trocar by one of the techniques described in Chapter 3. Insufflate the abdomen to 12 mm Hg and inspect the peritoneal cavity. Place four additional trocars, with one in each of the four abdominal quadrants, just lateral to the mammary glands at the lateral edge of the rectus abdominis muscle (Fig. 8-53).

Colotomy / Biopsy

Grasp and elevate the descending colon with Babcock forceps. Use endoscopic scissors to create a colotomy on the antimesenteric surface of the bowel. To obtain a

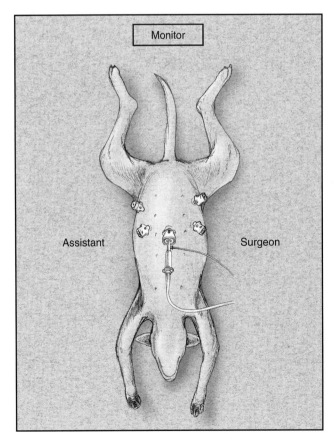

Fig. 8-53 Trocar sites for laparoscopic colon resection. The primary port is placed caudal to the umbilicus. One port is placed in each of the abdominal quadrants.

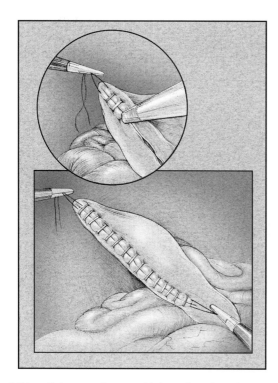

Fig. 8-54 Colotomy closure with box-shaped staples. A Lembert suture is inserted to begin inversion and provide traction on the wound edges.

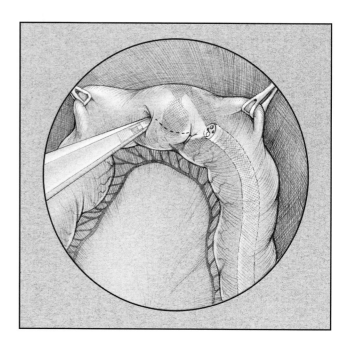

Fig. 8-55 Laparoscopy and colonoscopy are used to identify the site of a colonic polyp. The light from the endoscope is viewed through the wall of the colon. The site is marked with clips.

biopsy specimen, remove a portion of the antimesenteric surface of colon. Control bleeding with pressure or bipolar electrocautery. To initiate mucosal inversion, place a Lembert suture of size 4/0 polydiaxanone (PDS) at the distal end of the colotomy. Close the incision with one or two inverting suture layers or with box-shaped staples (Fig. 8-54).[14] If staples are used, the Lembert suture is placed under tension and the staples are applied approximately 5 mm apart. To facilitate inversion, place a second Lembert suture at the proximal end of the defect. When the defect has been closed, the sutures may be removed or left in place.

Laparoscopically Assisted Colonic Polypectomy

Remove colonic polyps by using a laparoscopic approach to access the colon and an endoscopic approach to assist in identifying the lesion.[15] After the abdomen is insufflated and the trocar and laparoscope are inserted, insert the colonoscope through the anus. Reduce the intensity of the laparoscope light source and observe the light of the colonoscope as it passes into the colon to the site of the lesion (Fig. 8-55). Use a laparoscopic instrument to indent the colon and place a clip to mark the location of the polyp. The endoscopist must avoid excessive insufflation of the colon because distended colon interferes

with laparoscopic vision. Elevate the marked colon with Babcock forceps and incise the colon with scissors near the site. Open the incision and insert Babcock forceps through the colotomy to grasp the polyp under endoscopic guidance. Remove the polyp from the colon laparoscopically. Use sutures, staples, or scissors and electrocautery to ligate the base of the polyp (Fig. 8-56). Close the colotomy incision with sutures or staples.

Colocolonic Anastomosis

Laparoscopically assisted (extracorporeal) and intracorporeal colocolonic stapled anastomoses can be performed. For an extracorporeal stapled anastomosis using the double-staple technique, identify, dissect, and ligate the blood supply to the proposed site of resection with clips or sutures (Fig. 8-57). Use electrocautery or the ultrasonic scalpel to control small blood vessels. Insert an endoscopic linear cutter through one of the caudal ports. Staple and transect the colon distal to the lesion, allowing an adequate margin if neoplasia is suspected (Fig. 8-58). Enlarge one of the caudal port sites and bring the proximal portion of the bowel outside the body. Resect the lesion and secure the anvil portion of the circular stapler with a purse-string suture or loop ligature in the proximal portion of colon (Fig. 8-59). Return the proximal segment

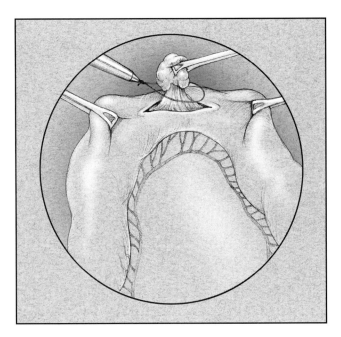

Fig. 8-56   A colotomy incision exposes the polyp. The base of a sessile polyp is ligated with a loop ligature.

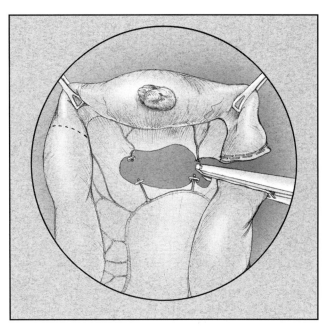

Fig. 8-58   Abdominal contamination is minimized by stapling and transecting the colon with an endoscopic linear cutter.

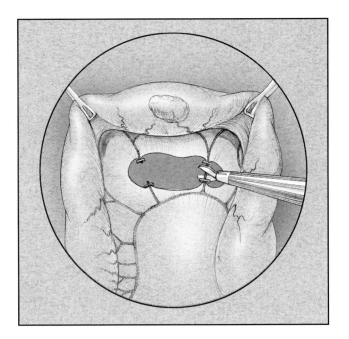

Fig. 8-57   To preserve blood supply to the descending colon, the vasa recta are ligated with clips and transected with scissors.

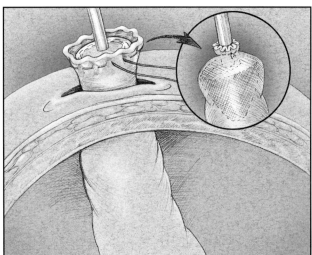

Fig. 8-59   The anvil portion of the circular stapler is secured in the proximal portion of bowel with a purse-string suture. The suture is tied around the anvil shaft.

containing the anvil to the abdomen. Suture the enlarged port site or reinsert the trocar and reestablish pneumoperitoneum. Insert the circular stapler through the anus. Extend the trocar tip of the circular stapler to emerge adjacent to the staple line in the distal portion of colon. With laparoscopic guidance, place the

anvil shaft from the proximal segment over the trocar in the distal segment. Align the anvil shaft, snap it into place, and test it for security (Fig. 8-60). Close the circular stapler, tighten it to the appropriate staple height setting, and fire the stapler to complete the anastomosis.

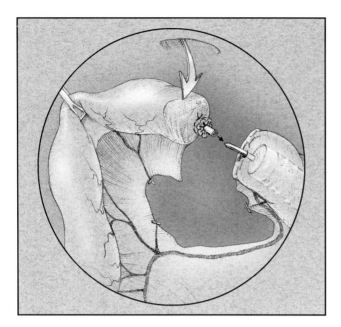

Fig. 8-60 The anvil shaft is joined with the trocar from the circular stapler. The instrument is closed and fired to perform the stapled end-to-end anastomosis.

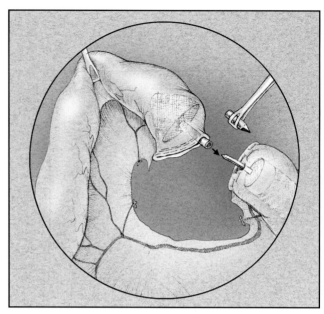

Fig. 8-62 In the triple-staple technique for intracorporeal anastomosis, a staple line closes the proximal segment of colon. An ancillary trocar tip on the anvil shaft is extended beside the staple line, and the trocar tip is removed. The anvil shaft is joined with the trocar from the circular stapler to perform the anastomosis.

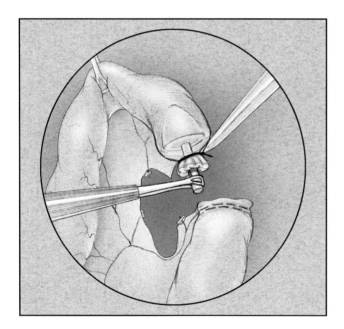

Fig. 8-61 An intracorporeal anastomosis does not require the proximal portion of bowel to be exteriorized. In the double-staple technique, the anvil is introduced into the proximal colon and secured with a loop ligature.

For an intracorporeal anastomosis using the double-staple technique, resect the lesion with two firings of the endoscopic linear cutter and remove it through one of the caudal ports. Using scissors, remove the staple line on the proximal portion of colon. Introduce the anvil of the circular stapler into the abdomen through a large port and direct it into the opened proximal segment of

the colon. Use a loop ligature or sew a purse-string suture to close the colon around the anvil shaft (Fig. 8-61). Insert the circular stapler through the anus. Extend the trocar tip of the circular stapler to emerge adjacent to the staple line in the distal portion of colon. With laparoscopic guidance, place the anvil shaft from the proximal segment over the trocar in the distal segment. Align the anvil shaft, snap it into place, and test it for security (see Fig. 8-60). Close the circular stapler, tighten it to the appropriate staple height setting, and fire the stapler to complete the anastomosis.

Intracorporeal anastomosis using the triple-staple technique is similar, except that the anvil shaft contains an ancillary trocar when it is introduced into the proximal portion of bowel.[16] A stapler is fired distal to the anvil shaft to close the proximal portion of bowel. The trocar of the anvil shaft is extended just beside the staple line, and the ancillary trocar is removed (Fig. 8-62). The remainder of the anastomosis is completed as previously described.

After the bowel is stapled, open the circular stapler and remove it from the colon. Examine the tissue doughnuts on the circular stapler for completeness. Test the colonic anastomosis for patency and leakage by filling the abdominal cavity with saline and occluding the colon proximal to the anastomosis. Instill air into the colon transanally and look for bubbles at the anastomotic site. The anastomosis can also be tested by distending the colon with povidone-iodine (Betadine) in saline and examining for fluid leakage (Fig. 8-63).

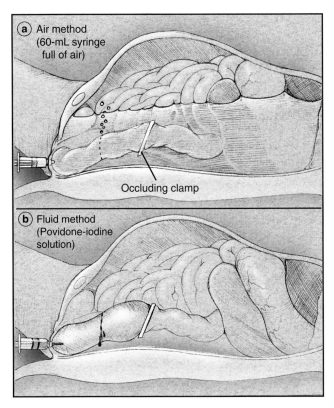

Fig. 8-63   Methods of evaluating the integrity of colonic anastomosis. Air is instilled transanally with the staple line submerged in saline to observe for bubbles (*a*). Fluid is instilled transanally, and the staple line is examined for leakage (*b*).

Ileocolonic Anastomosis

Ileocolonic anastomosis is performed if resection of the ascending colon is required. This procedure is difficult to perform laparoscopically. Identify the cecum and ileum by tracing the jejunum distally or the colon proximally. Isolate and ligate the vascular supply to the terminal part of the ileum, cecum, and ascending part of the colon with clips or sutures. Mobilize the ileum, cecum, and ascending part of the colon by transecting clipped vessels and dividing the mesentery. Transect the ileum with an endoscopic linear cutter. Resect the cecum and ascending colon with another firing of the endoscopic linear cutter. Insert a large trocar and remove the specimen from the abdomen.

Identify the staple line on the ileum and use scissors to remove it, leaving the distal portion of the ileum open. Insert the anvil and ancillary trocar of a circular stapler through the large trocar and into the open end of the ileum (Fig. 8-64, *a*). Extend the trocar through the antimesenteric border of the ileum and close the distal portion of the ileum with the endoscopic linear cutter. Use scissors to remove the staple line closing the colon to open the colonic lumen. Pass a circular stapler that has

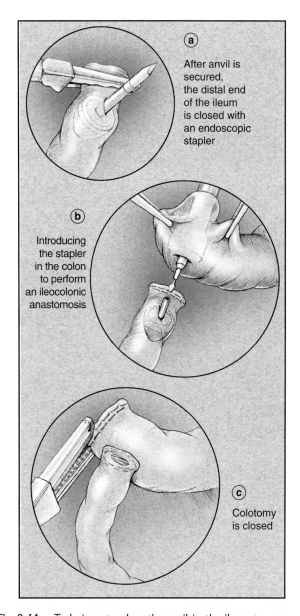

Fig. 8-64   Technique to place the anvil in the ileum to perform an ileocolonic anastomosis. After the anvil shaft is secured, the distal end of the ileum is closed with an endoscopic stapler (*a*). Introducing the stapler in the colon to perform an ileocolonic anastomosis (*b*). The colotomy is closed with an endoscopic stapler (*c*).

been sealed to prevent loss of pneumoperitoneum* through the large port. Introduce the circular stapler into the open end of the colon and extend the trocar point to exit on the antimesenteric border of the colon (Fig. 8-64, *b*). Attach the anvil shaft in the ileum to the circular stapler trocar shaft in the colon. Close and fire the stapler to create a circular side-to-side anastomosis of the ileum to the colon. Withdraw the circular stapler

---

*Stealth Circular Stapler, Ethicon Endo-Surgery, Inc, Cincinnati, Ohio 45242.

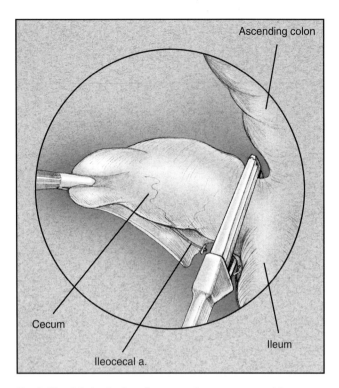

Fig. 8-65   Method of performing a laparoscopic typhlectomy with an endoscopic linear cutter.

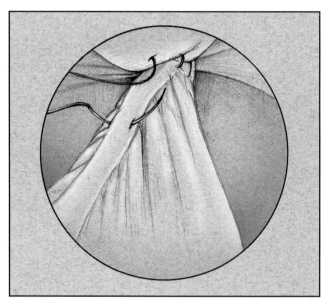

Fig. 8-66   Laparoscopic suturing techniques are used to place a simple continuous suture to secure the colon to the abdominal wall.

from the lumen of the colon and close the open lumen adjacent to the anastomosis with an endoscopic linear cutter (Fig. 8-64, *c*). Examine the tissue doughnuts on the circular stapler for completeness and test the anastomosis for patency and leakage.

Typhlectomy

Cecal tumors, granulomas, or parasitic lesions can be excised laparoscopically. If the cecum is inverted, cecal resection and ileocolostomy are performed. The cecum is identified by its attachments to the ileum by the ileocecal fold and to the colon by an accessory ileocecal fold. The blood supply is derived from the ileocecal artery, which is located in the ileocecal fold.

To perform typhlectomy, retract the tip of the cecum to tense the ileocecal fold. Incise and progressively dissect the peritoneum of the fold to identify the ileocecal artery. Ligate the branches of the ileocecal artery supplying the cecum while preserving the blood supply to the colon. Use electrocautery or ultrasonic energy to control hemorrhage from the dissection. When the cecum is free of its blood supply and mesenteric attachments, apply an endoscopic linear cutter across the base of the cecum to staple and transect the tissue (Fig. 8-65). Although some authors recommend oversewing the cecal stump, we have not found it to be necessary.[17] Wrap the cecal stump in omentum.

Closure

After the anastomosis is complete, lavage the abdominal cavity with sterile saline and aspirate the fluid. Wrap the anastomosis in omentum. Remove the trocar cannulas and suture the fascial incisions. Close the subcutaneous and subcuticular tissues with absorbable suture material.

Pull-Through Colonic Resection

Laparoscopic pull-through colonic resection is similar to the open approach except that the colon is mobilized laparoscopically. Although the technique has been performed successfully in acute studies in pigs, we are unaware of any survival studies in animals.[18]

Colopexy

Laparoscopic colopexy can be performed to reduce the tension applied to tissues after perineal herniorrhaphy or after unsuccessful treatment of rectal prolapse. Insufflate the abdomen and place the primary port at the umbilicus. Place two ports in the right caudal abdominal quadrant to facilitate suturing the descending colon to the abdominal wall to the left of midline. Place simple interrupted or continuous nonabsorbable sutures through the seromuscular layer of the colon and layers of the abdominal wall (Fig. 8-66).

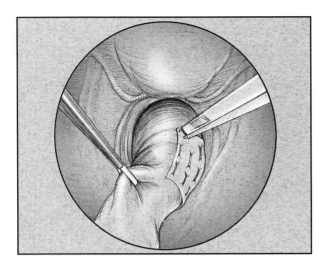

Fig. 8-67 Polypropylene mesh is secured with staples in the treatment of rectal prolapse.

Rectopexy

Children with cystic fibrosis or any condition leading to chronic constipation may suffer rectal prolapse.[19] For laparoscopic correction, the abdomen is insufflated and the primary port is placed at the umbilicus. Two additional 10-mm ports are placed on each side, lateral to the rectus abdominis muscle. The colon is moved aside to expose the sacral promontory. The mesentery is incised at the level of the sacral promontory, taking care not to injure the ureters or the iliac blood vessels. A strip of polypropylene mesh is inserted and tacked transversely to the presacral fascia dorsal to the colon. The mesh is wrapped around the colon. Tension is exerted on the colon until it is taut and there is no redundancy caudal to the mesh. The mesh is secured to the colon with staples or sutures and tested for security (Fig. 8-67). The ports are removed, and the wound is closed in two layers.

REFERENCES

1. Jacobs MD, Verdeja JC, Goldstein HS: Minimally invasive colon resection (laparoscopic colectomy). *Surg Laparosc Endosc* 1:144-150, 1991.
2. Allendorf JD et al: Better preservation of immune function after laparoscopic-assisted vs. open bowel resection in a murine model. *Dis Colon Rectum* 39:S67-S72, 1996.
3. Bohm B, Milson JW: Animal models as educational tools in laparoscopic colorectal surgery. *Surg Endosc* 8:707-713, 1994.
4. Kockerling F et al: Die laparosckopische tubulare rektum- und kolonresektion. *Zentralbl Chir* 117:103-110, 1992.
5. Olson KH et al: A comparative study of open, laparoscopic intracorporeal, and laparoscopic assisted low anterior resection and anastomosis in pigs. *Am Surg* 61:197-201, 1995.
6. Bessler M et al: Controlled trial of laparoscopic-assisted vs. open colon resection in a porcine model. *Surg Endosc* 10:732-735, 1996.
7. Reissman P et al: Adhesions formation after laparoscopic anterior resection in a porcine model: a pilot study. *Surg Laparosc Endosc* 6:136-139, 1996.
8. Hotokezaka M, Combs MJ, Schirmer BD: Recovery of gastrointestinal motility following open versus laparoscopic colon resection in dogs. *Dig Dis Sci* 41:705-710, 1996.
9. Bohm B et al: Laparoscopic oncologic total abdominal colectomy with intraperitoneal stapled anastomosis in a canine model. *J Laparoendosc Surg* 4:23-30, 1994.
10. Mathew G et al: Wound metastasis following laparoscopic and open surgery for abdominal cancer in a rat model. *Br J Surg* 83:1087-1090, 1996.
11. Allardyce R, Morreau P, Bagshaw P: Tumor cell distribution following laparoscopic colectomy in a porcine model. *Dis Colon Rectum* 39:S47-S52, 1996.
12. Jones DB et al: Impact of pneumoperitoneum on trocar site implantation of colon cancer in hamster model. *Dis Colon Rectum* 38:1182-1188, 1995.
13. Geis WP et al: Sequential psychomotor skills development in laparoscopic colon surgery. *Arch Surg* 129:206-212, 1994.
14. Cohen SM et al: An initial comparative study of two techniques of laparoscopic colonic anastomosis and mesenteric defect closure. *Surg Endosc* 8:130-134, 1994.
15. Ballantyne GH: Polypectomy. In Ballantyne GH, Leahy PF, Modlin IM, editors: Laparoscopic surgery, Philadelphia, 1994, WB Saunders.
16. Fleshman JW et al: Laparoscopic anterior resection of the rectum using a triple stapled intracorporeal anastomosis in the pig. *Surg Laparosc Endosc* 3:119-126, 1993.
17. Freeman LJ: Unpublished data. 1992-1996.
18. Ambroze WL et al: Laparoscopic assisted proctosigmoidectomy with extracorporeal transanal anastomosis. *Surg Endosc* 7:29-32, 1993.
19. Laparoscopic surgery for rectal prolapse. In Lobe TE, Schropp KP, editors: Pediatric laparoscopy and thoracoscopy, Philadelphia, 1994, WB Saunders.

Minimally Invasive Surgery of the Liver and Biliary System

RONALD J. KOLATA, LYNETTA J. FREEMAN

Laparoscopic approaches are ideal for examining the liver and biliary system in diagnostically challenging cases. Direct observation provides an opportunity to obtain a more reliable tissue sample than by ultrasound, computed tomography (CT)-guided percutaneous puncture, or blind fine-needle aspiration. The ability to detect small liver metastases and peritoneal seeding can prevent open laparotomy in inoperable conditions. Combining laparoscopy with intraoperative ultrasonography makes possible the detection and obtainment of biopsy specimens of lesions not visible on the surface. Laparoscopy and laparoscopic ultrasound can be used together to determine if a hepatic resection is feasible, establish the prognosis more accurately, and make decisions about adjuvant therapy. Laparoscopy can be used to determine whether bleeding from traumatic liver or splenic fractures has ceased, thereby avoiding laparotomy. With appropriate instrumentation, hemostasis of hepatic or splenic fractures can be achieved by using laparoscopic techniques. Evaluation of an animal with ascites is another potential indication for a minimally invasive approach to the liver.

Preoperative Preparation

Animals scheduled for liver biopsy should be fasted at least 12 hours to empty the stomach. As with open surgery, the animal's clotting ability should be evaluated before administering anesthesia. One-stage prothrombin time, activated partial thromboplastin time, and total platelet count are accepted tests of coagulation status. Animals predisposed to von Willebrand's disease should receive a von Willebrand factor assay. A source of fresh blood should be available to treat bleeding problems that may arise.

Laparoscopic Anatomy

The laparoscopic view of liver anatomy is essentially the same as or better than that obtained with open laparotomy. An orogastric tube is placed to aspirate fluid and gas from the stomach to ensure that a distended stomach does not restrict access to the liver. With the animal in dorsal recumbency and head-up position, the convex surface of the liver is easily viewed as it drapes over the stomach and intestines. A 30° laparoscope inserted through a port at the umbilicus provides visual access to the liver down to the vena cava (Fig. 8-68). In dogs, the midline structures are somewhat obscured by the falciform ligament. To view the concave surface and the hilum of the liver, the animal is positioned with its head down. Additional ports are required to retract the stomach and bowel. Tilting the animal to the right or left increases access to the contralateral lobes.

Surgical Procedures

LIVER BIOPSY

Surgical biopsy is performed to make or confirm a diagnosis of liver disease. Laparoscopic liver biopsy is a simple procedure, and 3-mm trocars and laparoscopic instruments make it even less invasive than previously described. Three techniques are used. A specimen can be taken from the edge of the liver or from a protruding mass with

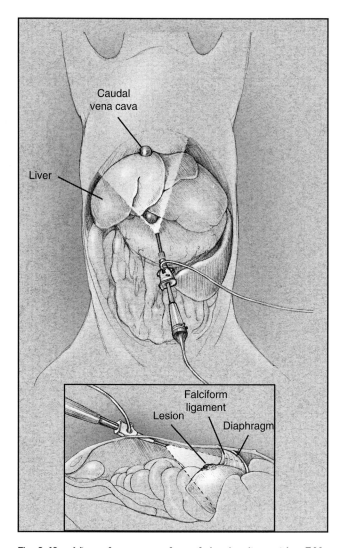

Fig. 8-68   View of convex surface of the dog liver with a 30° scope inserted at the umbilicus.

biopsy cup forceps. A pre-tied suture loop may be used to snare a portion of tissue, usually at the tissue edge. A needle-directed biopsy can be obtained by inserting the needle percutaneously or through the trocar. Instrumentation depends on the technique selected (Box 8-5).

For hepatic biopsy only, laparoscopy in small animals can be performed with sedation and local anesthesia or with general anesthesia. Dogs and cats are placed in left lateral recumbency because more of the liver surface is exposed through the right lateral midabdominal approach. Small animals can be placed in dorsal recumbency under general anesthesia, but fat in the falciform ligament often interferes with a thorough examination. In large animals, a standing approach and long biopsy forceps can be used to reach the right side of the liver.

Pneumoperitoneum is created, and the primary trocar is placed by one of the techniques described in Chapter 3. Special care should be taken when insufflating the abdomen in the presence of ascites. If the amount of as-

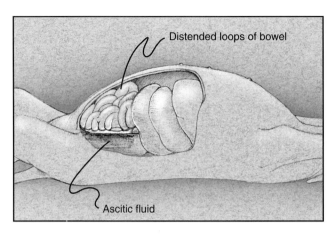

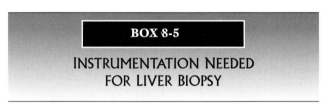

Fig. 8-69   Distended loops of small bowel floating on the surface of ascitic fluid.

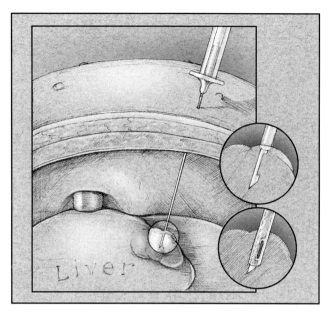

Fig. 8-70   Use of Tru-Cut needle to obtain a sample of a liver lesion for biopsy.

BOX 8-5

INSTRUMENTATION NEEDED FOR LIVER BIOPSY

1 to 3 trocars
Liver biopsy forceps
Tru-Cut biopsy needle
Endoloop loop ligatures
Electrocautery device
Aspiration and irrigation device
Hemostatic agent (Surgicel, Gelfoam, Thrombin)

TABLE 8-2

Laparoscopic Diagnosis of Hepatic Abnormalities*

ABNORMAL CONDITION	APPEARANCE
Hepatic lipidosis	Pale yellow color; friable, prominent portal triads
Steroid hepatopathy	Pale pink color; friable
Hepatic congestion	Enlarged, dark liver; distended hepatic sinusoids; "nutmeg" appearance
Neoplasia	Raised, discolored nodules. Cavitation or depression in center of lesion
Nodular hyperplasia	Raised nodules with yellow appearance. No depressions over the surface
Biliary tract disease	Prominent portal triads; greenish-black color; distended gallbladder and hepatic ducts
Cirrhosis	Irregular surface; small; firm on palpation; thickened, whitish liver capsule; multiple venous complexes

*Twedt DC: Laparoscopy of the liver and pancreas. In Tams T, editor: Small animal endoscopy, St. Louis, 1997, Mosby.

cites is significant, air-filled small bowel floats on the surface of the ascitic fluid (Fig. 8-69). The small bowel is close to the body wall and may be more easily injured during placement of a Veress needle and primary port. In addition, insufflating below the fluid level causes bubbles to form in the ascitic fluid. A Veress needle can be used to aspirate the ascitic fluid before insufflation, or an open technique for trocar placement can be used.

The liver is inspected, and the lesion is identified (Table 8-2). Biopsy should not be performed until the lesion has been inspected closely and palpated with a probe. Areas of increased vascularity, necrosis, and distended bile ducts should be avoided. Taking this step will avoid puncture of vascular malformations or hemangiosarcomas. For additional safety, insert a working port through which a surgical instrument attached to electrocautery can be used. Ensure that the tip of the instru-

ment will reach the proposed biopsy site. Be aware of adjacent structures to avoid accidental puncture of the diaphragm, stomach, or gastrointestinal tract, large blood vessels, or the gallbladder.

At least six types of tissue samples can be retrieved laparoscopically (Box 8-6). For fine-needle or Tru-Cut needle biopsies, the needle is inserted through the abdominal wall, directly above and perpendicular to the lesion. Under direct observation, the needle is inserted into the core of the lesion. In fine-needle biopsy, the syringe is aspirated; the barrel of a Tru-Cut needle is advanced to obtain the specimen (Fig. 8-70). Suspending

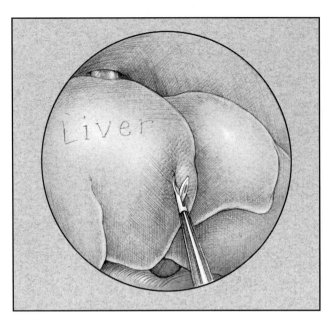

Fig. 8-71 Use of biopsy cup forceps to sample a lesion on the edge of the liver.

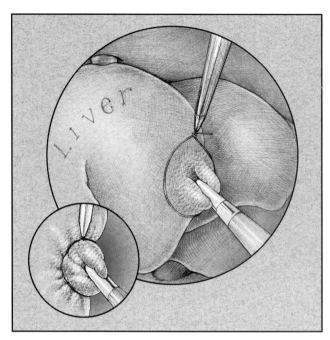

Fig. 8-72 Use of an Endoloop suture to obtain a biopsy specimen on the edge of a liver lobe. The suture uses the crush technique to obtain a sample and ligate the small ducts and vessels.

BOX 8-6

METHODS OF OBTAINING TISSUE SAMPLES LAPAROSCOPICALLY

Fine-needle aspiration
Tru-Cut needle biopsy
Excisional biopsy
Peritoneal washing
Aspiration of fluids (e.g., from gallbladder or hepatic cysts)
Brush cytology of visceral surfaces

---

ventilation during this step helps avoid tearing the hepatic capsule. The needle is removed, and pressure is applied to the liver surface with the suction/cautery probe. Additional biopsy specimens are taken as needed. Cautery is used if necessary to ensure hemostasis.

If generalized liver disease is present, marginal biopsy can be performed by excising a specimen from the edge of a lobe. An operating laparoscope with compatible biopsy forceps and an electrocautery probe can be used through a single 10-mm port or with an additional 5-mm port. The biopsy forceps are passed through the operative scope or the trocar and opened to straddle the lesion. The forceps are closed and gently rocked from side to side until the tissue is detached (Fig. 8-71). Keeping the forceps in place for a few seconds will re-

duce bleeding from the biopsy site. Control hemorrhage with electrocautery.

When using biopsy forceps that are not made specifically for endoscopic surgery, sealing the trocar to maintain pneumoperitoneum may be a problem. A seal that can accommodate instruments having diameters from 5 to 12 mm may allow use of some instruments with round shafts. Pneumoperitoneum can also be maintained by passing the instrument through a hole in a sterile surgical glove, placing the cuff of the glove over the body of the cannula, and securing it with a ligature. This technique prevents loss of pneumoperitoneum even though the seals and valves of the cannula are being compromised by an irregularly shaped instrument shaft.

Excisional biopsy can be performed by using an Endoloop as a snare suture. The Endoloop is introduced through a second 5-mm port, and the loop is positioned on the tissue. Grasping forceps are passed through the loop to pull the edge of tissue up and through the loop. The Endoloop is snapped at the scored area of the nylon cannula. Upward tension is applied to the suture as the cannula is slid forward to advance and tighten the loop, cut the parenchyma, and ligate the vessels and ducts (Fig. 8-72). The proximal end of the cannula is cut off, and the plastic cannula is removed from the trocar. Scissors are used to cut the suture and excise the tissue distal to the ligature.

Peritoneal washings are performed to detect free neoplastic cells in the peritoneal gutters. Peritoneal washings are also helpful in diagnosing septic or chemical peritonitis. Approximately 100 mL of saline is injected through an irrigation cannula in the peritoneal gutter. After mixing, the fluid is aspirated, centrifuged, and submitted for culture and cytologic examination. Aspiration of fluids from hepatic cysts helps determine whether the cyst is congenital, parasitic, or infectious. A long needle attached to a syringe is inserted percutaneously into the cyst. Congenital, benign hepatic cysts are treated in humans by aspirating the fluid, deroofing the cyst, and placing omentum in the cyst cavity to prevent reformation. Needle aspiration is also used to aspirate bile from the gallbladder for culture. Brush cytology can be used for surface lesions. Standard endoscopic brush cytology devices are inserted through a 5-mm or smaller trocar.

Animals with liver disease frequently have coagulation defects; thus careful attention should be paid to biopsy sites and trocar insertion sites. Hemostatic agents, such as Endo-Avitene, Surgicel, Gelfoam, or collagen sponge may be packed into or laid over the biopsy site.[1] If clotting abnormalities are present or suspected, thrombin solution can be used to moisten the hemostatic pledgets and augment their hemostatic potential. The abdominal cavity is lavaged with saline solution, and the fluid is aspirated before the trocars are removed. In animals with ascites, the port sites are closed in layers to prevent a chronic fluid leak.

Complications of liver biopsy include bile peritonitis, bleeding, and bacteremia.[2] Bile peritonitis occurs in people with obstructive jaundice. Serious bleeding is common in humans with cirrhosis, liver metastasis, and vascular tumors. Although most bleeding is acute, fatal hemorrhage has been reported as late as 13 days after biopsy. Care should be taken to ensure complete hemostasis. Bacteremia is reported in up to 13% of human patients; however, sepsis appears to be uncommon. Other potential complications include needle breakage and perforation of the gallbladder, stomach, or intestines with the biopsy needle. Accidental penetration of the diaphragm with the biopsy needle causes pneumothorax. In a report of more than 300 laparoscopic liver biopsies in animals, the overall complication rate was 3.3%.[3] Major complications included excessive bleeding during needle biopsy, laceration of a major blood vessel, and pneumothorax. Minor complications included subcutaneous emphysema and leakage of ascitic fluid into the subcutaneous space.

LOBECTOMY AND PARTIAL LOBECTOMY

Localized liver masses, such as abscesses, neoplasms, and lesions caused by trauma, can be removed by laparoscopic lobectomy or partial lobectomy. Instruments required for this procedure are listed in Box 8-7. In small dogs and cats, either of the left lobes can be removed

---

BOX 8-7

INSTRUMENTATION NEEDED FOR LOBECTOMY AND PARTIAL LOBECTOMY

3 to 5 trocars (either 5 or 10 mm, depending on patient size)
Endoscopic dissecting forceps
Endoscopic Kelly forceps
Liver retractor
Suction/irrigation/cautery cannula and probe
Endoscopic clip appliers
Endoloop loop ligature
Endopouch disposable specimen retrieval bag
UltraCision harmonic scalpel and accessories

---

with a single encircling ligature. In the right lobes or the quadrate lobe, dissection of the liver parenchyma from the vena cava is required before ligation.

The camera port is placed at the umbilicus, and additional working ports are inserted to provide optimal access to the area of interest. The right or left triangular ligament is transected to improve mobilization and access to the right or left hepatic lobes, respectively. Blunt dissection is performed across the lobe with the tips of a closed dissector or Kelly forceps, just as one uses a scalpel handle in open surgery. Small vessels and ducts are coagulated as they are encountered. Larger vessels and ducts are ligated with hemostatic clips or Endoloop sutures. The excised tissue is placed in a specimen retrieval bag for removal from the abdomen. The exposed surface of the liver may be covered with omentum, which can be secured with interrupted, absorbable sutures, taking large bites of the hepatic parenchyma and tying knots or using a Lapra-Ty suture clip.

The Pringle maneuver should be performed only as a last resort to control bleeding during laparoscopic liver resections. Researchers have shown that combining the Pringle maneuver with pneumoperitoneum is associated with decreased cardiac index and blood pressure, and elevated heart rate.[4]

Partial or complete lobectomy can also be performed with endoscopic staplers. The liver is incised on its convex surface and, if the jaw aperture allows, a 35- or 45-mm stapler is placed across the section of the lobe to be excised (Fig. 8-73). The stapler is closed, crushing the tissue between its jaws. Four to six rows of staples are applied, and the tissue is simultaneously cut between the middle rows. Depending on the amount of liver to be removed, one or more firings of the stapler may be required. Hemorrhage is controlled with electrocoagulation or hemostatic clips, after which the abdomen is

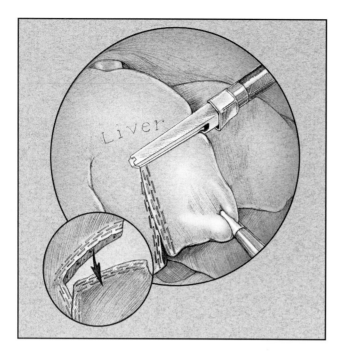

Fig. 8-73 Use of an endoscopic stapler to remove a partial lobe. The instrument is opened and positioned on tissue, closed, and fired to form the staples and transect the tissue.

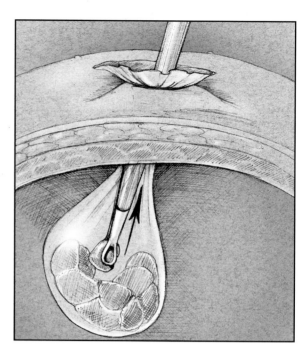

Fig. 8-74 Use of a disposable specimen retrieval bag, and morcellation of tissue inside the bag, for removal.

lavaged. The specimen is placed in a bag to allow safe retrieval from the abdomen. Large specimens should be removed by enlarging the umbilical trocar wound and pulling the mouth of the bag through the wound. Small pieces are cut from the specimen and removed until the entire bag and its contents can be removed (Fig. 8-74).

Investigators used an ultrasound dissector to perform laparoscopic liver lobe resections in 16 pigs.[5] Major blood vessels were clipped and bleeding surfaces were coagulated with an argon beam coagulator. After a 10-day survival period, there were wound infections in two pigs, a subphrenic abscess in one pig, and biloma in two pigs. Laparoscopic hepatic lobectomy should be considered experimental at this time.

BILIARY EVALUATION

The gallbladder, cystic duct, and extrahepatic ducts are located in the cranial right abdominal quadrant and can be evaluated from a ventral midline or right-side approach. Biliary obstruction is associated with distended gallbladder and cystic ducts, darkened liver, and bile staining. Bile can be aspirated from the gallbladder by inserting a 20-gauge spinal needle or Veress needle transabdominally. Samples are sent for aerobic and anaerobic bacterial culture and cytology. If necessary, a contrast cholecystocholangiogram can be performed under laparoscopic guidance by injecting 5 to 10 mL of radiopaque iodine contrast medium into the gallbladder. Passage of the contrast medium into the duodenum is monitored radiographically.

BOX 8-8

INSTRUMENTATION NEEDED FOR CHOLECYSTECTOMY

4 trocars (5 or 10 mm, depending on patient size and instrument compatibility)
Reducing caps for 10-mm trocars
2 grasping forceps
Dissecting forceps
Scissors
Hook cautery or UltraCision hook blade
Suction/irrigation/cautery cannula and probe
Endoscopic clip appliers
Endoloop loop ligature
Endopouch disposable specimen retrieval bag

CHOLECYSTECTOMY

Cholecystectomy is performed to treat cholelithiasis, cholecystitis, or gallbladder trauma with leakage of bile. In dogs, the gallbladder is to the right of midline, between the right medial lobe of the liver and the quadrate lobe. The cystic duct is joined by the hepatic ducts and carries bile to the common bile duct, which empties into the duodenum at the major duodenal papilla. Instrumentation needs are listed in Box 8-8.

The animal is placed in dorsal recumbency with its head up. Pneumoperitoneum is established in the us-

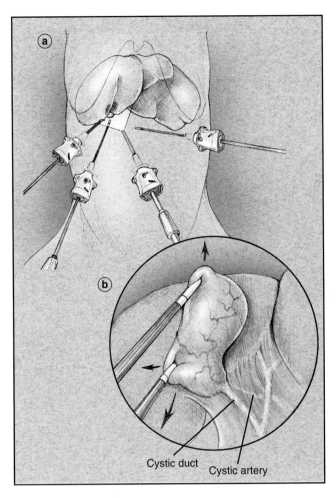

Fig. 8-75 Trocar placement for laparoscopic cholecystectomy in the dog (*a*). The gallbladder is held in tension (*b*).

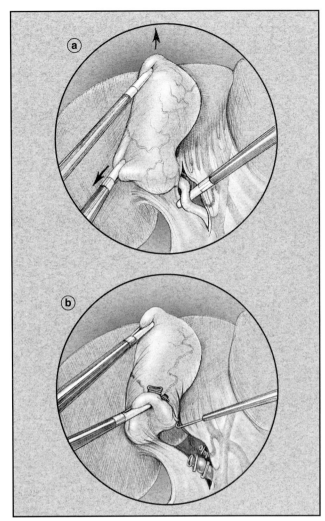

Fig. 8-76 Window behind cystic duct for placement of clips (*a*). Dissection of gallbladder from liver (*b*).

ual fashion. The trocars are inserted as indicated in Fig. 8-75, *a*. The camera port is placed at or near the umbilicus. Two ports for grasping and retracting are placed to the right of midline in the sagittal plane of the axilla. A port for dissecting and ligating instruments is placed to the left of midline, caudal to the costal arch. In large animals, it may be necessary to move this port closer to the midline. In dogs, removing the falciform ligament may be required to improve visibility and access to the gallbladder from the left side of the animal.

The apex and base of the gallbladder are grasped with instruments inserted through the right lateral ports. The apex of the gallbladder is lifted and reflected craniad. The base of the gallbladder is held in tension (see Fig. 8-75, *b*). The cystic duct is identified. Dissecting forceps are passed through the left port and behind cystic duct or between the cystic duct and artery to create a window for the clip applier (Fig. 8-76, *a*). The dis-

sector is removed, and a clip applier is inserted through the left port. Two clips are applied proximally and one distally on the cystic duct. The cystic artery is dissected, clipped, and divided. Some surgeons recommend the addition of an Endoloop ligature on the proximal segment of the cystic duct and artery in the event of clip displacement during the subsequent dissection.

The gallbladder is held by placing grasping forceps laterally at the level of the cystic duct and pulling upward. This creates a plane of tension between the hepatic gallbladder bed and the gallbladder. Dissection is begun by using a hook electrocautery device, a curved dissector, curved scissors, or an ultrasonic dissector (see Fig. 8-76, *b*). Dissection progresses toward the apex of the gallbladder. Smoke from the electrocautery device usually obscures vision. Smoke is aspirated by using suction on the electrocautery probes or by opening the insufflation port of one of the trocars. To free the apex of the gallbladder, it is sometimes necessary to flip the grasper holding the cystic duct portion of the gallbladder over the apex of the gallbladder. The clips and hepatic parenchyma are examined for bleeding before the gallbladder is freed from the liver.

The gallbladder is now ready to be removed from the abdominal cavity through a 10-mm port. The laparoscope is transferred to the 10-mm port in the cranial left quadrant. One of the grasping forceps is released and passed through the 10-mm umbilical port to grasp the cystic duct. The gallbladder and trocar cannula are removed simultaneously. Alternatively, the gallbladder can be placed in a specimen retrieval bag and removed by pulling the pouch partially into the port and pulling both the cannula and bag simultaneously. The trocar cannula is replaced. The liver is inspected for hemorrhage, and the abdomen is lavaged with sterile saline. The ports are removed and closed routinely.

Laparoscopic cholecystectomy was performed in 11 pigs.[6] At necropsy immediately after surgery in five pigs, there was no immediate evidence of injury to bile ducts, liver, or intestine. Six pigs were allowed to recover. One died 10 days after surgery as a result of bowel obstruction caused by adhesions. The remaining five were examined 1 month after surgery and showed no evidence of cholestasis. The hepatic enzyme values were normal.

Laparoscopic cholecystectomy resulted in faster return of intestinal motility than did open cholecystectomy in dogs.[7] After implanting electrodes on the jejunum to monitor electrical activity, researchers performed laparoscopic cholecystectomy in five dogs and open cholecystectomy in five dogs. Dogs that had undergone laparoscopy had return of intestinal motility in 5.5 hours; the time before intestinal motility returned was 46 hours in the dogs that had undergone laparotomy. Gastric emptying was delayed more than 2 hours after feeding in 6 dogs with open cholecystectomy, but not in 6 dogs with laparoscopic cholecystectomy.[8]

CHOLECYSTOENTEROSTOMY

Surgical anastomosis of the gallbladder to the intestine is performed when the common bile duct has been injured or is obstructed by neoplasia. Cholecystoenterostomy is an advanced laparoscopic procedure that requires considerable technical skills. The procedure should not be performed unless the surgeon has excellent suturing and knot-tying skills or has access to stapling instruments, or both. Instrumentation needed for cholecystoenterostomy is listed in Box 8-9.

A cholecystoenterostomy may be sutured or stapled. The laparoscopic approach and port placements are similar to those for cholecystectomy, except that a 12-mm port is necessary if an endoscopic stapler is used.

The descending duodenum is identified. A segment that can be brought up to the gallbladder without ten-

---

BOX 8-9

INSTRUMENTATION NEEDED FOR CHOLECYSTOENTEROSTOMY

4 to 6 trocars (5, 10, or 12 mm, depending on patient size and instrument compatibility)
Grasping forceps
Babcock forceps
Scissors with monopolar cautery
Sutures with pre-tied knots
Lapra-Ty suture clips and applier
35-mm endoscopic linear stapler
Suction/irrigation

---

sion is chosen for the anastomosis. The proposed incision site is tagged with a suture. The gallbladder is dissected from the hepatic fossa, taking care to preserve the cystic artery and cystic duct.

Depending on the size of the animal, 2- to 4-cm incisions are made in the antimesenteric surface of the duodenum and the peritoneal surface of the gallbladder. Traction sutures are placed at the proximal and distal ends of the proposed anastomosis. The sutures penetrate the gallbladder and duodenum, approximating the organs in the correct relationship and facilitating endoscopic suturing. The traction sutures can be grasped and held through additional ports by an assistant. Alternatively, sutures on Keith needles can be passed into the abdominal cavity percutaneously, placed through the gallbladder and duodenum, and passed out through the abdominal wall. The exteriorized ends of the suture can be used to position the gallbladder and duodenum to facilitate endoscopic suturing.

The sutured anastomosis is performed in the same way as an open anastomosis, but all suturing is done endoscopically. Knots are tied endoscopically or by tying them externally and using a knot pusher to snug them down. Using pre-tied knots and Lapra-Ty suture clips eliminates the need to tie knots and greatly facilitates the anastomosis.

When an endoscopic stapler is used, the gallbladder is mobilized as previously described. Traction sutures are placed at the apex of the gallbladder and at the proposed duodenal incision site. The apex of the gallbladder is grasped, and an irrigation and aspiration device with a monopolar electrosurgical tip is used to penetrate the gallbladder. Bile is aspirated, and the lumen of the gallbladder is lavaged and aspirated. A 2-cm incision is made on the antimesenteric border of the duodenum, and the duodenal contents are aspirated. A trocar site that will allow the endoscopic stapler to be inserted with its tip pointing orad is selected. The cartridge side of the linear

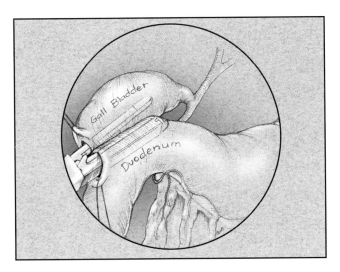

Fig. 8-77 Use of a stapler to perform a cholecystoduodenostomy with anvil in gallbladder and cartridge in duodenum. The gallbladder is mobilized from the liver bed before stapling.

cutter is inserted through an enterotomy into the lumen of the duodenum. The anvil jaw is inserted through an incision in the gallbladder, pointing toward the neck of the gallbladder (Fig. 8-77). With the linear cutter inserted in the duodenum and gallbladder, preplaced sutures are used to draw the gallbladder and duodenum back into the jaws. The instrument is closed and fired, stapling and transecting the tissue. A side-to-side anastomosis is created between the gallbladder and duodenum. When the stapler is removed, an opening remains where its jaws were inserted into the duodenum and gallbladder. This common opening is closed with sutures. Individual sutures with pre-tied knots, continuous sutures with Lapra-Ty suture clips, or intra- or extracorporeal ties are used. The surgical site is inspected and lavaged, and the trocars are removed. Port sites are inspected and closed.

At least four experimental studies evaluating the feasibility of laparoscopic cholecystojejunostomy have been conducted in swine. Over a 2-year period, surgeons in Scotland developed the Endoski needle to improve needle passage and a quick knotting technique using a single layer of sutures for a hand-sewn anastomosis.[9] Hand-sutured cholecystojejunostomy and gastrojejunostomy required approximately 1 hour more than the stapled/suture technique in 7 pigs.[10] All anastomoses were patent

and there was no change in liver function tests during the postoperative period. After ligation of the common bile duct with surgical clips in 20 pigs, a single-loop Roux-en-Y cholecystojejunostomy was compared to a double-loop Roux-en-Y with cholecystojejunostomy and gastrojejunostomy.[11] Twenty-eight days later, 19 pigs had patent and leak-free anastomoses. One pig was euthanatized on day 6 because of necrosis of the Roux-en-Y loop. Choledochojejunostomy was performed in 57 pigs to evaluate an absorbable stent and compare the anastomoses with ones made with suturing techniques.[12] The stent procedure required approximately 1 hour less operating time. During the postoperative period of 3 or 6 months, results did not differ. In expert hands, the technique is feasible; however, caution should be used in applying the results of the experimental studies to clinical cases in dogs and cats.

REFERENCES

1. Low RK, Moran ME, Goodnight JE Jr: Microfibrillary collagen hemostat during laparoscopically directed liver biopsy. *J Laparoendosc Surg* 3:415-420, 1993.
2. Nord HJ: Complications of laparoscopy. Endoscopy 24:693-700, 1992.
3. Twedt DC: Laparoscopy of the liver and pancreas. In Tams T, editor: Small animal endoscopy, St. Louis, 1997, Mosby.
4. Haberstroh J et al: Effects of the Pringle maneuver on hemodynamics during laparoscopic liver resection in the pig. *Eur Surg Res* 28:8-13, 1996.
5. Baer HU et al: Laparoscopic liver resection in the Large White pig: a comparison between waterjet dissector and ultrasound dissector. *Endosc Surg Allied Technol* 2:189-193, 1994.
6. Soper NJ et al: Safety and efficacy of laparoscopic cholecystectomy using monopolar electrocautery in the porcine model. *Surg Laparosc Endosc* 1:17-22, 1991.
7. Schippers E et al: Laparoscopic cholecystectomy: a minor abdominal trauma? *World J Surg* 17:539-542, 1993.
8. Hotokezaka M et al: Recovery of fasted and fed gastrointestinal motility after open versus laparoscopic cholecystectomy in dogs. *Ann Surg* 223:413-419, 1996.
9. Nathanson LK, Shimi S, Cuschieri A: Sutured laparoscopic cholecystojejunostomy evolved in an animal model. *J R Coll Surg Edinb* 37:215-220, 1992.
10. Patel AG et al: Palliation for pancreatic cancer: feasibility of laparoscopic cholecystojejunostomy and gastrojejunostomy in a porcine model. *Surg Endosc* 10:639-643, 1996.
11. Schob O et al: Experimenteller laparosckopisher bypass der gallenwegs- und duodenumobstruktion. *Schweiz Med Wochenschr* 124:1813-1820, 1994.
12. Schob O, Schmid R, Schlumpf R: Biliarer und gastroenteroaler bypass: laparoskopische moglichkeiten. *Swiss Surg* 4:S29-S32, 1996.

Minimally Invasive Pancreatic Surgery

LYNETTA J. FREEMAN

Although laparoscopic pancreatic biopsy is a well-established means of distinguishing between chronic pancreatitis and extrahepatic liver disease, therapeutic procedures to treat pancreatic disease in animals have not

been described.[1] The purpose of this section is to provide the reader with surgical approaches used in human surgery to address diseases of the pancreas and suggest where they may be applicable in veterinary medicine.

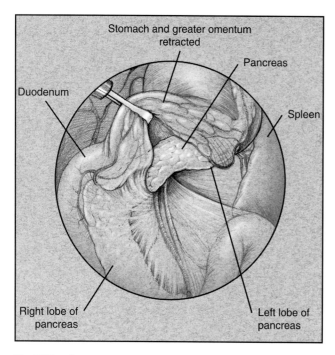

Fig. 8-78 Laparoscopic view of anatomy of the canine pancreas. The right lobe is identified in the mesoduodenum. Access to the left lobe is gained by making an opening into the omental bursa.

Advantages of a minimally invasive approach to diagnosing and treating pancreatic diseases in humans are shorter hospital stay and avoidance of unnecessary laparotomy. In debilitated patients, laparoscopic jejunostomy can be performed to facilitate nutritional support in the postoperative period. A few reports have documented abdominal wall or port site metastasis from pancreatic adenocarcinoma when a minimally invasive approach was used.[2,3]

As with other laparoscopic therapeutic procedures, the veterinary surgeon should be familiar with pancreatic anatomy and open surgery. He or she should be capable of performing any surgical procedure involving the pancreas and should be prepared to convert to an open procedure if necessary. Indications for conversion to an open procedure include inability to maintain the optical space, bleeding that cannot be controlled, excessive operative time, and tumor invasion.

Anatomy[4]

The pancreas is a retroperitoneal structure. The right lobe is situated between the two layers of the mesoduodenum adjacent to the duodenum, and the left lobe is in the deep leaf of the greater omentum (Fig. 8-78). The body of the pancreas unites the right and left lobes and is adjacent to the pylorus. The pancreatic ducts are in the central region of the lobes. The pancreatic duct drains the right lobe and opens into the common bile duct, or it enters the duo-

denum beside the common bile duct at the major duodenal papilla. The accessory pancreatic duct drains the left lobe and opens into the duodenum at the minor duodenal papilla. Blood supply to the right lobe is from branches of the cranial and caudal pancreaticoduodenal arteries. The left lobe is supplied by branches from the splenic, hepatic, gastroduodenal, and celiac arteries.

Instrumentation

Laparoscopic surgery can be performed with standard straight laparoscopic instruments. Box 8-10 lists other useful equipment. A laparoscopic ultrasound unit* is necessary to identify islet cell tumors and determine the extent of pancreatic cancer.

Preoperative Treatment

Preoperative treatment for the minimally invasive approach is the same as for an open procedure. Metabolic derangements and fluid and electrolyte imbalances must be corrected. An evaluation for metastatic disease is performed. Administration of glucocorticoids, anesthesia protocol, and monitoring for cardiac arrhythmias are performed in the same manner as for laparotomy. An orogastric tube is passed to decompress the stomach.

---

*Laparoscopic Ultrasonic Probe, 10 mm with 7.5 MHz frequency, Aloka, Tokyo, Japan.

BOX 8-10

INSTRUMENTATION NEEDED FOR LAPAROSCOPIC PANCREATIC SURGERY

30° laparoscope
3 to 5 trocars
Grasping forceps
Dissecting forceps
Endoscopic Babcock forceps
Endoscopic scissors
Biopsy cup forceps
Endoloop loop ligatures
Endoscopic surgical stapler
Needle holders
Clip applier
Tissue retractor
Irrigation/aspiration unit
Diagnostic laparoscopic ultrasound unit
UltraCision generator and laparoscopic hand pieces

Surgical Procedures

EXPLORATORY LAPAROSCOPY

Veterinary surgeons should consider performing laparoscopy to obtain pancreatic biopsy specimens, evaluate traumatic pancreatitis, and determine whether lesions that can be corrected surgically are present. Two approaches can be used to inspect the pancreas. The right midabdominal lateral approach is used to evaluate the right lobe of the pancreas and obtain biopsy specimens of the right lobe. The ventral midline approach is used with secondary operative ports to inspect both the right and left lobes and perform therapeutic procedures.

Right Lateral Approach[1]

Place the animal in left lateral recumbency. Prepare the right flank aseptically from the last rib to the iliac crest and from the dorsal to ventral midlines. Insert the primary trocar in the center of the prepared area. With this approach, the right lobe is identified adjacent to the duodenum. It can be traced proximally toward the left lobe. The duodenum is retracted ventrally to identify the portal vein, gallbladder, and common bile duct. The duodenum is retracted dorsally to view the ventral aspect of the right lobe. A limited view of the left lobe of the pancreas is obtained before it is lost in deeper structures.[1]

The normal pancreas is light pink and has a coarse nodular appearance. Acute pancreatitis may be characterized by adhesions, inflammation, and edema. Chronic pancreatitis may appear as irregular nodules with calcification, fibrosis, or necrotic tissue. Islet cell tumors are small and often difficult to find.[1]

Ventral Approach

Position the animal in dorsal recumbency and prepare the abdomen aseptically from the xiphoid to the pubis and laterally to the folds of the flank. Using the open technique, make a 1.5-cm skin incision at the umbilicus and continue through the linea alba. Remove as much of the falciform ligament as possible before placing the Hasson cannula. Secure the cannula to the abdominal fascia with two sutures. Place two secondary ports in the right and left caudal abdominal quadrants. Retract the omentum cranially and position it over the ventral surface of the stomach. Identify the duodenum and use grasping forceps to elevate the duodenum. Examine the right lobe of the pancreas, located in the mesoduodenum. To examine the left lobe of the pancreas, tilt the table so the animal's head is positioned upward (reverse Trendelenburg). Use Babcock forceps to elevate the greater curvature of the stomach. Make a window in an avascular part of the greater omentum caudal to the gastroepiploic vessels to enter the omental bursa. Retract the ventral leaf of the greater omentum over the stomach. Enter the lesser sac and examine the left lobe of the

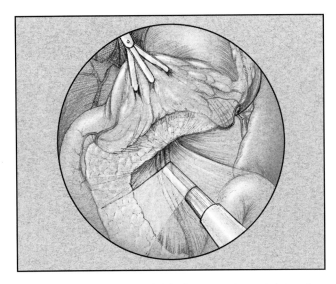

Fig. 8-79   A fan retractor holds the stomach craniad. An ultrasound probe scans the right lobe of the pancreas.

pancreas. Use a fan retractor if necessary to raise the stomach and expose the pancreas from the body to the splenic hilum. Examine the regional lymph nodes.

LAPAROSCOPIC STAGING OF PANCREATIC CANCER

Pancreatic cancer has been staged and islet cell tumors have been identified and resected in humans with a combination of laparoscopy and laparoscopic ultrasound imaging (Fig. 8-79).[5,6] Laparoscopic scans of the liver and pancreas and surrounding portal vein, hepatic artery, gastroduodenal artery, and regional lymph nodes provide colored maps and information on turbulent blood flow. If pancreatic tumors have metastasized to the liver or invaded the surrounding blood vessels, the patients may not be considered good candidates for surgical resection.

ISLET CELL TUMOR ENUCLEATION

Benign insulinomas in humans usually lie within the pancreatic fascia and are often intraparenchymal.[7] Ultrasonography reveals a well-defined hyperechoic lesion. If the lesion can be localized, the pancreatic parenchyma is incised at the site. The lesion bulges through the incision, and an ultrasonic scalpel is used to dissect and ligate the lesion from the surrounding pancreas. The specimen is placed in a plastic bag and removed through one of the ports. Frozen sections are submitted to ensure correct lesion identification before closure. The defect in the pancreas is closed with sutures. A drain is placed, and somatostatin is administered for three days.

PANCREATIC BIOPSY

Biopsy specimens are usually obtained from the margin of the pancreas to avoid transecting the pancreatic ducts.

Samples for cytology and microbiologic culture can be obtained by fine-needle aspiration. A long spinal needle is inserted percutaneously and a syringe is aspirated to obtain a sample. Tru-Cut* needles can be introduced percutaneously to obtain a core biopsy specimen of the pancreas. A wedge excision can be performed by dissecting between the nodules, and isolating and ligating the blood vessels and ducts with clips or sutures. The sample is then removed. Similar to the technique for performing liver biopsy, biopsy cup forceps can be used to grasp tissue and take a small sample of the pancreas.

PARTIAL PANCREATECTOMY

A larger portion of pancreas can be resected by dissection and ligation or by a suture fracture technique with loop ligatures.[8] The distal portion of either lobe can be removed by incising the peritoneum, isolating the blood supply, and using an Endoloop and scissors or endoscopic linear cutter to ligate and transect the pancreatic duct and vasculature (Fig. 8-80). The defect in the mesentery is apposed with sutures or staples.

DISTAL PANCREATECTOMY

Minimally invasive approaches are used in human surgery to perform pancreatic resections to treat cancer, intractable pain from chronic pancreatitis, pancreatic trauma, and islet cell tumors. Operative steps include entering the lesser sac and mobilizing the stomach, dissecting and ligating the splenic artery, mobilizing the pancreas from retroperitoneal structures, transecting the distal part of the pancreas with a surgical stapler, mobilizing the distal part of the pancreas en bloc with the spleen, removing the specimen, and placing drains to the pancreatic stump.[7]

Laparoscopic distal pancreatectomy was developed in six swine for surgeons to refine their techniques before performing the procedure in humans.[9] After insufflation to 12 mm Hg, five 10/12 mm ports were inserted. The primary port was placed caudal to the umbilicus, and other ports were placed in each of the abdominal quadrants. Babcock forceps were used to elevate the stomach, and the lesser sac was entered by creating a window in the omentum. The cranial mesenteric vein was identified, and a plane of dissection was created between the vein and the dorsal aspect of the pancreas. Dissection was continued until the proximal portion of the left lobe of the pancreas could be encircled with an endoscopic linear cutter. The linear cutter was closed and fired to staple and transect the proximal part of the left lobe of the pancreas. The distal part of the left lobe was elevated and dissected from its retroperitoneal attachments. Branches of the splenic artery and vein were clipped and divided to completely separate the pancreas. The excised segment

*Tru-Cut, C.R. Bard, Inc., Murray Hill, NJ. 07974.

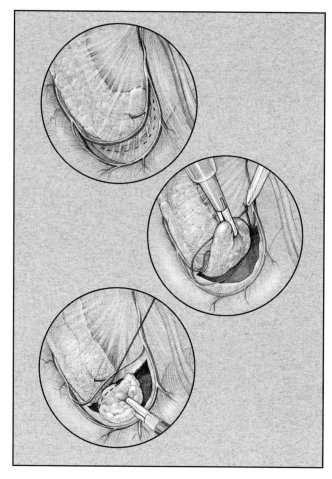

Fig. 8-80 Endoloop biopsy of the distal portion of the right pancreatic lobe.

was removed, and the abdomen was lavaged and closed. No drains were placed.

The surgical procedure required 1 to 1.5 hours. The animals had uncomplicated recoveries and tolerated liquid and solid food after surgery. They gained weight and were euthanized after 4 to 7 weeks. There were few adhesions and no evidence of pancreatitis or leakage.

CYST DRAINAGE

Pancreatic cysts can be drained laparoscopically.[10] Although 40% of small pancreatic pseudocysts in animals resolve without treatment,[8] laparoscopic techniques can be used to drain noninfected cystic structures. If the cyst is very large, it is possible to perform a cystoenteric anastomosis between the cyst and the stomach or an intestinal loop to provide permanent drainage.

LAVAGE AND DRAINAGE

Acute necrotizing or chronic pancreatitis with peritonitis and abscess formation requires careful lysis of adhesions;

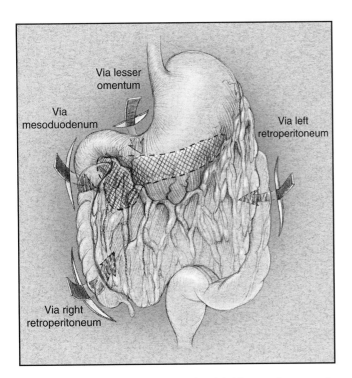

Fig. 8-81 Access to the pancreas for debridement, lavage, and drainage of a pancreatic abscess.

debridement; preservation of the vessels, nerves, and pancreatic ducts; and extensive lavage and drainage.[8] Because the pancreas is a retroperitoneal structure, approaches involve draining and debriding the retroperitoneal space.

Three approaches have been described to debride and remove necrotic tissue from an inflamed pancreas in humans, according to the extent of disease.[11] Early disease processes involving the area just around the pancreas were addressed by entering the retroperitoneal space through the abdominal cavity. The lesser sac was opened to gain immediate access to the pancreas as described previously. Additional approaches were made by incising and reflecting the peritoneum lateral to the colon and the descending duodenum (Fig. 8-81).

For early pancreatic necrosis with edema, a minimally invasive retroperitoneal approach was used to gain access to the area cranial to the kidney. With the patient in a lateral position, a small incision was made between the ribs and iliac crest. Blunt dissection was continued through the layers of muscle so a trocar could be positioned in the retroperitoneal space. With insufflation and dissection with the laparoscope, the area from the pancreas to the psoas muscle was dissected.

If significant adhesions from the pancreas to the stomach were present, a transgastric approach was used to drain and debride pancreatic abscesses or infected pseu-docysts. Trocars were placed inside the stomach, and the dorsal wall of the stomach was incised to gain access to the infected tissue.

The potential benefits of minimally invasive surgery to treat pancreatitis with peritonitis in animals are unknown. Lesions that involve substantial resection, lavage, and drainage are perhaps best managed by laparotomy and open peritoneal drainage.

BYPASS PROCEDURES

Humans with pancreatic cancer causing obstruction of the duodenum or bile duct have been successfully treated with laparoscopic procedures to bypass the obstruction.[12] Laparoscopic cholecystojejunostomy, choledochoenterostomy, and gastrojejunostomy have been performed. Surgical methods are discussed in the previous section.

Although a few clinical laparoscopic Whipple procedures (pancreaticoduodenectomy) have been performed in humans,[13] acceptance of the laparoscopic approach is unlikely even when performed by experienced laparoscopists.[14] The procedure takes several hours, requires multiple precise anastomoses, and does not result in shorter hospital stays.

REFERENCES

1. Twedt DC: Laparoscopy of the liver and pancreas. In Tams TR, editor: Small animal endoscopy, St. Louis, 1990, Mosby.
2. Iuppa A et al: Abdominal wall metastasis of pancreatic adenocarcinoma following laparoscopy. *Ann Ital Chir* 67:265-269, 1996.
3. Jorgensen JO, McCall JL, Morris DL: Port site seeding after laparoscopic ultrasonographic staging of pancreatic carcinoma. *Surgery* 117:118-119, 1995 (letter).
4. Evans HE, editor: Miller's anatomy of the dog, ed 3, Philadelphia, 1993, WB Saunders.
5. Gagner M, Pomp A, Herrera MF: Early experience with laparoscopic resections of islet cell tumors. *Surgery* 120:1051-1054, 1996.
6. Pietrabissa A et al: Laparoscopic exposure of the pancreas and staging of pancreatic cancer. *Semin Laparosc Surg* 3:3-9, 1996.
7. Cuschieri A: Laparoscopic pancreatic resections. *Semin Laparosc Surg* 3:15-20, 1996.
8. Harari J, Lincoln J: Surgery of the exocrine pancreas. In Slatter DH, editor: Textbook of small animal surgery, ed 2, Philadelphia, 1993, WB Saunders.
9. Soper NJ et al: Laparoscopic distal pancreatectomy in the porcine model. *Surg Endosc* 8:57-61, 1994.
10. Sanchez AW et al: Laparoscopic treatment of pancreatic serous cystadenoma. *Surg Laparosc Endosc* 4:304-307, 1994.
11. Gagner M: Laparoscopic treatment of acute necrotizing pancreatitis. *Semin Laparosc Surg* 3:21-28, 1996.
12. Fingerhut A, Cudeville C: Laparoscopic bypass for inoperable disease of the pancreas. *Semin Laparosc Surg* 3:10-14, 1996.
13. Gagner M, Pomp A: Laparoscopic pylorus-preserving pancreaticoduodenectomy. *Surg Endosc* 8:408-410, 1994.
14. Eubanks S, Schauer PR: Laparoscopic surgery. In Sabiston DC Jr., editor: Textbook of surgery: the biological basis of modern surgical practice, ed 15, Philadelphia, 1997, WB Saunders.

Minimally Invasive Surgery of the Large Animal Gastrointestinal System

STEVEN TROSTLE

Laparoscopy in large animals provides a minimally invasive approach to diagnosis and treatment of selected conditions of the gastrointestinal system. Although still evolving, laparoscopic procedures hold great promise for reducing postoperative morbidity as advances in techniques, instrumentation, and acceptance increase.

Special Considerations

Holding animals off feed for 24 to 36 hours before a laparoscopic procedure is performed enhances visibility in the abdominal cavity and facilitates laparoscopic manipulation by decreasing the gastrointestinal fill.[1-7] Intraabdominal pressures of 15 to 20 mm Hg provide adequate exposure with minimal cardiovascular impairment.[5,8] The volume of carbon dioxide (CO_2) required to achieve this initial intraabdominal pressure is 35 to 50 L.[4,5,7,9] Surgical or diagnostic procedures may require a total of 150 to 200 L CO_2.[4,5,7,9] An insufflator capable of maintaining a flow rate of 4 to 9 L CO_2 per minute is recommended.

Most laparoscopic instruments used in veterinary surgery were designed for use in humans. Because of the size of the abdominal cavity and viscera in large animals, a 10-mm scope and a 300 W light source are recommended to provide adequate illumination for direct viewing and video imaging.[4,7,9-11] Long hand instruments and a 57-cm laparoscope make it easier to observe and manipulate structures, particularly from the paralumbar fossa.[4,11] A 30° laparoscope is advantageous because rotating it can increase the visual field without moving the laparoscope.

Laparoscopic Anatomy

Successful laparoscopy involves knowledge of normal laparoscopic anatomy. The laparoscopic anatomy of the horse,[4,5] cow,[12] and llama[13] have been described in detail. Structures of the equine and bovine gastrointestinal systems visible from right and left paralumbar and ventral midline laparoscopic approaches are summarized in Tables 8-3 and 8-4.

HORSES

For standing laparoscopy, horses should be sedated and the paralumbar fossa blocked with regional or local anesthesia. The paralumbar fossa of a horse is smaller than that of a cow and limits placement of trocars and instrument ports. In horses, portions of the following structures are readily visible through the right paralumbar fossa: duodenum, caudate process and right lobes of liver, epiploic foramen, omental bursa, and base of the cecum (Fig. 8-82). Depending on the amount of ingesta in the stomach and right dorsal colon, the following structures can be seen: pyloric region of the stomach; gastrosplenic ligament; visceral surfaces of the left lateral, quadrate, and right lobes of the liver; common hepatic duct; and hepatoduodenal ligament.

The left paralumbar fossa provides laparoscopic access to the left lateral lobe of the liver with its associated esophageal notch and hepatic duct, caudodorsal blind sac of the stomach, spleen, renosplenic ligament, left kidney, descending colon, and lateral aspect of the transverse colon (Fig. 8-83). The following structures can be seen from either paralumbar fossa: jejunum, pelvic flexure of the ascending colon, descending colon, and rectum.

General anesthesia and assisted ventilation are necessary for horses to be placed in dorsal recumbency for ventral midline laparoscopy.[5,10] The laparoscope can be placed anywhere in the abdomen, but the umbilicus is the common landmark. Caution should be used in selecting the umbilicus as a trocar site in foals, young calves, and pigs. A patent urachus, remnant of the round ligament of the liver, or subclinical abscess from a previous umbilical infection, may be near the umbilicus. Body position affects the ability to see abdominal structures. Tilting the surgery table to elevate either the head or tail increases visibility of the cranial or caudal parts of the abdominal cavity. A 30° head-down (Trendelenburg) position helps expose the caudal parts of the abdominal cavity, whereas a 30° head-up (reverse Trendelenburg) position helps expose the cranial parts of the abdominal cavity. It is advisable to secure the horse to the surgery table with ropes to minimize sliding when the table is tilted. Gastrointestinal structures observed include the ascending colon, cecum, ileum, jejunum, stomach, spleen, and liver.

CATTLE

Cattle should be sedated and have local or regional anesthesia of the paralumbar fossa. From the left paralumbar fossa, the rumen is the most noticeable and space-

TABLE 8-3

Structures of the GI System Visible in Horses*

VISCERA	STANDING R-PLF†	STANDING L-LPF†	VENTRAL MIDLINE HEAD-DOWN POSITION†	VENTRAL MIDLINE HEAD-UP POSITION†
Stomach	+++	+++	0	++++
Pylorus	++−++++	0	0	0
Duodenum	++++	0	0	0
Jejunum	++++	+++	+++	+++
Ileum	+	0	0	++
Cecum	++++	0	++++	++++
Ascending colon				
Dorsal	++++	++++	++	++
Ventral	++	++	++++	++++
Transverse colon		++++	0	0
Descending colon	++++	++++	++++	+
Rectum	++++	++++	++++	+
Spleen	0	++++	+++	+++
Gastrosplenic ligament	0	++−++++	++	++
Renosplenic ligament	0	++++	0	0
Kidney				
Right	++++	0	0	0
Left	0	++++	0	0
Liver				
Left medial	++−++++	++++	++	++++
Left lateral	++−++++	++++	++	++++
Quadrate	++−++++	0	+	++++
Caudate	++++	0	0	0
Right lobes	++−++++	0	++	++++
Common hepatic duct	++−++++	++++	0	++
Hepatoduodenal ligament	++−++++	0	0	0
Epiploic foramen	++++	0	0	0

*Visibility of organs within the abdominal cavity varies with the amount of gastrointestinal fill and the length and angulation (0° vs. 30°) of the laparoscope.
†0 = <5%; + = 25%; ++ = 50%; +++ = 75%; ++++ = >90%.

TABLE 8-4

Structures of the GI System Observed in Cattle*

VISCERA	STANDING R-PLF†	STANDING L-PLF†	CRANIOVENTRAL MIDLINE†
Rumen	+++	++++	++++
Reticulum	0	0	++++
Abomasum	0	0	++++
Pylorus	++	0	++++
Duodenum	++++	0	0
Small intestine	++++	++++	0
Cecum	+++	0	0
Spiral colon	0	+	0
Descending colon	++++	0	0
Liver			
Right and caudate lobes	++++	0	0
Left lobe	0	0	+++
Spleen	0	++	++++
Pancreas	++++	0	0
Kidney			
Right	++++	0	0
Left	0	++++	0
Gallbladder	0	0	0

*Visibility of organs within the abdominal cavity varies with the amount of gastrointestinal fill and the length and angulation (0° vs. 30°) of the laparoscope.
†0 = <5%; + = 25%; ++ = 50%; +++ = 75%; ++++ = >90%.

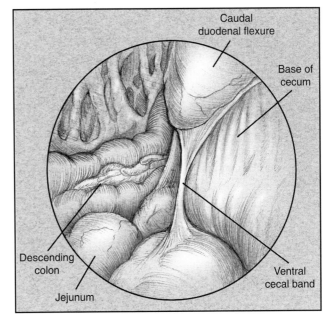

Fig. 8-82 Laparoscopic view from the right paralumbar fossa in a standing horse. The descending duodenum is readily identified. This procedure may be helpful in differentiating a strangulating small intestinal lesion from proximal duodenitis-jejunitis.

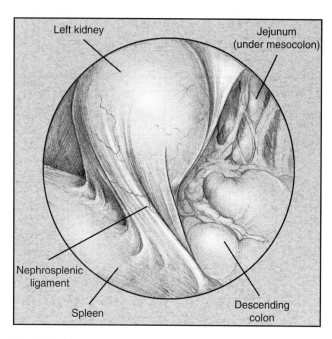

Left kidney

Jejunum
(under mesocolon)

Nephrosplenic
ligament

Spleen

Descending
colon

Fig. 8-83 Laparoscopic view from the left paralumbar fossa in a standing horse. The perirenal fat of the left kidney, renosplenic ligament, and spleen are readily identified.

occupying structure.[10] The spleen, left kidney, and small intestine caudomedial to the rumen are also visible. The reticulum may not be visible with a 33-cm 0° forward-viewing scope, but it can be seen with a 57-cm 30° laparoscope.

From the right paralumbar fossa, the descending duodenum, caudate and right liver lobes, right kidney, body and right lobe of the pancreas, free edge of the greater omentum, descending colon, jejunum, cecum, and spiral colon can be identified. The omental sling obscures the craniomedial aspect of the right paralumbar fossa, so the cystic duct and gallbladder may not be visible. Using a 30° laparoscope allows the practitioner to look around the omental sling.

Unlike horses, healthy cattle placed in dorsal recumbency require only sedation and not general anesthesia.[12] In dorsal recumbency a cranioventral approach 10 cm caudal to the xiphoid process is required because the omentum obscures the caudal part of the abdomen. The rumen, reticulum, abomasum, pylorus, and spleen are identifiable.

Laparoscopic Procedures of the Gastrointestinal System

DIAGNOSTICS
Initially, laparoscopy in large animals was used for inspection of the abdominal cavity.[4,5,10,12,13] Now, laparoscopic

surgical procedures are being developed as instrumentation and ingenuity continue to improve.* Laparoscopy is useful not only in diagnosing and treating disease, but also it can be used to help formulate plans for conventional surgical corrections.

Laparoscopy can be helpful in determining the extent and degree of metastatic disease as well as in obtaining biopsy specimens of tissues in question.[10] It can also be used to determine the extent and location of peritonitis.[11] When peritoneal fluid samples cannot be obtained by standard methods, peritoneal fluid aspirates or fibrin masses can be removed laparoscopically.[11] Confirmation and location of intraabdominal abscesses can also be performed laparoscopically. Abscesses can be aspirated to reduce their size and obtain specimens for bacterial culture.

Laparoscopy may be beneficial in evaluating the severity of rectal lacerations. Tears of the proximal portion of the rectum and distal descending colon are difficult to see or reach from either the rectum or by conventional ventral midline celiotomy. Although the procedure has not been reported, it is my opinion that standing laparoscopic techniques can be used to oversew grade III or lower rectal tears from within the abdomen. Laparoscopy can help differentiate surgical and medical diseases of the gastrointestinal system.[10] For example, by placing the laparoscope in the right paralumbar fossa, one can distinguish between proximal enteritis and strangulation of the small intestine.

BIOPSY
Biopsy of parenchymal organs, such as the liver, spleen, and kidney, has been performed laparoscopically.[10] Unlike percutaneous or ultrasound-guided percutaneous biopsy, laparoscopy allows direct inspection of the affected organ and selection of a biopsy specimen that is representative of the lesion. Specimens can be acquired by removing a full-thickness wedge resection with scissors or by using a biopsy instrument similar to conventional uterine biopsy forceps. Although hemorrhage from these biopsy sites is usually minimal, laparoscopic bipolar cautery forceps can be used to achieve hemostasis.

Full-thickness biopsy of hollow organs, such as bowel, is not recommended at this time because of inability to close the biopsy site rapidly to prevent contamination of the abdominal cavity.[10] An instrument that incises, removes tissue, and instantaneously closes the wound would be ideal. Using an automated stapling device may allow these procedures to be performed in the future. An alternative is to perform a laparoscopically assisted biopsy in which a loop of bowel is exteriorized through a mini-

---

*References 1-3, 6, 7, 9, 14, 15.

laparotomy incision. The specimen is obtained with standard techniques, and the defect is closed with sutures. The intestine is returned to the abdomen.

COLOPEXY[9]

Most laparoscopic surgical procedures developed for large animals have involved the urogenital system and the inguinal canal.[1-3,6,7,14,15] However, an experimental laparoscopic colopexy technique was developed to overcome the problems of performing a conventional colopexy in devitalized bowel.[9]

Laparoscopic colopexy is performed with the horse in dorsal recumbency under general anesthesia. After aseptic preparation and draping of the surgical field, a teat cannula is inserted into the abdominal cavity at the level of the umbilicus. After confirming peritoneal entry, the abdomen is insufflated with CO_2 to an intraabdominal pressure of 15 mm Hg. A 10-mm skin incision is made just cranial to the umbilicus to facilitate placement of a trocar (Fig. 8-84). A laparoscope is inserted into the cannula to observe placement of three instrument ports—one in the cranial and two in the caudal abdominal quadrants (see Fig. 8-84).

A 25-cm skin incision is made parallel to and 15 cm to the left of the linea alba. The assistant places laparoscopic Babcock forceps through the cranial instrument port. The lateral taenia of the left ventral colon is identified and brought to the proposed colopexy site. Suturing is started extraabdominally with size 2 nylon suture swaged to a large cutting needle. The suture tip is tagged with hemostatic forceps. The needle and suture are passed through the skin incision and through the external and internal fasciae into the abdominal cavity. The needle is grasped intraabdominally with in-line laparoscopic needle holders and guided through the seromuscular layer of the colon across the width of the taenia (Fig. 8-85). The needle is redirected to pass through the internal and external fasciae to exit in the skin incision. A continuous suture pattern is used for a length of 20 cm. This process is repeated with another strand of suture. The knots are tied and the colopexy is complete (Fig. 8-86).

The skin incision at the colopexy site and the laparoscopic port sites are closed in routine fashion. No complications were reported in the experimental study. The horses returned to unlimited physical activity 10 to 14 days after surgery and had a mature fibrous adhesion after 90 days.

LYSIS OF ADHESIONS

Laparoscopy has been used to evaluate adhesions between the abdominal wall and the reproductive tract after abdominal surgery.[10] Lysis of adhesions can be performed by gentle manipulation. Care should be taken

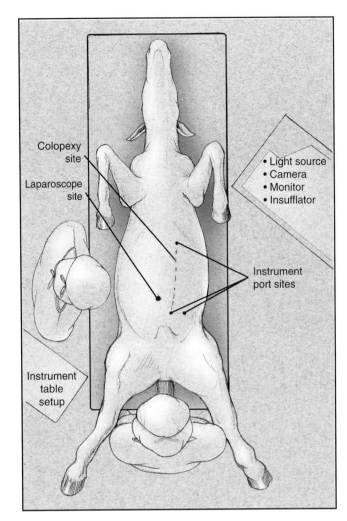

Fig. 8-84 Positioning of a horse and surgical instrumentation for laparoscopic colopexy.

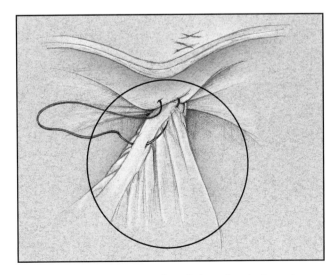

Fig. 8-85 Laparoscopic suturing of the colon during colopexy. Suture is being placed through the taenia of the lateral free band of the left ventral colon.

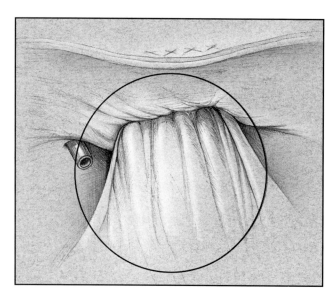

Fig. 8-86   Intraoperative view of a completed laparoscopic colopexy.

not to penetrate a hollow organ and cause contamination of the abdominal cavity.

Laparoscopic examination of adhesions involving the reticulum may be a useful way to evaluate and treat adhesions or abscesses associated with traumatic reticuloperitonitis in cattle.

Contraindications

One contraindication for laparoscopic examination in large animals is diaphragmatic hernia, in which insufflation of the abdominal cavity can cause pneumothorax. Even with assisted ventilation, the animal's respiratory function would be severely compromised.

Horses with distended abdominal viscera from strangulating or obstructive bowel disease should be approached cautiously because the bowel can be penetrated easily during insufflation or trocar placement. In these cases, an open technique is recommended for primary port placement.

Horses with lower airway respiratory disease may be at higher risk for laparoscopic abdominal procedures under general anesthesia. Horses with lower airway disease can have overperfusion of underventilated lung. This can be exacerbated by laparoscopic procedures because of the abdominal insufflation of CO_2 and the head-down (Trendelenburg) positioning.

REFERENCES

1. Fischer AT et al: Diagnostic laparoscopy in the horse. *J Am Vet Med Assoc* 189:289-292, 1986.
2. Fischer AT, Vachon AM: Laparoscopic cryptorchidectomy in horses. *J Am Vet Med Assoc* 201:1705-1708, 1992.
3. Fischer AT, Vachon AM, Klein SR: Laparoscopic inguinal herniorrhaphy in two stallions. *J Am Vet Med Assoc* 207:1599-1601, 1995.
4. Galuppo LD, Synder JR, Pascoe JR: Laparoscopic anatomy of the equine abdomen. *Am J Vet Res* 56:518-531, 1995.
5. Galuppo LD et al: Laparoscopic anatomy of the abdomen in dorsally recumbent horses. *Am J Vet Res* 57:923-931, 1996.
6. Klohnen A, Wilson DG: Laparoscopic repair of scrotal hernia in two foals. *Vet Surg* 25:414-416, 1996.
7. Ragle CA, Schneider RK: Ventral abdominal approach for laparoscopic ovariectomy in horses. *Vet Surg* 24:492-497, 1995.
8. Donaldson LD, Trostle SS, White NA: Cardiopulmonary changes during laparoscopic colopexy in dorsally recumbent horses anesthetized with halothane in oxygen. *Vet Surg* 25:181, 1996.
9. Trostle SS et al: Laparoscopic colopexy in horses. *Vet Surg* 27:56-63, 1998.
10. Fischer TA: Diagnostic laparoscopy. In Traub-Dargatz JL, Brown CM, editors: Equine endoscopy, St. Louis, 1990, Mosby.
11. Hendrickson DA, Wilson DG: Instrumentation and techniques for laparoscopic and thoracoscopic surgery in the horse. *Vet Clin North Am Equine Pract* 12:235-259, 1996.
12. Anderson DE, Gaughan EM, St. Jean G: Normal laparoscopic anatomy of the bovine abdomen. *Am J Vet Res* 54:1170-1176, 1993.
13. Yarbrough TB, Snyder JR, Harmon FA: Laparoscopic anatomy of the llama abdomen. *Vet Surg* 24:244-249, 1995.
14. Palmer SE: Standing laparoscopic laser technique for ovariectomy in five mares. *J Am Vet Med Assoc* 203:279-283, 1993.
15. Edwards RB, Ducharme NG, Hackett RP: Laparoscopic repair of a bladder rupture in a foal. *Vet Surg* 24:60-63, 1995.

C H A P T E R **9**

THERAPEUTIC VIDEO-ASSISTED THORACIC SURGERY

Laura Potter, Dean A. Hendrickson

Video-Assisted Thoracic Surgery

LAURA POTTER

Thoracoscopy is examination of the pleural cavity and its organs by means of an endoscope. The technique has been used to diagnose diseases of the thorax since 1910.[1] With the development of high-resolution microcameras, video optics, and fiberoptic light delivery systems, clear magnified images (up to sixteenfold) of the surgical field can now be transferred to a video screen. In combination with minimally invasive surgical instruments, the ability to perform advanced therapeutic procedures has been realized (Figs. 9-1 and 9-2). *Video-assisted thoracic surgery* (VATS) is a new term, recognized by the American Association for Thoracic Surgery and the Society of Thoracic Surgeons in 1991, for thoracoscopy reflecting these technologic advancements. VATS permits participation of all members of the surgical team (surgeon, assistant, anesthetist) and provides access to all regions of the thoracic cavity. VATS enables complex procedures to be performed in the thorax and expands the application of minimally invasive thoracic procedures from diagnosis to therapy, which is the focus of this chapter.

The purpose of VATS is to decrease the trauma of a conventional thoracotomy without reducing the operative exposure or diminishing a high standard of care. Potential benefits include rapid diagnosis and treatment, shorter convalescence, rapid return to full activity, and reduced postoperative pain and morbidity. VATS techniques will not supplant open surgical procedures but should become an increasingly essential part of the surgical armamentarium as we strive to improve veterinary patient care.

The surgeon's experience dictates the selection of animals for VATS procedures. The safety of the procedure depends on one's mastery of the surgical technique and effective monitoring of the animal under anesthesia. The principle absolute contraindication to VATS is inability to establish sufficient space in the thoracic cavity. Pleural adhesions from empyema or a previous thoracotomy are good examples. Relative contraindications include coagulopathies and significant gas exchange abnormalities.

Anesthesia Considerations

PREOPERATIVE PREPARATION

Preoperative anesthetic management is essentially the same for VATS as for a conventional thoracotomy. Animals are prepared for intraoperative monitoring by placing electrocardiogram (ECG) leads, at least one large-bore venous catheter, an indwelling arterial line, and a urinary catheter. Physiologic status during the procedure is monitored with an ECG, pulse oximeter, capnograph, continuous arterial line pressure, and urine output. Periodic blood gas analyses may also be indicated.

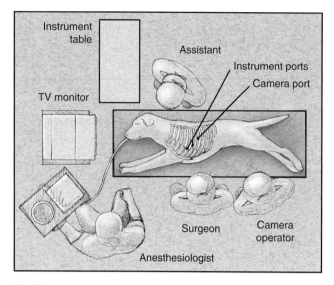

Fig. 9-1   Operating room setup for a video-assisted thoracic procedure in the cranial aspect of the thorax. The animal is in right lateral recumbency. The video monitor, anesthesia machine, and anesthetist are near the head of the animal. The surgeon, assistant surgeon, and camera operator face the video monitor. The instrument table is adjacent to the assistant surgeon.

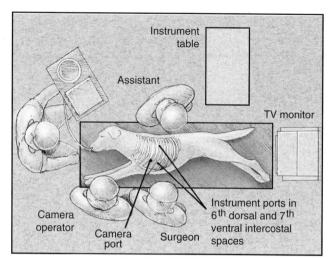

Fig. 9-2   Operating room setup for a video-assisted thoracic procedure in the caudal aspect of the thorax. The animal is in right lateral recumbency. The anesthetist and anesthesia machine are near the head of the animal. The surgeon, assistant surgeon, and camera operator face the video monitor at the end of the table. The instrument table is adjacent to the assistant surgeon.

Anesthetic considerations specific to VATS are a reflection of two techniques used to establish an optical cavity in the thorax: one-lung ventilation and carbon dioxide (CO_2) insufflation of the thorax.

THORACIC INSUFFLATION

Minimally invasive thoracic surgery differs from laparoscopic surgery in that CO_2 insufflation need not be practiced routinely. The thoracic cage creates a natural domed space when pneumothorax is established. Thoracic insufflation is used by some to limit ventilation of the lung and increase the working space in the hemithorax of interest. This technique may be adequate for minor procedures of short duration (e.g., pleural biopsies). In animals, possible complications of thoracic insufflation at low pressures (5 mm Hg) for short durations include significant hemodynamic compromise; impaired surgical exposure and a limited working space; and the risk of injury to a moving, partially ventilated lung and other thoracic structures (Fig. 9-3).[2,3] Specialized trocars with a gasket or flapper valve and sealed instruments with a round cross section are required to maintain insufflation pressure. Insufflation of the hemithorax at the beginning of a procedure to hasten evacuation of the lung is practiced by some, but in most cases it is not required.

ONE-LUNG VENTILATION

One-lung ventilation (*OLV*) refers to collapse of the lung in the operative hemithorax (usually the superior lung) and ventilation of the lung in the contralateral hemitho-

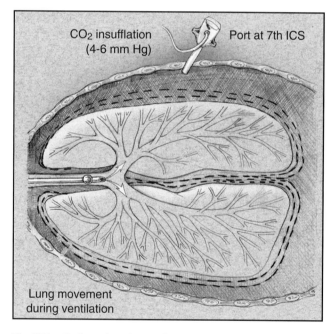

Fig. 9-3   Carbon dioxide insufflation (4 to 6 mm Hg pressure) of the operative hemithorax creates an optical cavity and limited operative space. The lung is being ventilated and will move into the optical space with each respiration (*dotted line*). *ICS,* Intercostal space.

rax (usually the inferior lung). One-lung ventilation provides a quiet surgical field and maximizes operative exposure (Fig. 9-4). It is mandatory for complete and safe vision in the operative hemithorax and safe manipulation of instruments during most therapeutic procedures.

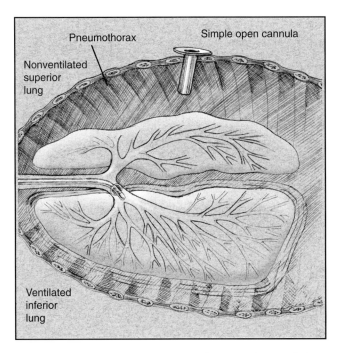

Fig. 9-4 Selective intubation and one-lung ventilation of the inferior lung. Atelectasis of the superior lung occurs with pneumothorax in the operative hemithorax. The optical space and working space are maximized. Motion is associated with ventilation of the inferior lung.

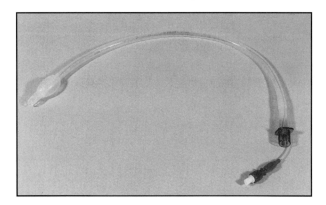

Fig. 9-5 A conventional 55-cm Silastic endotracheal tube can be used to selectively intubate most animals that weigh more than 20 kg.

BOX 9-1

RULES OF THUMB FOR ONE-LUNG VENTILATION (OLV) OF ANIMALS WEIGHING APPROXIMATELY 20 KG

Immediately after selective intubation:

a. Tidal volume $(V_T)/2 = 4$-5 mL/kg
b. Respiratory rate $(RR) \times 2 = 20$ breaths per minute (bpm)
c. Airway pressure $(P_{aw}) = 20$ cm H_2O

During the initial 30 minutes of OLV:

a. Slowly increase the V_T to approximately 10 mL/kg
b. Slowly decrease the RR to 10-12 bpm
c. Maintain a P_{aw} of 20 cm H_2O

Rules of thumb for managing anesthetized animals with OLV are listed in Box 9-1.

SELECTIVE ENDOBRONCHIAL INTUBATION

Selective endobronchial intubation in humans is performed with specialized double-lumen endotracheal tubes and endobronchial blockers. The tubes and blockers designed for humans often function poorly in animals

because of differences in the size of the tracheal lumen and location of the segmental bronchi. To selectively intubate most animals that weigh more than 20 kg, we routinely use a conventional 55-cm Silastic endotracheal tube (Fig. 9-5). For animals that weigh less than 20 kg, endotracheal tubes of an appropriate size are modified to accommodate the need for increased length (Fig. 9-6). Alternatively, endotracheal tubes with the desired dimensions can be specially ordered. Regardless of the type of endotracheal tube chosen, proper placement of the tube is essential to prevent ventilation of the lung in the operative hemithorax and maximize ventilation of the contralateral lung.

Technique

A pediatric flexible bronchoscope or general purpose 3-mm endoscope facilitates selective intubation of a primary bronchus. Selective endobronchial intubation should be performed after the animal has been fully instrumented and properly positioned on the operating table. The animal should be well oxygenated before the bronchoscope is introduced into the endotracheal tube and advanced to its distal end. The bronchoscope and endotracheal tube are advanced together until the tracheal bifurcation is identified through the bronchoscope or on the video monitor. The bronchoscope is advanced into the proximal portion of the selected primary bronchus. The endotracheal tube is guided over the bronchoscope into the bronchus. The Murphy hole (if one is present) is positioned to maximize ventilation by rotating the endotracheal tube (Figs. 9-7 and 9-8). The endotracheal tube is held in position while the bronchoscope is removed. The cuff is inflated gently, and the endotracheal tube is secured firmly to the patient.

If a bronchoscope is not available, selective intubation can be achieved by placing the animal in dorsal recumbency and directing the endotracheal tube toward the desired hemithorax. Repeated attempts may be

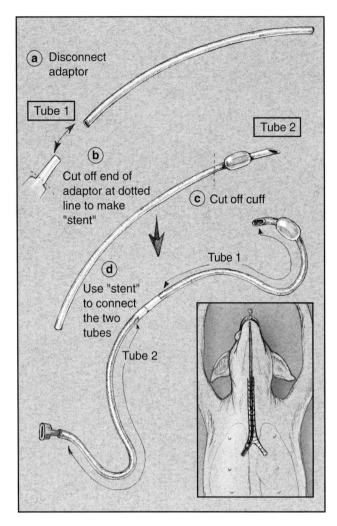

Fig. 9-6   For animals that weigh less than 20 kg, two endotracheal tubes of an appropriate size can be modified to provide the increased length required for selective intubation. The cuff and distal end of the first endotracheal tube are removed and discarded. The cut end is spliced to the tip of the second endotracheal tube's adaptor with a cyanoacrylate adhesive product. The cuff is inflated with an extension set.

required before the correct bronchus is intubated. The tendency with this technique is to advance the endotracheal tube too far into the bronchus. Proper endobronchial tube placement can be confirmed by observing more movement of the thoracic wall in the ventilated hemithorax than in the nonventilated hemithorax. One can also auscultate the thorax and hear more air movement in the ventilated hemithorax than in the nonventilated hemithorax.

When an animal has been selectively intubated properly, atelectasis of the lung in the operative hemithorax generally occurs within 5 minutes of establishing pneumothorax. If the lung in the operative hemithorax remains inflated, the endotracheal tube cuff may have expanded beyond the carina tracheae, blocking the bron-

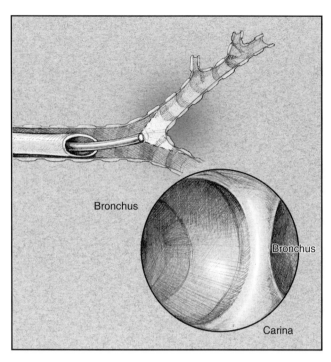

Fig. 9-7   The bronchoscope and endotracheal tube are passed through the trachea. When the tracheal carina is visible, the bronchoscope is advanced into the desired bronchus. The endotracheal tube is guided over the bronchoscope into the desired bronchus.

chus and preventing escape of residual air from the lung. If that is suspected, deflate the cuff and reinflate it slowly until it seals the selected bronchus.

Improper placement of the endotracheal tube can also prevent collapse of the lung in the operative hemithorax. The endotracheal tube may not have been advanced beyond the tracheal bifurcation, or it may not have been placed in the desired bronchus. The endotracheal tube may have been properly placed in the desired bronchus but backed out because of movement of the animal, surgical manipulations, or movement of the carina tracheae associated with ventilation. If a low SpO_2 reading is noted, ensure that the monitor is properly positioned over a moist, pink mucous membrane. Then assess the position of the endotracheal tube. It may have been advanced too far into the bronchus, or the Murphy hole (if one is present) is not being utilized.

At the completion of a VATS procedure, the endotracheal tube should be withdrawn from the bronchus into the trachea. Ventilation of the atelectatic lung can be observed directly before removal of the camera port.

VATS Surgical Instrumentation

ACCESS

Thoracic ports are rigid or flexible tubes devoid of gaskets or valves (Fig. 9-9; also see Fig. 1-27). They are placed through an intercostal space to facilitate instru-

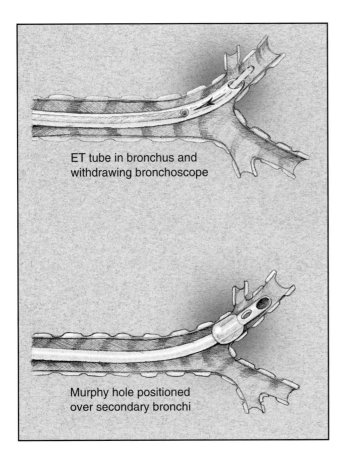

Fig. 9-8   The endotracheal tube is positioned in the proximal aspect of the desired bronchus. If present, the Murphy hole is positioned to permit ventilation of all of the lobar bronchi. The bronchoscope is withdrawn when the endotracheal tube is optimally placed.

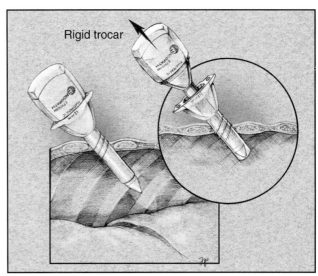

Fig. 9-9   A disposable, rigid thoracic trocar and blunt-tip obturator. There are no gaskets or flapper valves.

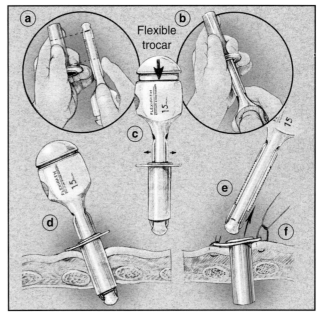

Fig. 9-10   Use of a disposable, flexible thoracic trocar. Estimate the thickness of the thoracic wall with Kelly forceps (a). Cut the flexible sleeve to the desired length (b). When the flexible trocar is inserted through the intercostal space, the cut end of the tube extends just beyond the parietal pleural surface of the thoracic wall to maximize the operative space (c). The outer flange of the trocar lies flush with the thoracic wall (d). Remove the obturator (e) and secure the flange to the chest wall with sutures or staples (f).

ment introduction and specimen removal, and to minimize trauma to the intercostal muscles, nerves, arteries, and veins. Rigid ports protect the camera lens from being smudged during introduction and manipulation, and they can be used as operating ports. Flexible ports are designed to minimize the length of sleeves protruding into the thorax and minimize damage to the intercostal bundle. The sleeve of a flexible port is cut to correspond with the estimated thickness of the thoracic wall. Flexible ports can be secured to the thoracic wall with staples or sutures (Fig. 9-10).

INSTRUMENTS

In all VATS procedures, a thoracotomy instrument pack should be available in case rapid conversion to an open procedure becomes necessary.

Specialized endoscopic graspers, forceps, scissors, tissue manipulators, and staplers are ideal for VATS procedures. Conventional instruments that can be inserted through a 1-cm intercostal incision or a flexible thoracic port, such as right-angle forceps and alligator forceps, can often be used. The ability to use conventional metal

instruments is reduced if thoracic insufflation is used to create the optical space. These instruments generally cannot be introduced through a trocar with a flapper valve or gasket. Exercise caution when using triangular lung clamps in a VATS procedure. Because of limited space, one is often required to roll the lung over the

BOX 9-2

SUGGESTED ENDOSCOPIC INSTRUMENTS FOR VIDEO-ASSISTED THORACIC SURGERY PROCEDURES IN SMALL ANIMALS*

1 10-mm endoscopic DeBakey forceps (21 cm)
1 10-mm endoscopic Glassman clamp
1 10-mm endoscopic Kelly forceps (21 cm)
2 10-mm endoscopic lung retractors (21 cm)
1 10-mm endoscopic right-angle forceps (21 cm)
1 10-mm endoscopic curved scissors (21 cm)
2 5-mm endoscopic curved dissectors
2 5-mm endoscopic graspers
1 5-mm endoscopic curved scissors (21 cm)
1 10/12 mm rigid thoracic trocar
4 15-mm flexible thoracic trocars
1 endoscopic clip applier
3 endoscopic cherry dissectors
3 endoscopic Kittner dissectors
1 Endoloop introducer
5 Endoloops
1 Endopouch (specimen retrieval bag) (2 × 2)
1 suction/irrigation unit

*Conventional metal instruments are not listed but should be available.

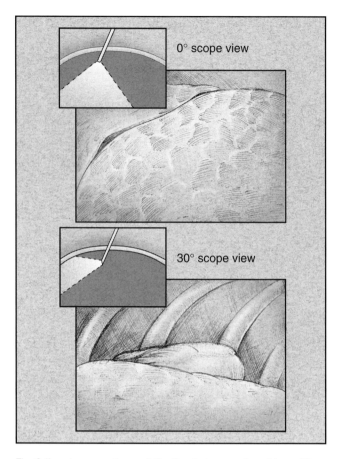

Fig. 9-11   A comparison of the fixed view produced by a 0° scope and the panoramic view produced with a 30° scope. The scopes were introduced through the same camera port at the same angle.

clamp. The sharp base of triangular lung clamps can cause parenchymal tearing and subsequent air leaks.

Instrumentation needed for selected surgical procedures is listed in Box 9-2.

SURGICAL VISUALIZATION

Rigid scopes angled at 30° or 45° permit a wide view and are preferable to 0° scopes for most VATS procedures in animals. Angled scopes reduce the "dead angle," which is particularly troublesome when examining the lateral thoracic wall (Fig. 9-11). Struggling to view a thoracic structure with a 0° scope placed at a low angle to the thoracic wall places excessive stress on the ribs bordering the camera port. The thoracic wall is depressed and deformed by the maneuver, impairing manipulation of instruments through adjacent operating ports (Fig. 9-12). Furthermore, the incidence of rib fractures, intercostal nerve damage, and postoperative pain increases.

The camera operator, who may be the primary surgeon or an assistant, has primary visual control of the procedure. It is imperative that he or she maintains proper orientation of the camera within the thorax. For example, if the animal is in lateral recumbency, the thoracic wall should be at the top of the video monitor. As each instrument is introduced into the thoracic cavity, the camera operator should offer a panoramic view. After the instrument has been guided to the operative site, an enhanced view is provided. This process is repeated each time an instrument is introduced into the thorax in order to avoid injury to intrathoracic structures. In essence, the camera operator coordinates the activities of the operative team.

Basic Surgical Procedures

Complications and frustration are minimized when the following basic surgical procedures are observed[4]:

1. Place the camera port and instrument ports at a distance from the lesion or intended surgical site sufficient to provide a panoramic view and allow room to manipulate the tissue. The camera port is routinely placed first in the sixth or seventh intercostal space, midway between the costochondral junction and the ventral border of the epaxial muscles (Fig. 9-13). To view the caudal part of

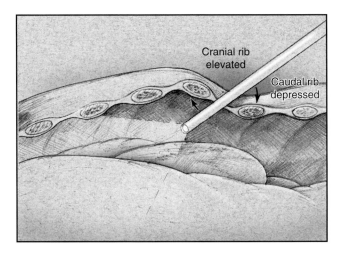

Fig. 9-12 To view the lateral thoracic wall, a 0° scope must be levered against the ribs at a very low angle. Adjacent rib fractures may occur. The thoracic wall is deformed, and manipulation of instruments through operating ports is impaired.

the thorax, move the camera to a port in the fourth or fifth intercostal space on the midlateral surface of the thorax (see Fig. 9-13).

2. Avoid placing trocars so close together that instruments interfere with each other during manipulations.

3. If possible, place the camera port and instrument ports within the same 180° arc to avoid creating paradoxical movement of instruments on the video monitor when an instrument is pointing toward the camera (Fig. 9-14). The camera and instruments should approach the lesion from the same general direction. In some VATS procedures, paradoxical motion cannot be avoided. With experience, the surgeon and assistant learn to compensate.

4. Manipulate instruments only when they are directly in view. Position or manipulate one instrument at a time.

5. Avoid synchronous, random, or rapid movements of instruments. Observing this rule minimizes the two most common complications in VATS procedures: inadvertent lung laceration and hemorrhage.

6. Consider the working length of the instruments and the space required to open instruments after they are introduced into the thorax. Open instruments while they are parallel to the lung surface (Fig. 9-15).

STANDARD THORACIC PORT LOCATIONS
The sixth or seventh intercostal space, midway between the costochondral junction and the ventral border of the

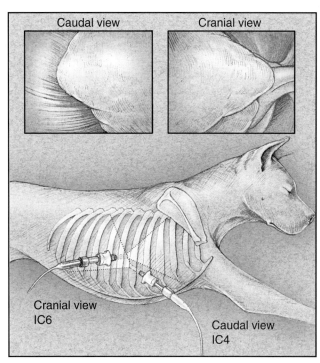

Fig. 9-13 The standard camera port location is at the sixth or seventh intercostal space (*ICS*) midway between the costochondral junction and the ventral border of the epaxial muscles. A panoramic view of the cranial and middle aspects of the thorax is achieved. A panoramic view of the caudal part of the thorax is achieved by placing the camera port at the fourth or fifth intercostal space on the midlateral surface of the thorax.

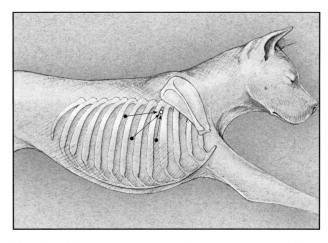

Fig. 9-14 Place instrument ports and the camera port within the same 180° arc to avoid creating paradoxical movement of the instruments on the video monitor.

epaxial muscles, is considered the *standard camera port site*. After the thorax has been explored, an operative port is placed in the fourth or fifth intercostal space at the level of the costochondral junction, which is considered a *standard operating port site* (Fig. 9-16). When a

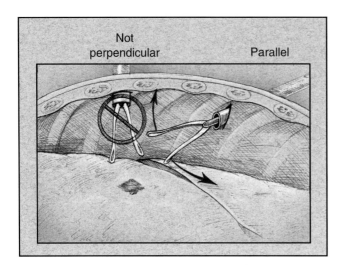

Fig. 9-15 The working length of an instrument may dictate where the operating port is placed with reference to the target anatomy. Open instruments while they are parallel to the surface of the lung.

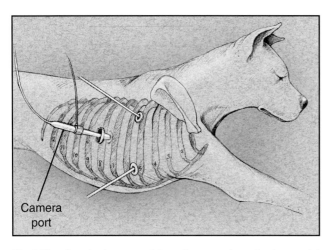

Fig. 9-16 Standard port positions for procedures in the cranial or middle parts of the thorax with the animal in lateral recumbency. The camera port is at the sixth or seventh intercostal space in the midlateral aspect of the thorax. Two operating ports are in the fifth intercostal space near the costochondral junction and ventral to the epaxial muscles dorsally. The three ports form a triangle.

caudal thoracic procedure is performed, the camera is moved from the standard camera port location at the sixth or seventh intercostal space to the operating port site at the fourth or fifth intercostal space (Fig. 9-17). A second operating port and any additional ports are placed under direct inspection, taking into consideration the location of the lesion and the surgical procedures to be performed (see Figs. 9-16 and 9-17).

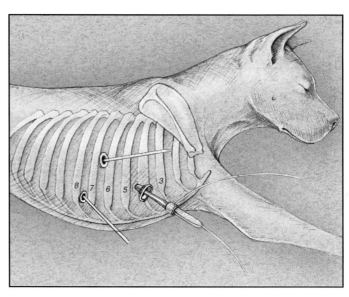

Fig. 9-17 Standard port positions for procedures in the caudal aspect of the thorax with the animal in lateral recumbency. The camera port is at the fourth or fifth intercostal space dorsal to the costochondral junction. Operating ports are at the seventh intercostal space near the costochondral junction and the sixth intercostal space at the midlateral aspect of the thorax. The three ports form a triangle.

THORACIC PORT INSERTION TECHNIQUES

Always place the camera port first. Locate the standard camera port site in the sixth or seventh intercostal space on the midlateral aspect of the thorax. Make a skin incision appropriate to the size of the port to be used. Insert Kelly forceps perpendicular to the thoracic wall, through the subcutaneous tissue, intercostal muscles, and parietal pleura. Control the depth of insertion with an index finger. Spread the tissues with the jaws of the Kelly forceps. Avoid creating a subcutaneous tunnel and inserting the Kelly forceps into the thorax at an angle, which would limit mobility of the instruments through the port (Fig. 9-18). Use direct digital palpation, if possible, to detect local adhesions. Tenuous adhesions can be broken down digitally. If significant pleural adhesions are present and a space cannot be created, consider an alternative site for the port or convert to a thoracotomy. In the absence of adhesions, insert the thoracic port and gently introduce the camera. Perform exploratory thoracoscopy. Place operating ports under direct observation, following basic surgical procedures.

In most cases, thoracic ports are not secured to the skin. This permits rapid removal of the port for introduction of a digit for palpation or standard metal instruments designed for open surgery.

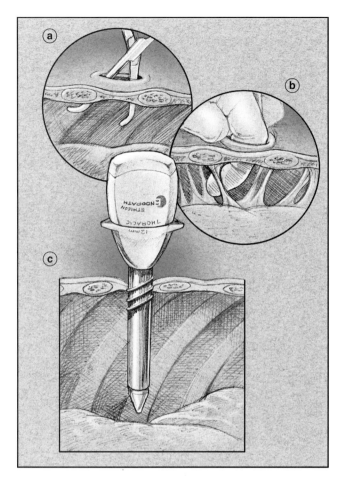

Fig. 9-18 Thoracic trocar insertion. To place a rigid thoracic port, make a skin incision of appropriate length over the desired intercostal space. Insert a Kelly forceps through the subcutaneous tissue, intercostal muscles, and parietal pleura perpendicular to the thoracic wall. Spread the tissue with the Kelly forceps to create a window into the thoracic cavity (*a*). Insert a digit to palpate for pleural adhesions (*b*). Gently insert the thoracic port with the blunt obturator (*c*).

Basic Surgical Approaches

The surgical approach is determined by the specific anatomy, manifestations of the disease process, knowledge of previous interventions, and the procedure to be performed. The most popular approaches are intercostal, paraxiphoid transdiaphragmatic, and thoracic inlet, singly or in combination. In select cases, or when mastering the VATS technique, one of these approaches is combined with a minithoracotomy. Thoracic radiographs obtained within the past 24 hours are important guides in planning the operative approach and port placement sites.

INTERCOSTAL APPROACH

The intercostal approach is the most common surgical approach in VATS. Position the animal in left or right lateral, oblique lateral, or dorsal recumbency as dictated by the procedure to be performed. Envision the location and number of ports required for the procedure before beginning placement. Consider if one will be working primarily in the cranial, middle, or caudal part of the thorax (see Fig. 9-13). Consider whether the working length of the instruments to be used will affect the operating port locations (see Fig. 9-15). Avoid the scapula, internal mammary artery, diaphragm, and epaxial muscles.

PARAXIPHOID TRANSDIAPHRAGMATIC APPROACH

The paraxiphoid transdiaphragmatic approach provides excellent visibility and access to ventral structures in the thorax and mediastinum, and access to the hilum of the lungs. It is usually used in combination with the intercostal approach for procedures such as partial pericardectomy.

Position the animal in dorsal recumbency. Make a skin incision to the right or left of the xiphoid process in the notch created with the caudocostal cartilages. Insert a rigid trocar with a sharp obturator through the abdominal wall, across the ventromedial segment of the pars sternalis muscle and into the selected hemithorax (Fig. 9-19). After penetrating the abdominal wall, reposition the trocar in the palm of the hand. Control insertion depth into the thoracic cavity with an index finger extended along the shaft of the trocar. Direct the trocar cranioventrad, lateral to the sternum. Remove the obturator and insert the camera. Inspect the thorax by advancing the camera cranially.

To avoid blind insertion of a paraxiphoid transdiaphragmatic port, place a port in the standard intercostal camera port site first. Inspect the ventral part of the diaphragm and insert the paraxiphoid transdiaphragmatic port under direct observation. Transferring the camera to the paraxiphoid transdiaphragmatic port allows the intercostal port to become an operating port (Fig. 9-20). Insert additional operative ports under direct inspection as required. If necessary, perforate the mediastinum to permit introduction of the camera into the opposite hemithorax.

THORACIC INLET APPROACH

The thoracic inlet approach is uncommon. It can be used to facilitate cranial mediastinum procedures such as thymectomy. It is usually used in combination with an intercostal approach.

Position the animal in dorsal recumbency. The port sites are left or right, between the lateral aspect of the

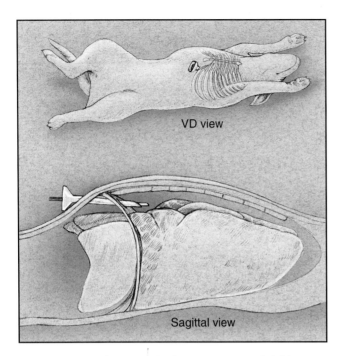

Fig. 9-19   Paraxiphoid transdiaphragmatic approach. Make a skin incision between the xiphoid process and the caudocostal cartilages. Direct the trocar cranioventrad, lateral to the sternum. Penetrate the diaphragm with the trocar sleeve.

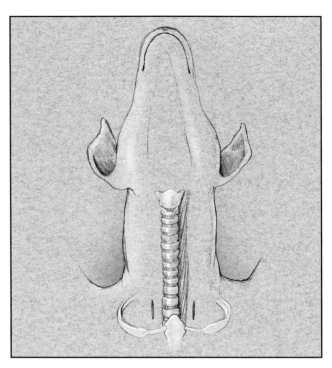

Fig. 9-21   The location for a thoracic inlet port is midway between the trachea medially and the medial aspect of the first rib laterally (external view).

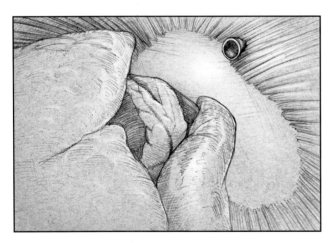

Fig. 9-20   A paraxiphoid transdiaphragmatic trocar is placed under direct vision. View the ventral diaphragm with the camera in the standard location at the sixth or seventh intercostal space at the midlateral aspect of the thorax. Observe the trocar sleeve penetrating the diaphragm.

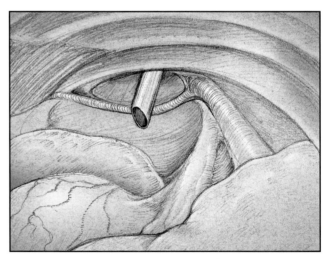

Fig. 9-22   Thoracoscopic view of the thoracic cavity with the camera inserted at the standard location and directed toward the thoracic inlet. The point of entry for a thoracic inlet port as seen from the pleural surface.

trachea and the medial aspect of the first rib (Fig. 9-21). Avoid blind introduction of a trocar through the thoracic inlet by placing the camera port in the standard intercostal camera port location first. Inspect the thoracic inlet from the pleural surface. Palpate the skin and underlying tissue

of the thoracic inlet to identify the location for the skin incision and the port insertion plane. Insert a trocar with a blunt obturator under direct observation, avoiding the internal thoracic artery and vein, brachiocephalic trunk, and common carotid artery (Fig. 9-22).

Surgical Preparation

OPERATIVE SETUP

A description of the operative setup, equipment, and instrumentation is provided in Chapter 1 and illustrated in Figs. 9-1 and 9-2.

PREOPERATIVE EVALUATION AND CARE

Preoperative evaluation of a VATS patient is identical to that of a thoracotomy patient. It should include a routine laboratory workup (i.e., complete blood count, electrolytes, blood urea nitrogen, creatinine, urinalysis, coagulation profile, ECG, and thoracic radiographs.

Clip, prepare aseptically, and drape the animal with sufficient margins to permit conversion to a standard thoracotomy or median sternotomy, if that should become necessary.

Suggested Approaches for Selected Surgical Procedures

PLEURA AND PLEURAL SPACE

The pleurae are serous membranes that cover the lungs and walls of the thoracic cavity, and form the mediastinum. The pleurae form two sacs, the left and right pleural cavities. For descriptive purposes, the pleurae are designated as *pulmonary*, covering the surface of the lungs, and *parietal*, forming the walls of the pleural cavities. The parietal pleura is further designated as *costal*, *mediastinal*, and *diaphragmatic*.[5]

VATS provides excellent visibility and access to all pleural surfaces. It can facilitate drainage of pleural effusion, drainage and debridement of empyema, pleurodesis, pleurectomy, ligation of the thoracic duct for chylothorax, and exploration and treatment of hemothorax.

Positioning and Port Placement

The choices of positioning and port placement generally depend on whether the condition is unilateral or bilateral. When a unilateral approach is indicated, position the animal in lateral recumbency with the camera port in the standard camera port location in the sixth or seventh intercostal space on the midlateral aspect of the thorax. Perform thoracoscopic exploration of the hemithorax. Place an operating port at the fifth intercostal space near the costochondral junction. Place additional operating ports as indicated by the lesion and the procedure to be performed.

If the condition warrants a bilateral approach, position the animal in dorsal recumbency. A bilateral intercostal approach or combined intercostal and paraxiphoid transdiaphragmatic approaches can be used (see Fig. 9-19).

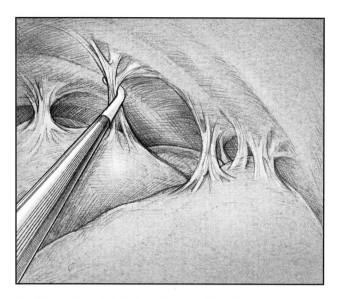

Fig. 9-23 Adhesiolysis is performed with a blunt probe or with scissors and an energy source.

Pleural Drainage

Biopsy and culture specimens are collected from selected sites. Pleural effusions, blood, and debris from the pleural space are evacuated under direct vision with a conventional curved-tip aspirator inserted through an operating port. Saline lavage is accomplished with a bulb syringe introduced through an operating port. In the treatment of hemothorax, blood clots can be aspirated or grasped and removed with a lung clamp, minimizing the potential for fibrothorax or infection. In the treatment of empyema, a multiloculated space is converted to a unilocular pleural space by performing adhesiolysis with a blunt probe or with scissors and an energy source (Fig. 9-23).

Reexpansion of lung lobes is confirmed visually after selective placement of thoracic drainage tube(s). Thoracic drainage tubes can be placed directly through a port site, but the incidence of an air leak or a sucking chest wound is increased. A thoracic drainage tube can be inserted through the skin incision at an existing port site and tunneled through the thoracic wall two intercostal spaces distant. If this technique is used, an airtight seal of the intercostal muscles at the port site must be achieved. Alternatively, the thoracic drainage tube can be inserted through a new incision in the standard fashion. The operating ports and camera port are removed. The port sites are closed in a standard three-layer closure.

Parietal Pleurectomy

Parietal pleurectomy is easily performed with VATS techniques, especially if the pleura is normal. To perform cranial partial parietal pleurectomy, place the camera port in the seventh intercostal space on the midlateral aspect of

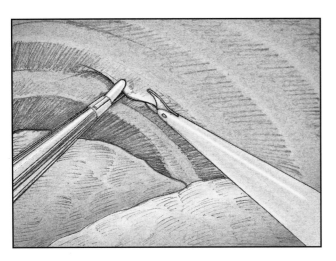

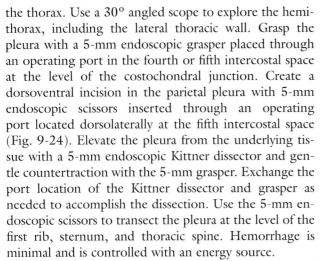

Fig. 9-24   To perform a cranial pleurectomy, a 30° scope is placed at the seventh intercostal space in the midlateral aspect of the thorax and directed cranially. Grasping forceps are placed through an operating port located at the fifth intercostal space near the costochondral junction. Scissors are introduced through a second operating port placed at the fifth intercostal space ventral to the epaxial muscles. A Kittner dissector is used to elevate the pleura.

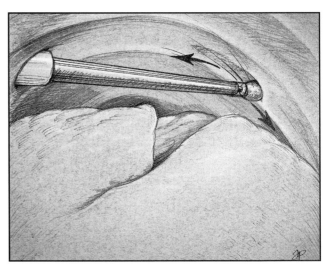

Fig. 9-25   Pleurodesis is performed with a gauze sponge or an endoscopic cherry dissector.

the thorax. Use a 30° angled scope to explore the hemithorax, including the lateral thoracic wall. Grasp the pleura with a 5-mm endoscopic grasper placed through an operating port in the fourth or fifth intercostal space at the level of the costochondral junction. Create a dorsoventral incision in the parietal pleura with 5-mm endoscopic scissors inserted through an operating port located dorsolaterally at the fifth intercostal space (Fig. 9-24). Elevate the pleura from the underlying tissue with a 5-mm endoscopic Kittner dissector and gentle countertraction with the 5-mm grasper. Exchange the port location of the Kittner dissector and grasper as needed to accomplish the dissection. Use the 5-mm endoscopic scissors to transect the pleura at the level of the first rib, sternum, and thoracic spine. Hemorrhage is minimal and is controlled with an energy source.

Caudal partial parietal pleurectomy can be performed by using the same technique with slightly different port locations. Place the camera through the port at the fourth or fifth intercostal space near the costochondral junction, directed toward the diaphragm. Use a grasper and Kittner dissector through ports at the sixth or seventh intercostal space. Elevate the parietal pleura from cranial to caudal to the level of the diaphragm.

Pleurodesis
Pleurodesis is the production of adhesions between the parietal and pulmonary pleurae. It can be a valuable treatment aid in animals with chronic pleural effusion or spontaneous pneumothorax. Pleurodesis is accomplished by mechanically abrading the pleural surfaces, or by instilling a pleural irritant (e.g., talc, tetracycline HCl, bleomycin).

Place a camera port in the seventh intercostal space on the midlateral aspect of the thorax. Perform thoracoscopic exploration of the hemithorax. Place an additional operating port in the fourth or fifth intercostal space at the level of the costochondral junction to permit insertion of an aspiration and irrigation device or a grasper-dissector, or to instill the pleurodesis agent. Ensure that all pleural fluid is completely drained and that the lung can expand fully. Instill the pleurodesis agent under direct inspection, covering all surfaces of the hemithorax.

Alternatively, the parietal pleural surface is abraded with a sponge on a grasper or an endoscopic cherry dissector (Fig. 9-25). The thoracic drainage tube is placed under direct inspection. Port sites are closed with a standard three-layer closure.

THE LUNGS
Intimate familiarity with topographic and hilar bronchopulmonary anatomy is required to plan and perform VATS procedures on the lungs. Anatomy of several domestic species is described and illustrated well in numerous texts, and therefore will not be described in detail here.[5-7] Consideration should be given to variations in lung lobation before placing operative ports for VATS lung procedures.

VATS approaches to the lung are attractive for evaluation and treatment of numerous pulmonary con-

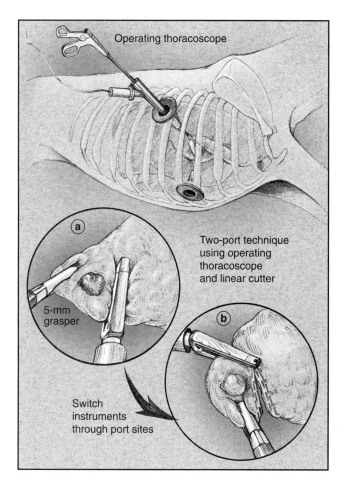

Fig. 9-26 A lung biopsy is performed using a two-port technique and an operating thoracoscope. An endoscopic grasper is placed through the operating thoracoscope port. An Endoloop or stapler is placed through the second operating port (a). Instruments are moved between ports as needed for access (b).

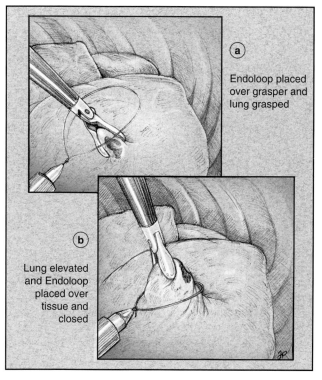

Fig. 9-27 Lung biopsy. To perform an Endoloop biopsy, place the camera port and two operating ports in the standard locations. The Endoloop is placed onto the shaft of an atraumatic grasper, and the lung tissue from which a sample will be taken for biopsy is elevated (a). Slip the Endoloop over the tissue and draw down the loop (b). The suture and tissue are transected with an endoscopic scissors.

ditions, such as diffuse infiltrative lung disease, primary spontaneous pneumothorax, lung lacerations secondary to blunt and penetrating trauma, and excision of pulmonary nodules.[8-12] Video-assisted lobectomies can be performed, although specific indications are unclear in animals and remain controversial in humans.[4,13-15]

Port Placement

For each of the pulmonary procedures described, the animal is usually positioned in lateral recumbency. The camera port is placed in the sixth or seventh intercostal space on the midlateral aspect of the thorax. The first operating port is placed in the fourth or fifth intercostal space near the costochondral junction. Additional ports are placed according to the location of the target lesion and the procedure to be performed.

Biopsy

The following technique can be used to obtain biopsy specimens in cases of diffuse lung disease, and to resect small pulmonary blebs, or bullae, in cases of primary spontaneous pneumothorax.[7,10]

A three-port technique is usually used. If an operating thoracoscope is available, lung biopsies can be accomplished with a two-port technique (Fig. 9-26). Locate the lesion with preoperative radiographs and thoracoscopic exploration. Slip a pre-tied Endoloop suture onto the shaft of an atraumatic grasper. Elevate the lung with a grasper and pass the suture loop from the shaft of the grasper onto the selected tissue. Secure the knot. Transect the tissue specimen distal to the knot and retrieve it through the thoracic port (Fig. 9-27).

Place a thoracic drainage tube in the standard fashion. Close all port sites routinely.

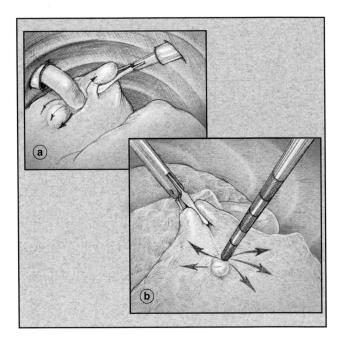

Fig. 9-28 Two methods of locating lung lesions. Use a grasper to elevate the lung lobe to digitally locate a lung lesion (*a*). Pass a blunt probe over the surface of the lung to detect nodules (*b*).

Partial Lobectomy and Wedge Resection

Indications for performing partial lobectomy or wedge resection include the treatment of bullous disease that is too large to resect with the Endoloop technique, iatrogenic or traumatic lung lacerations, and excision of pulmonary nodules. Recurrence of tumors after VATS resection of malignant pulmonary nodules has been reported in the pulmonary staple line, pleura, and subcutaneous tissues along the port tract.[13] Such retrospective studies reveal flaws in current techniques for removing malignant tumors of the thorax. The chance of tumor recurrence is decreased by utilizing a wide margin of resection and not carrying tumor cells through the thoracic incisions. Using thoracic ports during instrument introduction and removal, and using a specimen retrieval bag to remove the resected tissue from the thoracic cavity, may minimize the chances of tumor dissemination.

Use a two- or three-port technique, as described for lung biopsies (see Figs. 9-26 and 9-27). Place the camera port and first operating port in the standard locations. Explore the thorax and identify the lesion. Place the third port according to the location of the lesion and the basic principles of port placement.

One of the greatest shortcomings of VATS for resection of a pulmonary nodule is difficulty in identifying the location of the nodule without palpating the lung when the lesion is not videoscopically apparent. Techniques that facilitate nodule location include inserting a finger through the operating port site and digitally palpating the underlying lung. If the distance from the tip of the finger to the pulmonary parenchyma is too great, insert an additional operating port in a selected location, and elevate the lung lobes to the finger with a lung grasper (Fig. 9-28). One can also pass a blunt probe over the surface of the lung to detect nodular inconsistency in the pulmonary parenchyma (see Fig. 9-28). In humans, a preoperative high-resolution computed tomography (CT) scan with guided placement of a wire or color marker is used by some to identify lesions.[7,16]

Partial lobectomy or wedge resection is most easily performed if the animal is large enough to accommodate an endoscopic linear cutter with a 12-mm shaft diameter. The endoscopic stapler must be introduced into the thorax through an operating port far enough from the lesion so that the jaw of the stapler can be fully opened and maneuvered onto the lung (Fig. 9-29). Several applications of the endocutter may be required. Alternating the port locations of the grasper and endocutter may be helpful. The excised portion of lung is removed from the thorax in a specimen retrieval bag (Fig. 9-30). This method is most applicable for lesions at the margins and apex of the lung. When the lesion is on the broad, flat, costal surface, excision can be more difficult. An alternative technique in this situation is to grasp the lung gently near the lesion and elevate it to form a "tongue" of tissue. Place the endoscopic stapler at the base of the tissue tongue and resect the lesion (Fig. 9-31).

In animals too small for an endoscopic stapler, a combination of minithoracotomy and VATS can be employed. The camera port and first operating ports are placed in the standard locations. When the lesion is identified, a minithoracotomy is performed over the lung lobe containing the lesion. The lung lobe is delivered through the minithoracotomy by videoscopic guidance and an endoscopic grasper. A linear cutter or linear stapler is used to resect the lesion, as in an open case (Fig. 9-32). With this technique, the partial lobectomy can be accomplished through a significantly smaller thoracotomy incision and without spreading the ribs.

After removal of the specimen, the staple lines are inspected for hemorrhage. The lung is tested for leaks in the standard fashion by submerging the transection site in saline. If the animal is selectively intubated, the endotracheal tube must be repositioned to ventilate both lungs.

A thoracic drainage tube is inserted in the standard fashion. All port sites are closed routinely.

Lobectomy

VATS lobectomy is a technically challenging procedure and should be attempted only by an experienced thoracoscopic surgeon. VATS lobectomies are performed by

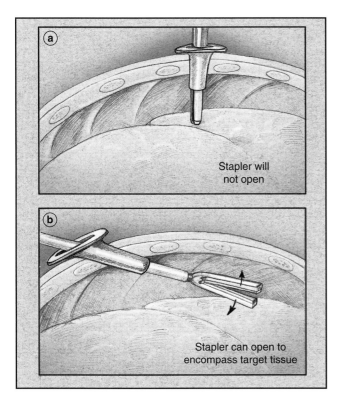

Fig. 9-29   The working length of an endoscopic stapler requires that the device be introduced into the thorax at a distance from the target lesion (*a*). The jaws of the stapler must lie completely within the thorax before they will open to encompass the target tissue (*b*).

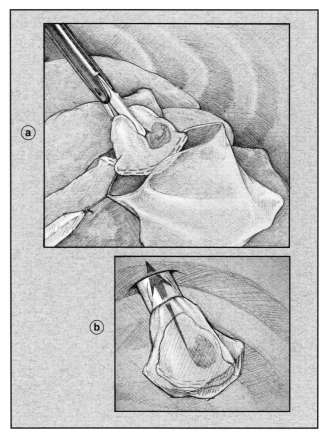

Fig. 9-30   Specimen removal. The excised portion of lung is placed in a specimen bag that has been introduced into the thorax. The mouth of the specimen bag is closed with a drawstring (*a*). The bag is removed from the thorax through an intercostal opening (*b*).

some thoracic surgeons in selected human patients.[17] The principle advantages of lobectomy over standard thoracotomy are less pain and morbidity, decreased length of hospitalization, and more rapid return to normal activities. The procedure is most readily accomplished when ligation and transection of the pulmonary artery, vein, and bronchus are performed with an endoscopic linear stapler. Human patients are usually large enough for introduction and manipulation of the stapler around the hilar structures.

The indications for performing a VATS lobectomy in animals are unclear, and the procedure is technically challenging. Use of an endoscopic linear stapler for hilar ligation is extremely difficult in most animals with small intercostal spaces and a laterally flattened thoracic cage, which provides limited intrathoracic space. The angle of approach to the hilum is usually too steep to place an endoscopic stapler appropriately.

A VATS lobectomy can be performed in animals, with slight modification of the operative techniques used in thoracotomy procedures. Four ports are usually required to facilitate introduction of a lung retractor.

Position the animal in lateral recumbency with the sternum elevated 3 to 4 inches. Place the camera port and first operating port in the standard locations. Inspect the thoracic cavity and locate the third and fourth ports to facilitate retraction and dissection of the desired lung lobe (Fig. 9-33). If the lung has an incomplete fissure, complete the fissure with an endoscopic stapler or electrocautery. Divide the pulmonary ligament if removing a caudal lobe. Expose the pulmonary artery supplying the lobe with a combination of blunt and sharp dissection. Pass a silk suture around the vessel. Tie an extracorporeal knot and slide it into position with a knot pusher (Fig. 9-34). It is imperative that no significant traction or "sawing" action be applied to the suture during formation of the extracorporeal knot and manipulation of the knot into position. Place a second ligature distal to the first one in a similar fashion. Place an endoscopic clip proximal to the proximal ligature and divide the vessel

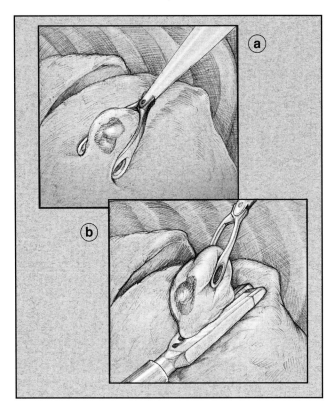

Fig. 9-31 A tongue of tissue is created by elevating tissue from the broad surface of the lung (*a*). An endoscopic stapler is fired at the base of the tongue of tissue (*b*).

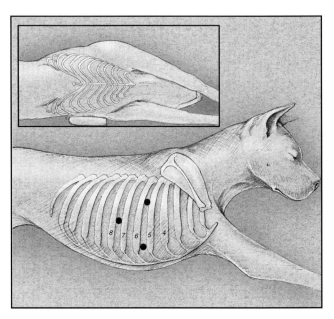

Fig. 9-33 Camera and operating port locations for a lobectomy.

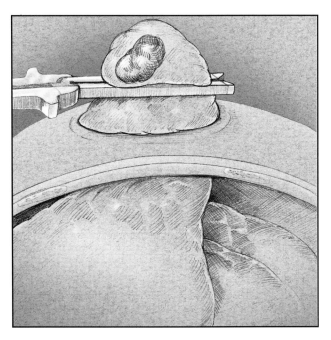

Fig. 9-32 The lung lobe is delivered through a minithoracotomy under videoscopic guidance. A linear stapler is used to transect the tissue.

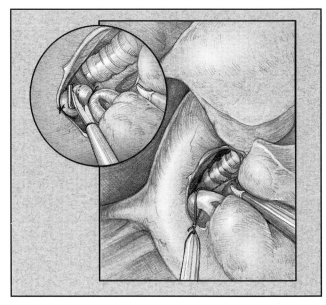

Fig. 9-34 An extracorporeal knot is positioned on the pulmonary artery with a knot pusher. Two sutures and an endoscopic ligating clip are placed on the pulmonary artery. The vessel is transected between the ligating clip and the distal suture.

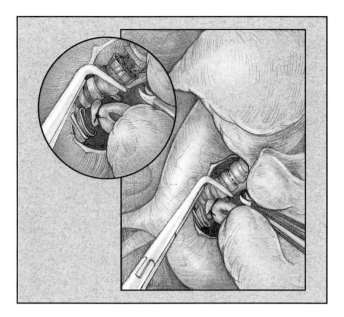

Fig. 9-35 The bronchus is cross-clamped with right-angle forceps and transected with endoscopic scissors. The bronchial stump is closed with interrupted or continuous sutures.

with scissors. Repeat this process on the pulmonary vein(s). Bluntly dissect the lobar bronchus. Cross-clamp the bronchus with a right-angle forceps and transect the bronchus with scissors. Close the proximal stump with interrupted or continuous sutures (Fig. 9-35). Place the excised lobe in a tissue retrieval bag placed through a port. Remove the port and bring the end of the bag through the port site. Cut the neck of the bag open and cut and remove fragments of the lobe from the bag until the bag and remaining lung can be withdrawn from the port site. Inspect the thorax for bleeding. Ventilate the lung and submerge the bronchial stump in saline to check for air leaks. Place additional sutures as required if an air leak is detected. Place a thoracic drainage tube and close all port sites.

THE PERICARDIUM

The pericardium comprises an outer fibrous layer and an inner serous layer. The fibrous layer envelops the heart and covers the proximal portion of the great vessels. The apex of the fibrous pericardium continues to the diaphragm and is identified as the sternopericardial ligament. The serous pericardium consists of two layers: parietal and visceral. The parietal serous layer is fused to the fibrous pericardium. The visceral serous layer is closely adherent to the surface of the heart and is called the epicardium. The parietal and visceral serous pericardial layers enclose a potential space, the pericardial cav-

ity, which normally contains a few milliliters of clear lubricating fluid.

Surgery for effusive pericardial disease is performed primarily to relieve the clinical signs and obtain tissue for cytologic, histopathologic, and microbiologic analyses. Surgery is usually performed after medical treatment, and repeated pericardiocentesis fails to resolve the effusion. Partial pericardectomy may decrease the likelihood of subsequent chronic constrictive pericarditis.

Open surgical approaches to the pericardial sac for partial pericardectomy include intercostal thoracotomy and median sternotomy. Intercostal thoracotomy provides limited access to the base of the heart. Although median sternotomy provides adequate access to all aspects of the pericardial sac, a potential complication is drainage of effusion through the sternotomy incision.

A VATS partial pericardectomy technique developed in four healthy dogs to evaluate thoracic instruments and ports was deemed feasible.[18] Postoperative pain was minimal, and recovery was uncomplicated. The trachea, phrenic nerves, lungs, and heart were unaffected, and there was no evidence of postoperative hemorrhage. In two dogs, there were mild to moderate fibrous adhesions of the right apical lung lobe to the thymus and the thymus to the adjacent ventral parietal pleura.

Port Placement

Clip and surgically prepare the animal as for a median sternotomy. Position the animal in dorsal recumbency, rolled slightly toward the right side. Selectively intubate the right principal bronchus. Place a camera port at the left sixth or seventh intercostal space on the midlateral aspect of the thorax. Inspect the left hemithorax. Identify the course of the left phrenic nerve over the base of the heart to its diaphragmatic attachment. Place an operating port under direct vision at the second or third intercostal space in the axilla. Place a third operating port under direct vision at the left paraxiphoid transdiaphragmatic position, directed into the left hemithorax (Fig. 9-36).

Partial Pericardectomy

Insert a 30° angled scope through the paraxiphoid transdiaphragmatic port and inspect the left cranial quadrant of the pericardial sac. Insert endoscopic DeBakey scissors and endoscopic graspers through the other two operating ports and begin transection of the pericardial sac at the left cranial quadrant, avoiding the phrenic nerve and left atrial appendage (Fig. 9-37). Proceed around the base of the left side of the heart, alternating placement of the DeBakey forceps and scissors in the two operating ports as needed. To approach the caudal aspect of the base of the heart, place the camera in the port at the second or third intercostal space. Insert the DeBakey for-

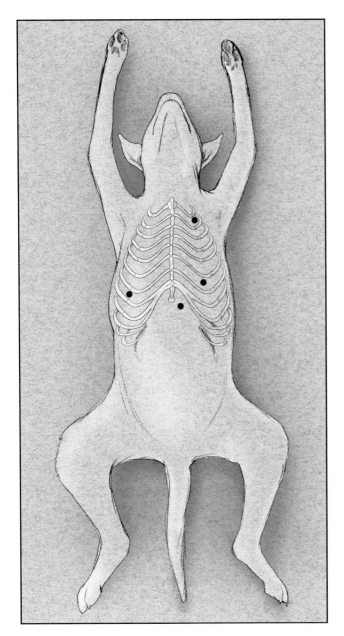

Fig. 9-36 Port placement for partial pericardectomy. The camera port is in the standard position. Operating ports are in the second or third intercostal space in the axilla and in the left paraxiphoid transdiaphragmatic position.

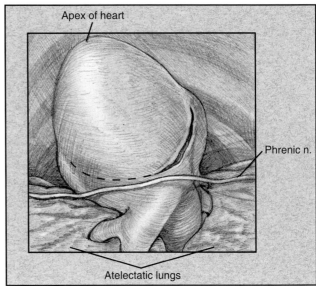

Fig. 9-37 Begin the partial pericardectomy in the left cranial quadrant. Avoid the phrenic nerve and left atrial appendage.

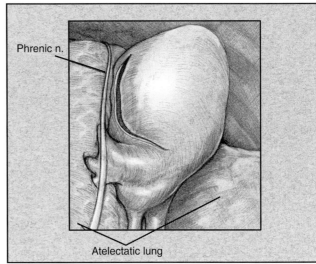

Fig. 9-38 The camera is placed in the port at the second or third intercostal space. The pericardectomy is continued around the base of the heart from left lateral to caudal.

ceps and scissors through the other two operating ports as required to transect the caudal aspect of the pericardial sac (Fig. 9-38). Continue transecting the pericardial sac from caudal to cranial on the right side of the heart. This is facilitated by rolling the animal slightly toward the left. If vision is obscured by ventilation of the right lung, consider selectively intubating the left principal bronchus. Place an operating port in the right second or

third intercostal space and complete the partial pericardectomy in the right cranial quadrant.

If infectious pericarditis is suspected, consider placing the pericardial sac in a tissue retrieval bag within the thoracic cavity to avoid contaminating the trocar insertion site. Remove the bag through a trocar site. It may be necessary to enlarge the incision. Alternatively, pull the opening of the tissue retrieval bag through the thoracic

Lung Biopsy

Position: Left lateral recumbency; Optical port: IC 6, midlateral thorax. Working ports: IC 4, dorsally and ventrally situated.

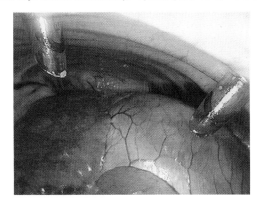

Plate 1 Thoracoscopic view of the cranial part of the porcine right hemithorax. Although one-lung ventilation was used, a small positive pressure of CO_2 (4 mm Hg) was introduced to assist in collapsing the lung to provide an adequate optical cavity. Hemodynamic parameters must be monitored continuously.

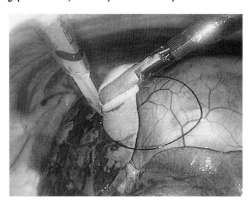

Plate 2 An Endoloop suture is used to obtain a lung specimen for biopsy. PDS material is preferred for pulmonary procedures because it slides easily. The lung is grasped gently through the loop and elevated. Atelectasis is beginning to be observed in the nonventilated lung (darker areas).

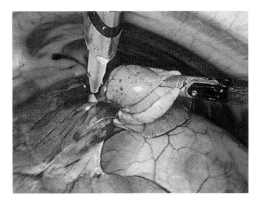

Plate 3 The loop is tightened by advancing the nylon cannula while external tension is applied to the suture. Generally, obtaining specimens for biopsy with a loop is reserved for tissues less than 1 cm in diameter.

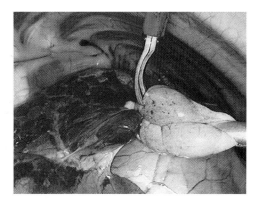

Plate 4 After the loop is tightened sufficiently, the nylon cannula is removed and endoscopic scissors are introduced through the same port. Tissue is transected distal to the ligature and removed by removing the trocar and tissue simultaneously.

Pericardial Biopsy

Position: Left lateral recumbency; Optical port: IC 6, midlateral thorax. Working ports: IC 4, dorsally and ventrally situated.

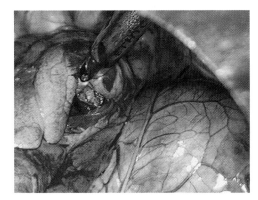

Plate 5 The collapsed lung is gently retracted dorsally to expose the pericardium covering the base of the heart. The right phrenic nerve is identified so that it can be avoided when specimens are taken for biopsy.

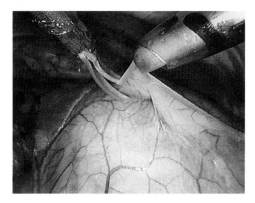

Plate 6 With scissors in the dorsal port and grasping forceps in the ventral port, the pericardium is grasped and elevated. The parietal pleura and visceral pericardium are two distinct layers that may be separated by adipose tissue. When both are grasped, they can be cut together. If not, each layer must be grasped, elevated, and incised.

Pericardial Biopsy—cont'd

Position: Left lateral recumbency; Optical port: IC 6, midlateral thorax. Working ports: IC 4, dorsally and ventrally situated.

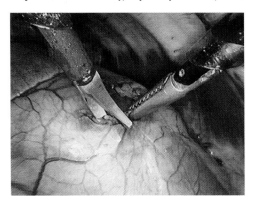

Plate 7 Tips of endoscopic scissors are visualized so that cutting can be timed with heart movement to avoid accidental cutting of the atria. Bleeding from vessels in the pericardium is self-limiting. As the forceps or scissors contact the heart, premature ventricular contractions may occur.

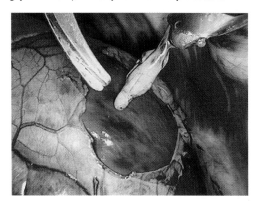

Plate 8 The specimen is removed through one of the ports. The procedure can be continued to perform a partial or total pericardectomy. In humans, removal of a postage-stamp–size portion of pericardium provides symptomatic relief of cardiac tamponade, and the pericardium does not appear to reseal.

Liver Biopsy

Position: Left lateral recumbency; Optical port: Midlateral abdomen. Working ports: Cranioventrally and caudodorsally situated.

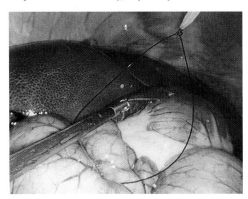

Plate 9 Laparoscopic view of cranial portion of porcine abdomen. Endoloop technique for obtaining a liver biopsy specimen. The Endoloop is introduced through a 5-mm port and positioned over the proposed site.

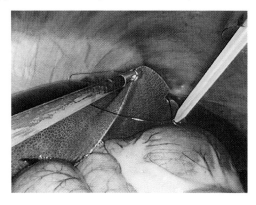

Plate 10 Grasping forceps are inserted through the loop and positioned to elevate the tissue.

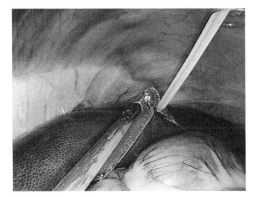

Plate 11 The loop is tightened by advancing the nylon cannula while external tension is applied to the suture. The loop is tightened to indent, but not completely crush, the tissue.

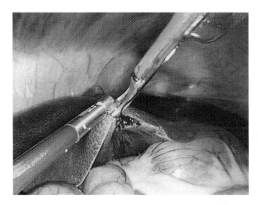

Plate 12 The nylon cannula is removed, and less tension is applied to the suture. Endoscopic scissors cut the tissue and then the suture. The biopsy specimen is removed through one of the ports.

Renal Biopsy

Position: Left lateral recumbency; Optical port: Midlateral abdomen. Working ports: Cranioventrally and caudodorsally situated.

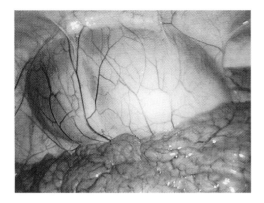

Plate 13 Laparoscopic anatomy of normal right porcine kidney. The kidney is covered by parietal peritoneum. Loops of small intestine are situated medial to the kidney and must be avoided during the procedure.

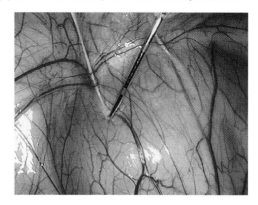

Plate 14 A 21-gauge biopsy needle is introduced percutaneously through the abdominal wall. The needle is directed into the renal cortex away from the renal hilus. Suspending ventilation temporarily while the biopsy specimen is obtained helps prevent abdominal wall movement, which causes a larger needle tract.

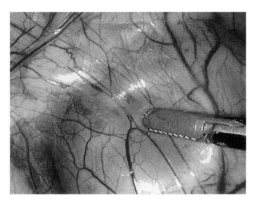

Plate 15 Following tissue removal, a small hematoma is seen in the retroperitoneal space at the point of needle insertion. Pressure is applied to the site to obtain hemostasis.

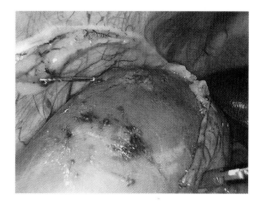

Plate 16 For better visualization of the renal parenchyma, the peritoneum can be incised and reflected medially. Unless the kidney is excessively mobile, closure of the peritoneum is not necessary following the procedure.

Pancreatic Biopsy

Position: Left lateral recumbency; Optical port: Midlateral abdomen. Working ports: Cranioventrally and caudodorsally situated.

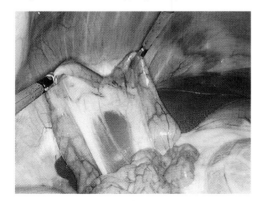

Plate 17 Normal anatomy of the porcine duodenum and right lobe of the pancreas. Two 5-mm grasping forceps suspend the duodenum. A window is created in the mesoduodenum with endoscopic scissors.

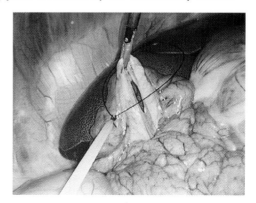

Plate 18 An Endoloop is introduced, and 5-mm forceps are passed through the loop to gently grasp the margin of the pancreas. The tissue is elevated while the loop is tightened.

Pancreatic Biopsy—cont'd

Position: Left lateral recumbency; Optical port: Midlateral abdomen. Working ports: Cranioventrally and caudodorsally situated.

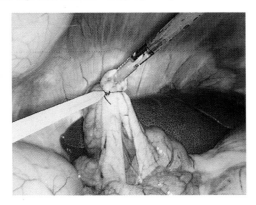

Plate 19 The nylon cannula is used to push a pre-tied knot to close the loop. To ensure accurate placement of the loop, the tip of the cannula is positioned just beneath the proposed site from which a biopsy specimen will be obtained.

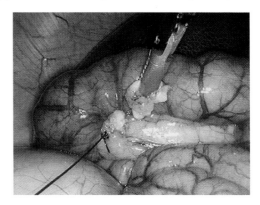

Plate 20 The cannula is removed, and endoscopic scissors are introduced beside the suture. The tissue sample is cut free and removed from the abdomen. The suture is then cut.

Experimental Minimally Invasive Thyroidectomy

Position: Dorsal recumbency; Optical port: Midline cervical area. Working ports: Caudolaterally situated.

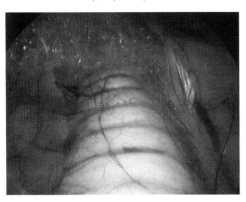

Plate 21 A balloon-tipped trocar is introduced into the pretracheal space through a small incision in the midcervical area in the dog. The balloon takes the path of least resistance as dissection progresses, sparing blood vessels and nerves. The tracheal rings are visualized through the wall of the balloon.

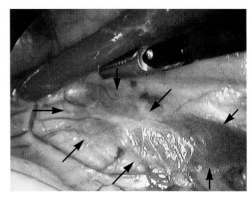

Plate 22 The balloon is deflated and removed, and a trocar is placed so that the space can be maintained with very low pressures of CO_2 insufflation (≈ 4 mm Hg). The left thyroid gland *(arrows)*, carotid artery, and vagosympathetic trunk and sternothyroideus muscle are easily identified.

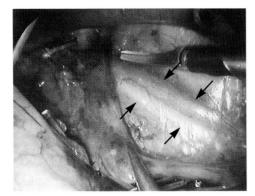

Plate 23 The thyroid gland is mobilized with a combination of sharp and blunt dissection, using endoscopic scissors and grasping forceps through 5-mm ports. The carotid artery and vagosympathetic trunk are easily identified *(arrows)*.

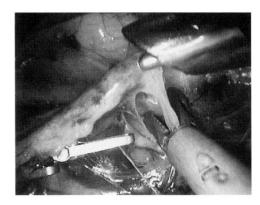

Plate 24 Thyroid branches from the carotid artery to the thyroid gland are isolated and ligated with a 5-mm endoscopic multiple-clip applier. When the gland is fully mobilized, it is removed through one of the ports.

Adrenalectomy

Position: Dorsal recumbency; Optical port: Umbilicus.

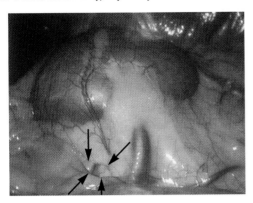

Plate 25 Laparoscopic anatomy of the normal canine left adrenal gland *(arrows)*. The gland lies beneath the parietal peritoneum cranial to the renal vein. The spleen is retracted cranially and the bowel is retracted medially as described in the legend for Plate 29.

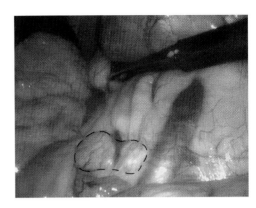

Plate 26 Endoscopic Babcock forceps are used to bluntly retract the kidney laterally to improve exposure of the adrenal gland *(dashed line)*. The gland is pink and is definitively identified by the phrenicoabdominal vein, which courses over the ventral surface.

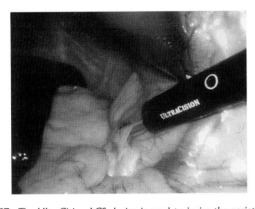

Plate 27 The UltraCision LCS device is used to incise the parietal peritoneum. Ultrasonic energy creates minimal lateral thermal damage and preserves surrounding structures.

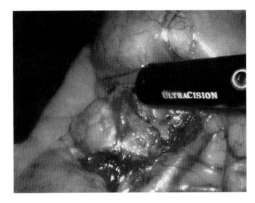

Plate 28 Continuing the dissection of the adrenal gland, the phrenicoabdominal vein is ligated with ultrasonic energy. When the gland is mobilized completely, it can be removed through one of the 10-mm trocars.

Renal Anatomy

Position: Dorsal recumbency; Optical port: Umbilicus.

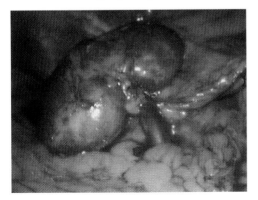

Plate 29 Normal laparoscopic anatomy of the canine left kidney. The animal is tilted to the right to allow gravity to retract bowel, and the head is placed down so that the spleen moves craniad. The ureter is identified under the parietal peritoneum with forceps. The peritoneum over the kidney has been reflected.

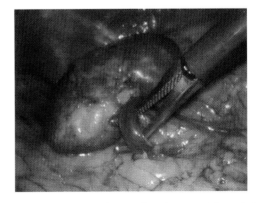

Plate 30 The renal vein is isolated with endoscopic right-angle forceps. Care is taken to avoid excessive tension during dissection. A 30° scope improves visualization.

Renal Anatomy—cont'd

Position: Dorsal recumbency; Optical port: Umbilicus.

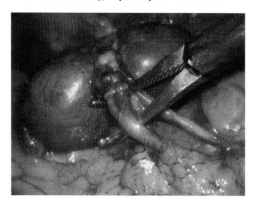

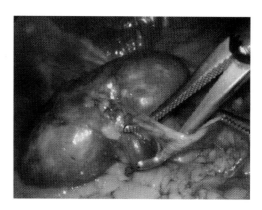

Plate 31 The renal artery is dissected. Near the kidney, the artery appears to branch. Dissection must be performed proximally to ensure that the entire arterial supply is ligated. Although not apparent in this view, if only one branch of the renal artery is ligated, only half of the kidney will appear blanched. Dissection must be continued to identify and ligate other branches.

Plate 32 The ureter is identified and mobilized as far distally as possible. Each of the structures are then ligated with endoscopic clips or staples.

wall. Cut the end of the bag open and carefully remove the pericardial sac from the bag with Allis forceps.

Inspect the thorax for points of hemorrhage. Hemorrhage is controlled with electrocautery or other energy source. Endoscopic Kittner dissectors are helpful for dissection and blunt retraction during this procedure.

Place a thoracic drain tube. Close the port sites in a standard three-layer closure.

Complications

The most common complications in VATS procedures are inadvertent lung injuries and hemorrhage.

Inadvertent lung injuries usually occur during insertion or removal of instruments through operating ports. Teamwork between the surgeon, assistant, and camera operator is imperative during these maneuvers. Lung injuries also occur when instruments are introduced into the thorax and left unattended. A member of the surgical team may inadvertently bump the instrument handle or hastily remove it, not realizing what is adjacent or what may be clasped in the end effector. Avoid leaving instruments unattended.

Depending on the severity, inadvertent lung injuries are usually managed by insertion of a thoracic drainage tube or resection with an Endoloop ligature or stapler.

Hemorrhage generally is managed in VATS procedures just as it is in thoracotomies. For immediate control, place direct pressure on the bleeding vessel or structure with an endoscopic cherry dissector, Kittner dissector, or grasper. If bleeding persists, provide tamponade with a 2-inch square gauze sponge held in a grasper. Do not release the sponge from the grasper while it is in the thoracic cavity. Use suction and irrigation to clear the field. Assess the severity of the injury and determine a course of action. Often, discrete placement of endoscopic clips or sutures is sufficient. Magnification on the video screen often makes the amount of hemorrhage appear greater than it is. With experience, the bleeding site can usually be controlled without converting to a thoracotomy.

An example of endoscopic hemorrhage control is our experience with surgeons learning to perform partial pericardectomy. The left atrial appendage is often inadvertently incised with the endoscopic scissors during its excursion beneath the pericardial sac. Hemorrhage is profuse but readily controlled by placing a grasper over the bleeding site on the atrial appendage. The thorax is evacuated of blood, and optimal vision restored. An Endoloop ligature can be placed over the handle of the grasper and guided down the shaft of the instrument into the thoracic cavity. The Endoloop suture is manip-ulated over the tissue held by the grasper and closed to ligate the lacerated site.

One should always be ready to convert to an open procedure if hemorrhage cannot be controlled.

Postoperative Care

Although the incisions are small, VATS procedures are identical to procedures performed through a conventional thoracotomy. Therefore, the same level of postoperative care should be provided.

REFERENCES

1. Jacobaeus HC: The practical importance of thoracoscopy in surgery of the chest. *Surg Gynecol Obstet* 32:493-496, 1921.
2. Hill RC et al: Selective lung ventilation during thoracoscopy: effects of insufflation on hemodynamics. *Ann Thorac Surg* 61:945-948, 1996.
3. Jones DR et al: Effects of insufflation on hemodynamics during thoracoscopy. *Ann Thorac Surg* 55:1379-1382, 1993.
4. Landreneau RJ et al: Video-assisted thoracic surgery: basic technical concepts and intercostal approach strategies. *Ann Thorac Surg* 54:800-807, 1992.
5. Evans HE, editor: Miller's anatomy of the dog, ed 3, Philadelphia, 1993, WB Saunders.
6. Slatter D, editor: Textbook of small animal surgery, ed 2, Philadelphia, 1993, WB Saunders.
7. Hare, WCD: General respiratory system. In Getty R et al, editors: Sisson and Grossman's the anatomy of the domestic animals, ed 5, Philadelphia, 1975, WB Saunders.
8. Rothenberg SS et al: The safety and efficacy of thoracoscopic lung biopsy for diagnosis and treatment in infants and children. *J Pediatr Surg* 31:100-104, 1996.
9. McLaughlin MJ, McLaughlin BH: Thoracoscopic ablation of blebs using PDS-Endoloop in recurrent spontaneous pneumothorax. *Surg Laparosc Endosc* 1:263-264, 1991.
10. Wong MS et al: Videothoracoscopy: an effective method for evaluating and managing thoracic trauma patients. *Surg Endosc* 10:118-121, 1996.
11. Landreneau RJ et al: Thoracoscopic management of benign pulmonary lesions. *Chest Surg Clin N Am* 3:249-262, 1993.
12. Sisler GE: Malignant tumors of the lung: role of video-assisted thoracic surgery. *Chest Surg Clin N Am* 3:307-318, 1993.
13. Downey RJ et al: Dissemination of malignant tumors after video-assisted thoracic surgery: a report of twenty-one cases. *J Thorac Cardiovasc Surg* 111:954-960, 1996.
14. Kohno T, Murakami T, Wakabayashi A: Anatomic lobectomy of the lung by means of thoracoscopy: an experimental study. *J Thorac Cardiovasc Surg* 105: 729-731, 1993.
15. Rossi L, Litwin DEM, Gowda K: Anatomic thoracoscopic lobectomy (ATL) without minithoracotomy: preliminary experience. *Surg Laparosc Endosc* 6:49-55, 1996.
16. Nomori H, Horio H: Colored collagen is a long-lasting point marker for small pulmonary nodules in thoracoscopic operations. *Ann Thorac Surg* 61:1070-1073, 1996.
17. McKenna R: VATS lobectomy with mediastinal lymph node sampling or dissection. *Chest Surg Clin N Am* 5:279-292, 1995.
18. Potter LA: Unpublished data; abstract, presented at ACVS 1995.

Thoracoscopic Surgery in Horses

DEAN A. HENDRICKSON

For the past 10 years, equine practitioners have used pleuroscopy to diagnose intrathoracic disease. A flexible or rigid endoscope is introduced into the thoracic cavity through a chest drain site or one of the intercostal spaces to examine the parietal and visceral pleural surfaces. The procedure is used to assist in identifying the cause of pleural effusion.[1,2] Biopsy specimens are obtained with endoscopic biopsy forceps, rongeurs, or uterine biopsy forceps.[3-5] Thoracoscopic surgical techniques have not yet been widely applied to horses.

Indications

Minimally invasive techniques allow veterinarians to examine more of the pleural cavity and its contents than is possible with a standard thoracotomy. Even with proper radiographic and ultrasound examinations, the diagnosis of pleural effusion often remains elusive. Thoracoscopy allows surgeons to identify intrathoracic masses, abscesses, adhesions, and primary or metastatic neoplasms of the thoracic cavity. The technique can be used to evaluate chronic pleuropneumonia that has not responded to therapy. Other indications for thoracoscopy include identification of diaphragmatic hernias, drainage of abscesses, and lung biopsies.

Surgical Approaches

Two approaches are used for thoracoscopic surgery in horses. Standing thoracoscopy can be performed while the animal is sedated. The horse must be able to tolerate pneumothorax without experiencing respiratory distress. Thoracoscopy can also be performed with the animal under general anesthesia with positive pressure ventilation. Techniques for one-lung ventilation have not been developed for horses, so ventilation must be controlled to allow sufficient space for examination and therapeutic procedures.

STANDING THORACOSCOPY
Preoperative Preparation
The horse need not be fasted. Administration of antibiotics and nonsteroidal antiinflammatory drugs is determined by the surgeon's preference and the disease process present.

Physical examination, including auscultation and percussion, and radiographic and ultrasound evaluations are performed to identify the proper side and site of entry.

> ### BOX 9-3
>
> ## INSTRUMENTATION FOR EQUINE THORACOSCOPY
>
> 1 30-mm rigid telescope
> 1 10-mm endoscopic lung clamp
> 1 5-mm endoscopic grasper
> 1 5-mm endoscopic curved scissors (21 cm)
> 1 10/12 mm rigid thoracic trocar
> 2 15-mm flexible thoracic trocars
> 2 Endoloops
> 1 Endopouch (specimen retrieval bag) (2 × 2)
> 1 suction/irrigation unit
> 1 chest tube
> 1 Heimlich valve

Instrumentation for equine thoracoscopy is listed in Box 9-3. Rigid scopes usually provide more light, a clearer image, and a larger field of view than flexible endoscopes. If a rigid scope is used, a 30° viewing angle provides better visibility of the thoracic cavity. Flexible endoscopes must be cleaned and disinfected properly to prevent postoperative wound infections.[2]

Anesthesia
Some horses may allow thoracoscopic examination after local infiltration of the skin, subcutaneous tissue, intercostal muscles, and parietal pleura with 2% lidocaine or 2% mepivacaine. If necessary, the horse can be sedated with xylazine (0.5 mg/kg intravenously [IV]) or detomidine (0.02 mg/kg IV), alone or with butorphanol (0.05 mg/kg).

Positioning
Place the horse in "stocks" and tie its tail to one of its legs or to the stocks to keep the tail out of the surgical field. When sedation is required, support the horse's head by suspending it from the top of the stocks. Clip and prepare the surgical field for aseptic surgery (Fig. 9-39). Drape the field to allow access to the lateral surface of the thorax. Place the video monitor in front of the horse. The surgeon and assistant stand on the same side of the animal.

Surgical Technique
It is advisable to determine if a horse can tolerate unilateral pneumothorax or if an incomplete mediastinum

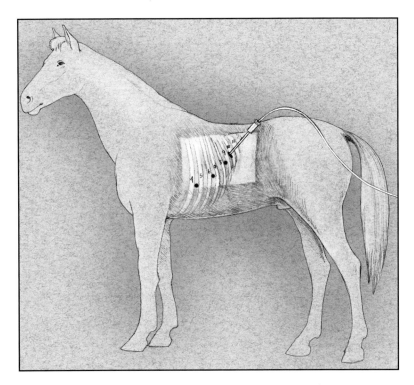

Fig. 9-39   Left side of a horse prepared aseptically for standing thoracoscopic surgery.

would make the procedure impossible. Insert a chest tube and open it to allow air to enter the thorax. If the respiratory rate increases or the horse becomes anxious, evacuate air from the chest with a vacuum pump and attach a Heimlich valve to the chest tube. If the horse cannot tolerate unilateral pneumothorax but could tolerate general anesthesia, it may be best to perform the procedure under general anesthesia with positive pressure ventilation.

Once it is established that the horse can tolerate pneumothorax, proceed with cannula placement. Make an approach through an intercostal space near the suspected lesion. The tenth intercostal space at the midlateral aspect of the thorax is used for diagnostic procedures involving the caudal part of the mediastinum.[6] The thickest part of the lung is at the level of the eighth intercostal space.[7] The left cardiac notch is at the third to sixth intercostal spaces, and the right cardiac notch is at the third to fourth intercostal spaces, ventrally.[7] Collapsing one lung allows a better view of the pleural cavity.

Make a 2-cm incision through the skin and subcutaneous tissue. Dissect through the intercostal muscles and penetrate the parietal pleura with Kelly forceps. Insert a teat cannula in the pleural space to drain any pleural effusion not removed through the previously placed chest tube. Insert a fingertip to ensure that there are no adhesions between the lung and chest wall. Insert a blunt trocar cannula to protect the telescope from bending and

---

BOX 9-4

EQUINE ANATOMIC STRUCTURES VISIBLE DURING THORACOSCOPY

RIGHT HEMITHORAX	LEFT HEMITHORAX
Aorta	Aorta
Azygos vein	Intercostal vessels
Intercostal vessels	Subclavian vessels
Esophagus	Internal thoracic vessels
Apical lung lobe	Thymus
Diaphragmatic lung lobes	Apical lung lobe
Pulmonary ligament	Diaphragmatic lung lobe
Ribs	Pulmonary ligament
Intercostal muscles	Ribs
Thoracic vertebral bodies	Intercostal muscles
Cardiac notch	Thoracic vertebral bodies
Heart	Cardiac notch
Pericardium	Heart
Diaphragm	Pericardium
	Diaphragm

the intercostal artery, vein, and nerve from trauma. Insufflation of the thoracic cavity is not necessary, so airtight trocar cannulas are not required. If additional ports are needed, flexible trocar cannulas can be used. Insert the telescope and examine the thoracic cavity (Box 9-4).[2]

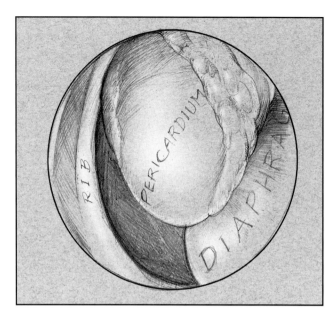

Fig. 9-40 Intrathoracic view of a standing horse undergoing thoracoscopic surgery, left side.

Use grasping forceps to harvest fibrin or exudate from the surface of lesions for microbiologic culture. Alternatively, insert a uterine culture swab through a trocar cannula to obtain a sample of fluid for culture (Fig. 9-40). Open pockets of pleural fluid or abscesses to allow drainage. Under endoscopic guidance, place drainage tubes to allow thorough drainage of the pleural space.

Lung Biopsy

Biopsy forceps can be introduced through a flexible endoscope to obtain small biopsy samples. Uterine biopsy forceps or Ferris Smith rongeurs can be passed through small intercostal incisions to obtain samples of suspected lesions. Bleeding can be controlled with bipolar electrocautery.

A biopsy specimen can be obtained from the periphery of the lung by using an Endoloop suture through a 15-mm flexible port. Slip a pre-tied Endoloop suture onto the shaft of a surgical instrument. Introduce the instrument through the port to grasp and elevate the lung. Pass the suture loop from the shaft of the instrument over the selected tissue below the instrument. Tighten the loop. Introduce scissors through the same port and transect the tissue specimen distal to the loop ligature. Remove the tissue, cut the suture 3 mm from the knot, and remove the scissors.

An automated stapling device can be used to obtain a biopsy specimen from the margin of a lung lobe. Introduce the stapler through a port located far enough from the lesion for the stapler to be opened and positioned on tissue. Close the instrument on the tissue and fire it to staple and transect the tissue. Reload, reposi-

tion, and fire the instrument as many times as necessary to perform the resection. Remove the tissue by placing it in a plastic bag or bring it directly through one of the thoracic ports.

Closure

After the examination or surgery has been performed, aspirate as much air as possible from the thoracic cavity. If necessary, insert a chest tube to permit continued evacuation of air from the thoracic cavity. Close the intercostal muscles with an absorbable, simple interrupted or cruciate suture. Close the skin incision with a cruciate suture of a monofilament, nonabsorbable suture material.

Results

Standing thoracoscopy can be performed with no adverse consequences.[1,2,6] If the other side of the thorax requires examination, it is preferable to wait at least 2 days to allow reinflation of the lung and reduce the stress of a prolonged procedure. Clinically normal horses have been examined several times without ill effect. The following conditions have been identified thoracoscopically: metastasis of gastric squamous cell carcinoma, pleural cholangiocellular carcinoma, fungal granulomatous pneumonia, bacterial pleuritis, and disseminated hemangiosarcoma.

Complications

Complications may include pneumothorax, infection, laceration of a lung, and pain.[2] Pneumothorax can occur after biopsy if the lung is not sealed adequately. Depending on the severity of the pneumothorax, air is aspirated through a teat cannula with a vacuum line or through a chest tube with three-bottle suction or a Heimlich valve. Infection can occur if endoscopes are inadequately sanitized, the disease process spreads to the surgical site, or proper antibiotic therapy is not used. Pulmonary laceration was reported when a transected syringe case was used as a trocar cannula.[2] Atraumatic entry technique, blunt-tipped trocars, and cautious tissue handling and intrathoracic manipulations are precautions to take to avoid lung injury.

Although most horses tolerate thoracoscopic surgery with local anesthesia and mild sedation, manipulation near the mediastinum, vessels, and nerves can cause pain.[2] Intrapleural instillation of local anesthetic agents could be considered in horses that appear to be particularly sensitive. Analgesics, such as phenylbutazone, are usually administered after surgery.

THORACOSCOPY WITH GENERAL ANESTHESIA

General anesthesia is used when assisted ventilation is necessary or when access to both sides of the thorax is desired during one operative procedure. General anesthesia facilitates positioning animals in lateral or dorsal recumbency to provide better access to the pericardium or ventral parts of the thorax. With its minimally invasive approach, thoracoscopy allows a surgeon to perform a thorough examination, obtain biopsy and culture specimens, and perform limited therapeutic procedures such as partial pericardectomy.

Preoperative Preparation

Fast the horse for 24 to 48 hours to decrease the volume of intestinal contents and reduce pressure on the diaphragm. Follow accepted standards for administering antibiotics and nonsteroidal antiinflammatory drugs.

Anesthesia

Anesthetize the horse as for any thoracic procedure. Provide assisted ventilation. To my knowledge, selective intubation of the horse has not been described, but the technique will be beneficial when it has been developed.

Positioning

After the horse is anesthetized, position it in dorsal or lateral recumbency. I prefer lateral recumbency for most procedures. Dorsal recumbency is used if access to both sides of the chest is required. Tie the horse to the table to minimize slippage if it becomes necessary to tilt the table. Prepare and drape the surgical site aseptically. Position the video monitor at the side of the surgery table opposite the surgeon. The surgeon and assistant stand on the same side of the animal.

Surgical Technique

Approach the lesion through the nearest intercostal space. Examine the thoracic cavity and obtain biopsy and culture samples as described previously.

Partial Pericardectomy

Partial pericardectomy is performed to obtain biopsy specimens for microbiologic culture and histologic examination in cases of chronic pericardial effusion. If medical treatment and repeated pericardiocentesis fail to resolve the condition, partial pericardectomy may be performed to decrease the likelihood of subsequent chronic constrictive pericarditis.

Place the port for the telescope at the sixth or seventh intercostal space on the left side or the fourth or fifth intercostal space on the right side, midway between the dorsal and ventral midlines. Place two additional ports for triangulation of the operative site. On the left side, identify the course of the phrenic nerve over the base of the heart. Remove only the ventral half of the pericardial sac. Insert endoscopic scissors and grasping forceps through the operating ports and begin transecting the pericardial sac below the phrenic nerve. Proceed around the base of the left side of the heart, avoiding the left atrial appendage. Alternate placement of the scope, forceps, and scissors in the operating ports as needed. Continue transecting the pericardial sac from caudal to cranial on the other side of the heart. Tilting the horse slightly may facilitate access to the opposite side of the heart. Remove the specimen through one of the ports.

Closure

Evacuate air from the chest. Consider placing a chest tube to allow continued evacuation of air and fluid from the thoracic cavity. Close the port sites as previously described.

Results

Partial pericardectomy has been performed in one horse.[8] The horse was positioned in dorsal recumbency, and ports were inserted in each side of the thorax for the scissors and telescope. Access to the pericardium was sufficient to remove the ventral portion of the pericardium without major complications. The technique should be considered experimental at this time.

Complications

In addition to the previously mentioned complications, horses anesthetized for pleural disease require close monitoring. Tissue oxygenation and perfusion should be monitored carefully because concurrent disease compromises the respiratory capacity, especially during anesthesia.

REFERENCES

1. Mackey VS: Equine pleuropneumonia: radiology—diagnostic ultrasound—pleuroscopy. Proceedings of the Twenty-ninth Annual Convention of the American Association of Equine Practitioners, Las Vegas, 1983.
2. Mansmann RA, Bernard-Strother S: Pleuroscopy in horses. *Mod Vet Prac* 66:9-17, 1985.
3. Mueller PO et al: Antemortem diagnosis of cholangiocellular carcinoma in a horse. *J Am Vet Med Assoc* 201:899-901, 1992.
4. Rossier Y, Sweeney CR, Hamir AN: Pleuroscopic diagnosis of disseminated hemangiosarcoma in a horse. *J Am Vet Med Assoc* 196:1639-1640, 1990.
5. Ford TS et al: Pleuroscopic diagnosis of gastroesophageal squamous cell carcinoma in a horse. *J Am Vet Med Assoc* 190: 1556-1558, 1987.
6. Mackey VS, Wheat JD: Endoscopic examination of the equine thorax. *Equine Vet J* 17:140-142, 1985.
7. Hare WCD: Equine respiratory system. In Getty R et al, editors: Sisson and Grossman's the anatomy of the domestic animals, ed 5, Philadelphia, 1975, WB Saunders.
8. Hendrickson DA: Unpublished data. 1996.

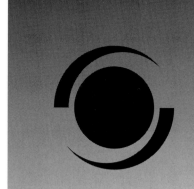

C H A P T E R 10

MINIMALLY INVASIVE SURGERY OF THE HEMOLYMPHATIC SYSTEM

Lynetta J. Freeman, Laura Potter

Laparoscopic Splenectomy

Lynetta J. Freeman

Laparoscopic splenectomy in adults and children provides smaller incisions, less postoperative pain, shorter hospital stays, more rapid recovery, and less blood loss than does open splenectomy. Because of the technical difficulties in manipulating and extracting a solid organ and the potential for significant hemorrhage, the laparoscopic approach should be applied only in selected cases. Laparoscopic splenectomy should be performed by experienced laparoscopists who are well trained in dissection, manipulation, and hemostasis and who have access to vascular staplers and coagulation methods. The relatively low number of splenectomies performed in animals may make it difficult for veterinary surgeons to progress along the learning curve for this procedure.

Anatomy

Knowledge of splenic anatomy is essential to prevent ischemic injury to the left limb of the pancreas (Fig. 10-1). The splenic artery arises from the celiac artery and branches off to the stomach as the left gastroepiploic artery and to the pancreas before entering the hilus of the spleen. Ligating the splenic artery proximal to the pancreatic branches may

cause ischemia of the left limb of the pancreas.[1] However, ligating the splenic artery distal to the pancreatic branches does not lead to ischemia of the greater curvature of the stomach.[2] The short gastric arteries and veins run from the head of the spleen to the greater curvature of the stomach within the gastrosplenic ligament. Vessels in the splenocolic ligament run from the tail of the spleen to the transverse colon. At the tail of the spleen, branches are given off to supply the greater omentum.

Indications

Neoplasia, splenic torsion, and trauma are the most common indications for splenectomy in dogs.[1] In humans, splenectomy is performed most often to treat idiopathic thrombocytopenic purpura (ITP), hereditary spherocytosis, and hemolytic anemia, or for staging Hodgkin's lymphoma.[3] Many patients with acquired immunodeficiency syndrome (AIDS) have ITP, which responds to splenectomy. Although these diseases are rarely diagnosed or treated extensively in animals, laparoscopic splenectomy may provide benefit in selected cases. An ideal indication for the laparoscopic approach is elective

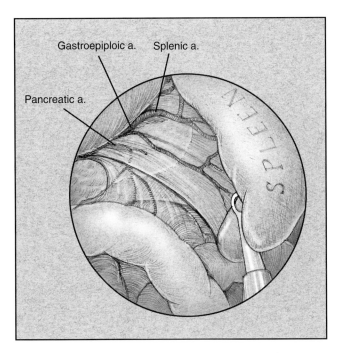

Fig. 10-1 Surgical anatomy of the canine spleen. The gastrosplenic ligament and short gastric vessels, splenic artery with gastroepiploic and pancreatic branches, and splenocolic ligament with branches to the greater omentum are visible.

splenectomy in blood donor dogs to prevent transmission of *Haemobartonella* infection.

Hemangiosarcoma is the most common canine splenic neoplasm. Splenectomy is performed as a palliative procedure to remove a source of intraabdominal hemorrhage. Splenectomy usually does not affect the survival time.[1] Perhaps in these animals, a minimally invasive partial splenectomy would cause less immunologic stress and would assist in returning the animals to their owners sooner. The procedure could be associated with increased risk of peritoneal or trocar site seeding if the specimen were not managed properly during extraction.

Splenic torsion occurs either as an acute or a chronic condition in large breeds of dogs. The acute condition is probably not amenable to a minimally invasive approach because the animal is in shock, the spleen is enlarged, and the anatomy of the twisted vasculature is confusing. Exploratory laparoscopy may be indicated to confirm and perhaps treat chronic splenic torsion. A combined splenectomy and prophylactic gastropexy could be performed through a laparoscopic approach.

Exploratory laparoscopy may be of benefit in trauma cases to confirm a diagnosis of, and potentially treat, splenic injuries.[4] Laparoscopy may also reduce the rate of unnecessary laparotomy by excluding significant intraabdominal trauma. Abdominal paracentesis and peritoneal lavage have been used routinely to confirm hemorrhage. In one study in humans, laparoscopy had higher specificity, a higher positive predictive value, and a lower unnecessary laparotomy rate than did peritoneal lavage.[5] Exploratory laparoscopy should also be considered when an animal has unexplained episodic hypotension, significant pelvic injuries, or full-thickness penetration of the abdominal wall such as stab, gunshot, or bite wounds.

Contraindications

Contraindications to a laparoscopic approach may include previous cranial abdominal surgery and severe obesity. Adhesions from previous surgery and excessive adipose tissue make hilar dissection difficult. The presence of a huge spleen is a relative contraindication, because it may be more easily injured during trocar placement and more difficult to retract for hilar dissection. An enlarged spleen obscures the visual field and is more difficult to extract. Preoperative splenic artery embolization has been described in humans to reduce blood loss significantly and make splenectomy easier to perform.[6]

Preoperative Treatment

Preoperative treatment of an animal for the laparoscopic approach is similar to that for open splenectomy. The hemodynamic and cardiovascular status of the animal is assessed and corrected. An orogastric tube is inserted to decompress the stomach.

Surgical Approaches

Two laparoscopic approaches have been described. In the ventral approach, the animal is positioned in dorsal recumbency. The ventral approach provides better access to the entire abdomen and allows for easier conversion to an open laparotomy if that becomes necessary. The animal can be tilted 45° to the right to facilitate access to and ligation of the short gastric vessels.

In the lateral approach, the animal is positioned in right lateral recumbency. The lateral approach is preferred for pediatric splenectomy[7] and was determined in one study in humans to facilitate the procedure by reducing the operative time and the number of trocars required to complete the procedure.[8] Because the anatomy of the human spleen is different from animals, caution should be used in applying the results of these studies to animals. Instrumentation requirements are listed in Box 10-1.

BOX 10-1

SUGGESTED ENDOSCOPIC INSTRUMENTS FOR LAPAROSCOPIC SPLENECTOMY PROCEDURES IN SMALL ANIMALS*

2 5-mm endoscopic curved dissectors
2 5-mm endoscopic grasping forceps
1 5-mm endoscopic curved scissors
1 10/12 mm Hasson trocar
4 5-mm or 10/12 mm trocars with reducing caps
1 endoscopic clip applier
3 endoscopic cherry dissectors
1 bipolar forceps and electrocautery cord
1 endoscopic linear cutter with vascular reloading units (3)
2 Endoloops
1 Endopouch (specimen retrieval bag)
1 electrosurgical generator (bipolar and monopolar capability)
1 suction/irrigation unit

*Conventional metal instruments are not listed but should be available.

Surgical Procedures

SPLENIC BIOPSY/SPLENECTOMY/PARTIAL SPLENECTOMY

In an anesthetized patient, the tail of the spleen is frequently located just beneath the umbilicus. An open approach for initial port placement is safest. A visual examination is performed before the spleen is identified. If desired, a percutaneous fine-needle biopsy or punch biopsy may be obtained as described for liver biopsy in Chapter 8.

Secondary ports are placed in an arc to provide the best access to the hilus of the spleen (Fig. 10-2). The first ports are placed in the right upper and right lower quadrants. An additional port may be required in the left upper quadrant. Depending on the distance from the umbilicus to the spleen, the camera port may be at the umbilicus or in the right lower quadrant. A retractor is inserted through the left lower quadrant to retract the tip of the spleen to the left side of the abdomen. The vessels to the greater omentum are identified and ligated with clips or cauterized (Fig. 10-3). Dissection is continued through the gastrocolic ligament to identify and ligate additional branches to the greater omentum.

To gain better access to the splenic hilus, the animal can be rotated 45° to the right. The camera is placed at the umbilical port. A vascular linear cutter is inserted in the right lower quadrant port and positioned on the splenic artery and vein adjacent to the hilus. The instrument is fired to staple and transect the tissue, simultane-

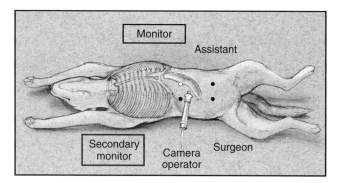

Fig. 10-2   Positioning and port placement for laparoscopic splenectomy. The animal is tilted 45° to the right.

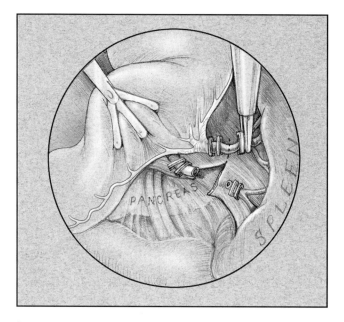

Fig. 10-3   Ligation of the splenic vessels with clips. Operative view.

ously ligating the splenic artery and vein (Fig. 10-4). Additional stapling may be required. Electrocautery is used as required to control bleeding around staple penetration sites. As dissection progresses, the epiploic branches and short gastric artery and vein are identified, isolated, and ligated.

Partial splenectomy or a large splenic biopsy can be performed by isolating the blood supply to the portion of spleen to be removed. The linear cutter is opened and placed across the splenic parenchyma, including the hilus. The stapler is closed and fired to staple and transect the spleen. Bleeding is minimal and is controlled with an energy source.

Care should be taken not to grasp the spleen with Babcock or grasping forceps because the capsule is friable and bleeding will occur. Likewise, instrument insertion and removal should be monitored carefully to avoid

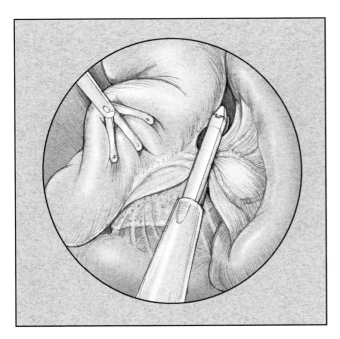

Fig. 10-4 Ligation of the splenic pedicle with the vascular stapler. Operative view.

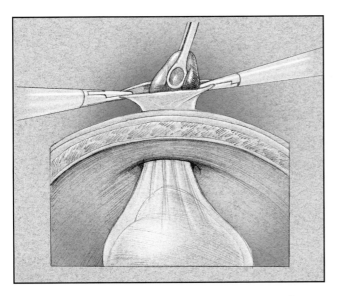

Fig. 10-5 Morcellating tissue inside a bag with sponge forceps allows the specimen to be removed through a smaller port.

inadvertent splenic puncture. A large disposable specimen retrieval bag is introduced at the umbilical port. The spleen is placed in the bag, and the neck of the bag is brought to the exterior through the midline incision. Sponge forceps, a suction device, or a finger tip is placed in the bag to morcellate the spleen (Fig. 10-5). Pieces are extracted until the bag can be removed. The trocar is replaced, and the pedicles are examined to ensure hemostasis. The abdomen is lavaged, and the port sites are closed routinely.

Evaluation of Trauma

Diagnostic laparoscopy is performed to evaluate blunt or penetrating abdominal injuries and to assess and treat splenic hemorrhage. Although splenic injuries are relatively rare, they are easily located with laparoscopy. A 10/12 mm trocar is inserted at the umbilicus by the open technique. After insertion of the laparoscope, the injury is usually located by finding bluish-tinged omentum adhered to the spleen, raised by a pool of clotted blood. The presence of severe, active hemorrhage or significant injuries to the liver, diaphragm, or intestine are indications for an open laparotomy. If the injury appears to be confined to the spleen, secondary ports are placed as described for splenectomy. Clots and blood surrounding the spleen are aspirated with a large-bore suction cannula. The extent of damage is assessed. Small tears in the splenic capsule are controlled with topical hemostatic agents, such as Gelfoam,* Avitene,† or cellulose sponges, alone or in combination with thrombin. If fibrin glue is available, it can be used effectively to control hemorrhage.[9] Extensive tears can be resected by performing a partial or total splenectomy, as previously described.

Other Applications

The spleen has been used experimentally as a site for transplantation of hepatocytes in swine.[10] The goal is to provide therapy for liver insufficiency and heritable disorders of liver metabolism as an alternative to organ transplantation. To date, researchers have been unsuccessful in transplanting more than 2% of the original liver mass laparoscopically without significant complications, including adhesion formation and portal vein thrombosis.

Results

Laparoscopic splenectomy has been reported in more than 200 human clinical cases. Of those cases, 81% to 100% were able to be completed laparoscopically. Spleen size, bleeding, obesity, and equipment failure were listed as reasons for conversion. The complication rate and long-term cure rate for ITP are similar to those for open splenectomy.

Animal studies have been conducted with swine as a training model for laparoscopic splenectomy in humans. An acute study was performed in seven pigs to refine the port placement and the technique for human surgery.[11] The procedure was performed successfully with minimal

---

*The Upjohn Co, 7000 Portage Road, Kalamazoo, Mich. 49001-0102.
†MedChem Products, Inc, 232 W. Cummings Pk, Woburn, Mass. 01801-6346.

bleeding. Others performed the procedure successfully in 10 of 12 pigs (83%).[12] Five of the pigs suffered a splenic injury that resulted in an average blood loss of 80 mL. Laparoscopic partial splenic resection was performed successfully in 20 pigs.[13] The first two pigs bled from the splenic parenchyma and hilus because of the surgeons' unfamiliarity with porcine anatomy. Hemisplenectomy was successful in all animals. Because none of these studies involved a postoperative observation period, the procedure should be considered experimental at this time. With increasing experience and access to instrumentation, the technical feasibility of these procedures will be proved in veterinary surgery.

REFERENCES

1. Lipowitz AJ, Blue J: Spleen. In Slatter D, editor: Textbook of small animal surgery, ed 2, Philadelphia, 1993, WB Saunders.
2. Hosgood G et al: Splenectomy in the dog by ligation of the splenic and short gastric arteries. Vet Surg 18:110-113, 1989.
3. Friedman RL et al: Laparoscopic splenectomy for ITP: the gold standard. Surg Endosc 10:991-995, 1996.
4. Targarona EM, Trias M: Laparoscopic treatment of splenic injuries. Semin Laparosc Surg 3:44-49, 1996.
5. Cuschieri A et al: Diagnosis of significant abdominal trauma after road traffic accidents: preliminary results of a multicentre trial comparing minilaparoscopy with peritoneal lavage. Ann R Coll Surg Engl 70:153-155, 1988.
6. Poulin E et al: Splenectomy by celioscopy: experience of 20 cases. Ann Chir 47:832-837, 1993.
7. Fitzgerald PG et al: Pediatric laparoscopic splenectomy using the lateral approach. Surg Endosc 10:859-861, 1996.
8. Trias M, Targarona EM, Balague C: Laparoscopic splenectomy: an evolving technique. A comparison between anterior and lateral approaches. Surg Endosc 10:389-392, 1996.
9. Salvino CK: Laparoscopic injection of fibrin glue to arrest intraparenchymal abdominal hemorrhage: an experimental study. J Trauma 35:762-766, 1993.
10. Rosenthal RJ et al: Techniques for intrasplenic hepatocyte transplantation in the large animal model. Surg Endosc 10:1075-1079, 1996.
11. Thibault C et al: Laparoscopic splenectomy: operative technique and preliminary report. Surg Laparosc Endosc 2:248-253, 1992.
12. Gossot D et al: Laparoscopic splenectomy: initial laboratory experience. Endosc Surg Allied Technol 1:26-28, 1993.
13. Uranus S et al: Laparoscopic partial splenic resection. Surg Laparosc Endosc 5:133-136, 1995.

Thoracoscopic Thymectomy

LAURA POTTER

Video-assisted thoracic surgery (VATS) has emerged as a viable alternative approach for the treatment of many disorders of the thorax, including spontaneous pneumothorax, empyema, and chest trauma.[1-4] The excellent view of intrathoracic structures supports VATS as a tool for the diagnosis and treatment of selected mediastinal disorders. Thymic resections for thymoma, cysts, and myasthenia gravis, and excision of ectopic mediastinal thyroid glands, lymph nodes, and neurogenic tumors have been performed.[5] The precise role of VATS in these procedures is still being defined.

The appropriateness of performing mediastinal surgery using a VATS approach is determined by the surgeon's experience and the nature of the disease process. VATS should not be used if the visibility, operative technique, or extent of a resection is compromised.

An accepted surgical approach for thymectomy in humans involves a transverse cervical incision in combination with median sternotomy. In 1992 we determined that using a VATS technique for thymectomy was feasible in dogs.[6] In attempting to identify a less invasive method for complete surgical removal of the thymus gland for the treatment of humans with myasthenia gravis, we developed a VATS technique in dogs. Clinical application of the procedure in animals is currently undefined.

Developing the Technique

Before beginning a human clinical study, techniques for thoracoscopic thymectomy were developed in dogs. Four mongrel dogs that weighed approximately 18 kg were used. The surgical approach was designed to mimic the combined transverse cervical and median sternotomy approach used in humans for complete thymectomy. That technique required tracing each of the two upper poles of the thymus into the lower neck to the level of the thyroid glands and removing all of the mediastinal and perithymic fat and lymphatic tissue to the level of the diaphragm. In the experimental study in dogs the entire thymus was removed, including mediastinal fat and lymphatic tissue from the level of the phrenic nerves to the sternum and from the thoracic inlet to the diaphragm.

Selective endobronchial intubation of the right mainstem bronchus was performed under bronchoscopic guidance. After completion of the procedure in the left hemithorax, the left mainstem bronchus was intubated to permit surgical access to the right hemithorax. Access to and visibility of the thoracic anatomy were excellent. Inserting instruments through the thoracic inlet facilitated retraction and dissection during the procedure and allowed extraction of the gland from the thoracic cavity.

It is anticipated that a surgical approach to the right hemithorax would not be required in a clinical case because, in dogs, the right thymic lobe can be reached easily from the left side.

After surgery, the dogs were humanely euthanized, and the thoracic cavities were examined via median sternotomy. The thymus had been excised completely in all of the dogs. Damage to vital structures was not apparent, except in one dog in which the left phrenic nerve had been transected at the level of the first rib. Although the VATS approach to thymectomy was feasible, this study did not include a postoperative observation period. Therefore, the procedure in dogs should be considered experimental at this time.

Indications

The most common indication for surgery of the thymus in dogs and cats is neoplasia. In those species, thymoma is the most common primary tumor of the thymus. In theory, the best candidates for video-assisted thoracoscopic thymectomy are those that appear radiographically to have a well-encapsulated, small to medium anterior mediastinal mass. However, because most thymic tumors in animals are large at the time of hospital admission, median sternotomy is usually required. A thoracoscopic approach to the thymus for intrathymic cell transplantation and inoculation studies in beagle dogs has been reported.[7]

Anatomy

The thymus is a light pinkish-gray, lobulated gland, which lies in the precardial mediastinal space, primarily in the left cranioventral part of the thoracic cavity. Two lobes are individually encapsulated, although they are difficult to separate. In dogs, the left lobe extends from the thoracic inlet to the fifth rib. The right lobe extends from the cranial pericardial space laterally.[8] The thymus extends dorsally to the phrenic nerves, cranial vena cava, and trachea. The principal blood supply to each lobe is from one or two thymic branches from the ipsilateral internal thoracic artery. Arterial branches from the brachiocephalic artery and subclavian artery may also be present. Lymph drainage from the gland is to the cranial mediastinal and sternal lymph nodes.

Procedure

POSITIONING AND PORT PLACEMENT

The entire thorax and ventral cervical region are clipped and prepared for surgery. The dog is positioned on the operating table in dorsal recumbency with a roll under the caudal cervical region to elevate the thoracic inlet.

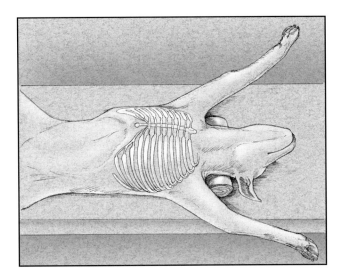

Fig. 10-6   Positioning for thoracoscopic thymectomy.

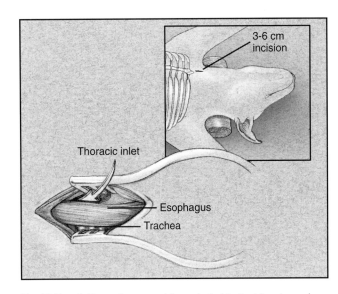

Fig. 10-7   A 3- to 6-cm caudal cervical skin incision is made to gain access to the thoracic inlet.

The right mainstem bronchus is selectively intubated under bronchoscopic guidance. The forelimbs are gently abducted (Fig. 10-6).

A 3- to 6-cm caudal cervical skin incision is made to gain access to the thoracic inlet (Fig. 10-7). The trachea and esophagus are retracted to the left. A camera port is inserted in the left sixth intercostal space, on the midlateral aspect of the thorax. Operating ports are placed, under direct vision, in the third intercostal space in the axilla and in the fifth intercostal space at the level of the costochondral junction (Fig. 10-8).

OPERATIVE PROCEDURE

Perforate the left cranial mediastinal pleura near its sternal attachment and transect the pleura to allow access to the

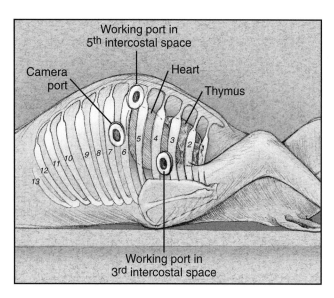

Fig. 10-8   Port placement for thoracoscopic thymectomy.

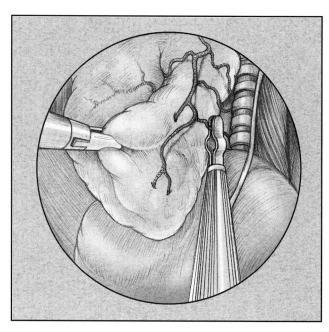

Fig. 10-10   Thymic arterial branches from the left subclavian artery are coagulated with bipolar forceps.

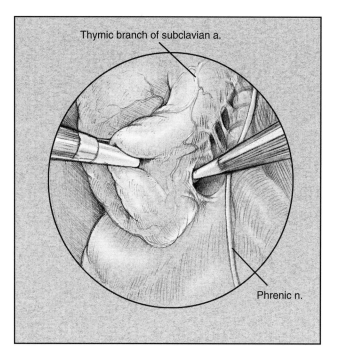

Fig. 10-9   Dissection is begun at the caudal pole of the left lobe of the thymus.

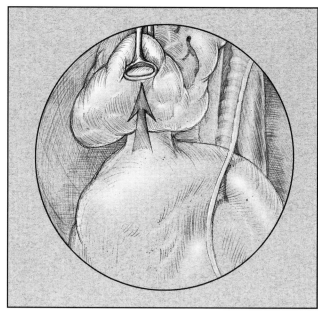

Fig. 10-11   The left lobe of the thymus is dissected to the thoracic inlet.

thymus in the precardial space. Begin the dissection at the caudal pole of the left lobe of the thymus (Fig. 10-9). Using a combination of blunt dissection with endoscopic Kittner dissectors and sharp dissection with endoscopic scissors, separate the left lobe from the phrenic nerve, cranial vena cava, and trachea, and retract it toward the midline. Proceed carefully to avoid invading the delicate

connective tissue capsule surrounding the gland. Identify thymic arterial branches from the left subclavian artery and coagulate them with bipolar forceps (Fig. 10-10). Insert sponge forceps through the thoracic inlet to grasp and retract the thymus. Continue dissection to the level of the thoracic inlet (Fig. 10-11). Bluntly dissect attachments to the sternum. Thymic arterial branches from the internal thoracic artery are coagulated with bipolar forceps and transected with endoscopic scissors.

The right lobe of the thymus is easily exposed and dissected from the left hemithorax. When all attachments are free, the thymus is extracted from the thorax through the thoracic inlet.

REFERENCES

1. Hazelrigg SR et al: Thoracoscopic stapled resection for spontaneous pneumothorax. *J Thorac Cardiovasc Surg* 105:389-392, 1993.
2. Bertrand PC et al: Immediate and long-term results after surgical treatment of primary spontaneous pneumothorax by VATS. *Ann Thorac Surg* 61:1641-1645, 1996.
3. Mackinlay TA et al: VATS debridement versus thoracotomy in the treatment of loculated postpneumonia empyema. *Ann Thorac Surg* 61:1626-1630, 1996.
4. Lang-Lazdunski L et al: Role of videothoracoscopy in chest trauma. *Ann Thorac Surg* 63:327-333, 1997.
5. Hazelrigg SR, Mack MJ, Landreneau RJ: Video-assisted thoracic surgery for mediastinal disease. *Chest Surg Clin N Am* 3(2):283-287, 1993.
6. Potter L: Unpublished data. 1992.
7. Schachner RD et al: A minimally invasive technique for intrathymic cell transplantation in the dog. *Cell Transplant* 3:349-350, 1994.
8. Evan HE, editor: Miller's anatomy of the dog, ed 3, Philadelphia, 1993, WB Saunders.

Minimally Invasive Adrenalectomy

LYNETTA J. FREEMAN

Adrenalectomy is usually performed on high-risk patients who, because of hyperadrenocorticism, have poor wound healing.[1] Open procedures involve either a midline laparotomy with unilateral or bilateral paracostal incisions, or an extensive muscle-cutting approach to the retroperitoneum. A minimally invasive approach with a small wound is ideal for adrenalectomy because adrenal masses are usually small and may be benign, and no reconstructive procedures are necessary.[2] However, minimally invasive adrenalectomy is a technically challenging procedure. The less invasive approach should be reserved for experienced laparoscopists with excellent knowledge of anatomy and advanced technical skills in delicate tissue handling and hemostasis.

Laparoscopic and retroperitoneal adrenalectomy approaches have been developed in swine so that surgeons may refine their techniques before performing these procedures in humans.[3-5] A considerable number of clinical laparoscopic adrenalectomies have been performed on humans and the procedure is considered safe and effective when performed by experienced laparoscopists. Although the operative times are initially longer, the laparoscopic approach is associated with less blood loss, less pain, and better cosmetic results; further, patients recover and are able to return to work faster.[6] No significant complications have resulted from using the minimally invasive approach.

Anatomy

The adrenal glands are retroperitoneal, adjacent to the kidney (Fig. 10-12). Their exact location varies by species. The right adrenal gland is close to the caudal vena cava. The left is adjacent to the aorta. In dogs, both

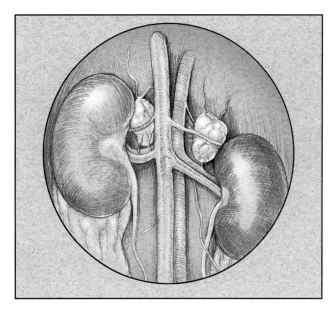

Fig. 10-12   Anatomy of the left and right adrenal glands.

glands are dorsal to the phrenicoabdominal vein and ventral to the phrenicoabdominal artery.

Contraindications and Indications

Small benign lesions of the adrenal glands are ideal for the minimally invasive approach. With increasing experience, surgeons can apply the procedure to larger, more extensive lesions. Contraindications are evidence of a tumor, such as a pheochromocytoma, invading the caudal vena cava, or any other contraindication for laparoscopy. Indications for conversion to an open procedure include inability to maintain the optical space, bleeding that cannot be controlled, excessive operative time, and tumor invasion.

Preoperative Treatment

Preoperative treatment for laparoscopic adrenalectomy is the same as for an open procedure. Metabolic derangements and fluid and electrolyte imbalances must be corrected. An evaluation for metastatic disease is performed. Administration of glucocorticoids, anesthesia, and monitoring for cardiac arrhythmias are performed in the same manner as for open adrenalectomy.

Surgical Approaches

The following are three approaches used for minimally invasive adrenalectomy:
1. Ventral transabdominal, in which the animal is positioned in dorsal recumbency and tilted from side to side
2. Lateral transabdominal, in which the animal is positioned in lateral recumbency with the affected side up
3. Retroperitoneal, in which the animal is positioned in lateral recumbency with the affected side up.

Two methods of establishing the optical cavity for a retroperitoneal approach (pneumoretroperitoneum) have been described.[3,4] Selection of the surgical approach depends on whether the condition is unilateral or bilateral, whether liver biopsies are planned, and the surgeon's preference.

VENTRAL TRANSABDOMINAL APPROACH

The transabdominal approach with the animal in dorsal recumbency facilitates exploration of the abdomen, including evaluation of the liver for metastatic disease. With proper retraction, this approach gives the same view as a midline laparotomy with bilateral paracostal incisions. The ventral approach gives access to both adrenal glands without significantly repositioning and redraping the animal. The transabdominal approaches provide the largest optical space. One disadvantage is that the colon, spleen, pancreas, and liver require retraction for optimal visibility.

The primary 10-mm port is placed at the umbilicus by methods described in Chapter 3. After insertion of a 30° laparoscope, visual exploration of the abdomen is performed. The leaves of the surgery table are adjusted to provide a 30° to 60° tilt to the side opposite the adrenal gland being removed. The animal is placed in head-up position to permit the intestines to retract into the pelvis. Two additional 5-mm ports are placed to access the right adrenal gland. One is right of the midline (to avoid the falciform ligament), midway between the xiphoid process and umbilicus. Another is placed in the right lower

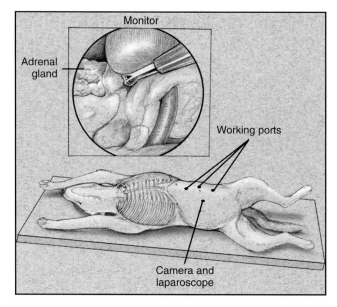

Fig. 10-13   Port placement for ventral transabdominal approach to left adrenal gland.

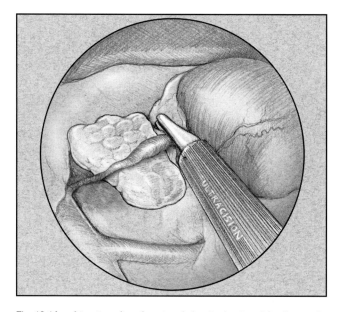

Fig. 10-14   Ligating the phrenicoabdominal vein with ultrasonic energy preserves the renal vasculature.

quadrant at the lateral edge of the rectus abdominis muscle. A 10-mm port is placed midway between the umbilicus and right kidney. For access to the left adrenal, a mirror image of port placement is used (Fig. 10-13).

The surgeon uses the two cranial ports to grasp and elevate the peritoneum lateral to the adrenal gland. The peritoneum over the adrenal gland is incised with scissors or an ultrasonic scalpel. Dissection is performed as in an open adrenalectomy, between the adrenal gland and the caudal vena cava or aorta and along the phrenicoabdominal vein lying over the gland (Fig. 10-14). The vein is

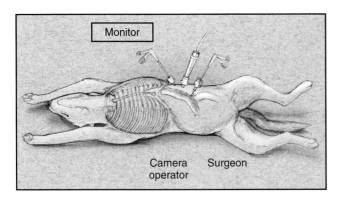

Fig. 10-15 Port placement for the lateral transabdominal approach to the left adrenal gland.

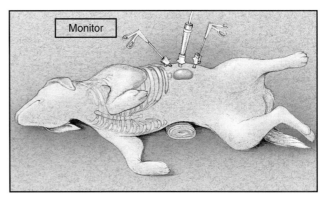

Fig. 10-16 Port placement for the retroperitoneal approach to the left adrenal gland.

isolated, ligated with vascular clips, and transected. With careful blunt dissection, all vascular branches are clipped and ligated until the adrenal gland is completely mobilized. The renal vasculature is identified and preserved. In the case of tumor, care is taken not to invade the capsule of the gland to prevent abdominal seeding. The gland is removed through the 10-mm port. The surgical site is irrigated and inspected before closure of the port sites.

LATERAL TRANSABDOMINAL

The lateral transabdominal approach[3] provides a larger optical space for better access to a single adrenal gland by improved organ retraction. Bilateral adrenalectomy requires repositioning and redraping.

To access the left adrenal gland, the animal is placed in right lateral recumbency. A roll of towels is placed behind the last rib to increase the space between the last rib and the iliac crest. A Veress needle is used to insufflate the abdomen to 12 to 14 mm Hg pressure. The Veress needle is placed caudal to the last rib, midway between the dorsal spine and ventral midline, to avoid injuring the spleen. A 5- or 10-mm trocar, depending on scope size, is placed approximately 1 cm caudal to the last rib at the same level the Veress needle was inserted. A 30° laparoscope is used. Three other 5- or 10-mm ports are placed to provide access to the adrenal gland (Fig. 10-15). The spleen and large bowel are retracted medially, and the animal is placed head-up to allow gravity to retract the bowel. Dissection and ligation proceed as previously described.

RETROPERITONEAL

A minimally invasive retroperitoneal approach to adrenalectomy has been described in pigs.[4,5] The retroperitoneal approach has the advantages of minimizing trauma to the bowel, pancreas, spleen, liver, and colon and reducing the risk of intraabdominal adhesions. The optical space is much smaller and the procedure is tech-

nically more challenging than either of the transperitoneal approaches. The peritoneum of pigs is thicker and less adherent than the peritoneum of dogs and cats; therefore, the approach may be more feasible in pigs. Penetration of the peritoneum into the abdominal cavity is almost inevitable because the adrenal capsule is adherent to peritoneum. Insufflation of gas in the retroperitoneal space may carry a low risk of mediastinal emphysema, causing pneumothorax or pneumomediastinum.[4] There have been isolated reports of mediastinal emphysema with retroperitoneal insufflation during colonoscopy, culdoscopy, and fulguration of bladder tumors in humans.[7-9] We have not observed pneumothorax or pneumomediastinum during retroperitoneoscopy in any of the research studies conducted in our laboratories.[10]

Two approaches have been described for gaining access to the retroperitoneal space. Retroperitoneal CO_2 insufflation in pigs was accomplished by a technique similar to a pneumographic technique in radiology.[4] Pneumography was developed to outline the kidney and adrenal glands for the detection of tumors before the introduction of computed tomography (CT) scans.[11] The technique has been used experimentally in dogs.[12]

Fluoroscopy is used to help locate the retroperitoneal space.[4] Using cystoscopic techniques, a urethral catheter is placed on the side of the proposed adrenalectomy. Dye is injected to outline the ureter and kidney. Under fluoroscopic guidance in two views, a Veress needle is directed into the retroperitoneal space just caudal to the kidney. CO_2 is instilled to insufflate the space and establish the optical cavity. Trocars are placed in a diamond configuration over the proposed surgical site (Fig. 10-16). Dissection, ligation, and removal are performed as previously described. Potential complications from this approach are injuries to the kidney, retroperitoneal vessels, or abdominal viscera during Veress needle insertion and trocar placement. It is possible for a trocar to penetrate the diaphragm and cause pneumothorax.

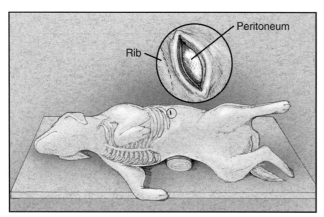

Fig. 10-17   Dissection is carried out through the layers of the abdominal wall. The peritoneum is not penetrated.

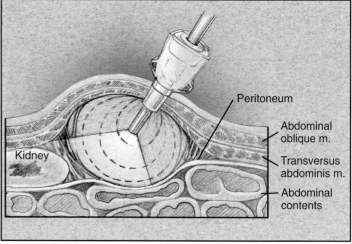

Fig. 10-18   The balloon is inflated in the retroperitoneal space.

A second method for establishing pneumoperitoneum makes use of a trocar with an attached balloon.[5] The animal is placed in lateral recumbency over a roll to elevate the flank. A 1-cm incision is made 2 cm caudal to the last rib, midway between the dorsal and ventral midlines. Dissection is continued in a muscle-splitting approach until the peritoneum is identified but not penetrated (Fig. 10-17). Finger dissection is used to create a small pocket between the peritoneum and transverse fascia, large enough for insertion of the tip of the trocar with the attached balloon. A 10-mm port with attached balloon is placed through the incision into the retroperitoneal space. A 0°, 10-mm laparoscope is inserted into the trocar, and the balloon is filled with air. Balloon inflation and progressive dissection of the retroperitoneal space are monitored with the laparoscope (Fig. 10-18). Pressure from the inflated balloon provides hemostasis. The balloon is then deflated, and the trocar and balloon are removed. A 10-mm blunt trocar is placed and secured. The retroperitoneal space is insufflated with 12 to 14 mm Hg pressure.

Three additional 5- or 10-mm ports are placed in the retroperitoneal space under direct vision. Two are placed caudal to the last rib, dorsal and ventral to the primary port. One port is placed caudal to the primary port at approximately the same level. Dissection, ligation, and removal are performed as described previously.

The balloon trocar eliminates the need for cystoscopy, cannulation of the ureter, and fluoroscopy. The initial dissection must be performed cautiously to prevent peritoneal tearing. The retroperitoneal approach provides a direct view of the adrenal gland, but perspective seems somewhat distorted to a surgeon accustomed to seeing the adrenal gland from the laparotomy approach. In ad-

dition, the optical space is smaller and the angles of dissection are more limited.

Results

Laparoscopic adrenalectomy is a feasible procedure with minimal complications. Operative times improve with surgical experience. More time is required to dissect the right adrenal gland, because it is adherent to the vena cava and the adrenal veins are shorter. Operative times in pigs were 60 to 90 minutes for left adrenalectomy and 60 to 160 minutes for right adrenalectomy, depending on whether the lateral or the retroperitoneal approach was used.[3-5] The lateral approach had the shorter operative times.

Tachycardia was reported in one of the studies during manipulation of a normal gland.[5] The investigators administered an unspecified amount of labetalol intravenously in the remaining animals to "blunt the epinephrine surge caused by manipulating the adrenal gland."[5] Labetalol is an adrenergic receptor blocking agent that has both selective alpha$_1$- and nonselective beta-blocking actions.[13] Tachycardia was not observed in the subsequent procedures.

At least one laparoscopic adrenalectomy has been performed clinically in a dog.[14] The right adrenal gland was removed with the ventral transabdominal approach. Operative time was less than 2 hours. No complications were encountered.

REFERENCES

1. Birchard SJ: Adrenalectomy. In Slatter D, editor: Textbook of small animal surgery, ed 2, vol II, Philadelphia, 1993, WB Saunders.

2. Lee DW, Chung SC: Laparoscopic adrenalectomy. *Int Surg* 80:311-314, 1995.
3. Park A, Gagner M: A porcine model for laparoscopic adrenalectomy. *Surg Endosc* 9:807-810, 1995.
4. Brunt LM et al: Retroperitoneal endoscopic adrenalectomy: an experimental study. *Surg Laparosc Endosc* 3:300-306, 1993.
5. Hoenig DM et al: Direct retroperitoneoscopic adrenalectomy in the porcine model. *J Laparoendosc Surg* 5:385-388, 1995.
6. Brunt LM et al: Laparoscopic adrenalectomy compared to open adrenalectomy for benign adrenal neoplasms. *J Am Coll Surg* 183:1-10, 1996.
7. Schmidt G, Borsch G, Wegener M: Subcutaneous emphysema and pneumothorax complicating diagnostic colonoscopy. *Dis Colon Rectum* 29:136-138, 1986.
8. Fortier QE: Retroperitoneal, mediastinal, and cervical emphysema following culdoscopy. *Fertil Steril* 5:173-181, 1954.
9. Sivak BJ: Surgical emphysema: report of a case and a review. *Anesth Analg* 43:415-417, 1964.
10. Freeman LJ: Unpublished data. 1994.
11. Saxton HM, Strickland B: Presacral pneumography. In Saxton HM, editor: Practical procedures in diagnostic radiology, London, 1972, HK Lewis.
12. Kaplan LE, Johnston GR, Hardy RM: Retroperitoneoscopy in dogs. *Gastrointest Endosc* 25:13-15, 1979.
13. Physicians' desk reference, ed 49, Ronald Arky, medical consultant, Montvale, NJ, 1995, Medical Economics.
14. McCarthy T: Personal communication. 1997.

Thyroidectomy/Parathyroidectomy

LYNETTA J. FREEMAN

Minimally invasive access to the thyroid and parathyroid glands was investigated in pigs, dogs, and goats to create, perform, and evaluate surgical procedures in small optical cavities. One goal was to develop techniques that would provide intraoperative vision, instrumentation for fine dissection, and improved cosmetic results in humans undergoing parathyroidectomy. Acute studies were performed to explore the feasibility of such techniques.[1] Although minimally invasive approaches to the thyroid and parathyroid glands did not appear to offer distinct advantages over the conventional open approach and are not recommended at this time, the experimental procedure will be described in this chapter as an aid to those who would continue such investigations.

Anatomy

The thyroid gland consists of two lobes adjacent to the trachea. Two parathyroid glands are associated with each lobe. One is internal to the capsule of the thyroid gland at the caudal and medial aspect of the lobe. The external parathyroid gland is outside the lobe at the cranial portion of the gland. The parathyroid gland is identified by its color, which is lighter than the thyroid.

Surgical Approach

A pig was positioned in dorsal recumbency with inhalation anesthesia provided by endotracheal intubation. A roll was placed beneath the neck. A 10-mm midline skin incision was made approximately 1 cm caudal to the thyroid cartilage (Fig. 10-19). The incision was deepened between the sternohyoid and sternothyroid muscles until the tracheal rings were identified. The approach was similar to that used in tracheostomy tube placement. A

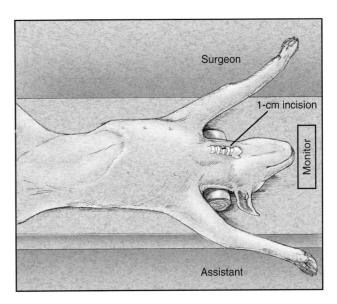

Fig. 10-19 A 1-cm incision on the ventral aspect of the cervical region.

pouch large enough to accommodate a balloon-tipped trocar was created by digital dissection between the trachea and the sternothyroid muscle (Fig. 10-20). A trocar was inserted into the pouch, and the balloon was inflated to approximately the size of a softball. Care was taken not to collapse the endotracheal tube. The laparoscope was inserted into the balloon-tipped trocar to view the progress of the dissection. The balloon was palpated externally and somewhat "forced" to dissect caudally, although this was difficult because the balloon took the path of least resistance in the tissue. The balloon was left inflated for approximately 1 minute to achieve hemostasis before it was deflated. The cannula was removed.

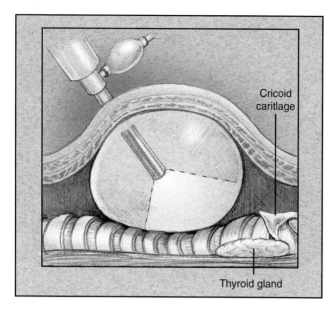

Fig. 10-20   Cross section of a balloon-tipped trocar being inflated in the pretracheal space.

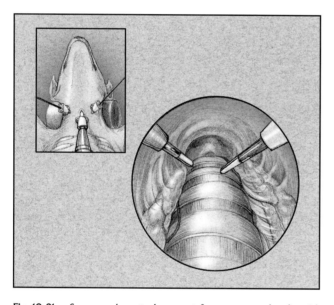

Fig. 10-21   Scope and port placement for access to the thyroid gland. The internal view is shown on the video monitor.

At this point, several means for maintaining an optical cavity were attempted. A trocar was placed on midline and secured with sutures to facilitate insufflation with CO_2. Radiographic evidence of pneumomediastinum was present when pressures reached 12 mm Hg. Manual retraction appeared to be safer; however, the optical cavity was not as large as with insufflation. Manual retraction allowed the use of standard operating instruments, because it was not necessary to prevent gas loss.

A lack of conventional landmarks made orientation difficult. A 5-mm, 30° arthroscope provided adequate

light and visibility of the operative field. After the thyroid gland was identified, two additional 5-mm or smaller ports were placed to allow introduction of grasping and dissecting forceps and endoscopic scissors (Fig. 10-21). Pediatric instrumentation with the shorter handles were preferred for the dissection. An energy source, such as electrosurgery or the ultrasonic scalpel, was used to control bleeding. Care was taken to identify and preserve the recurrent laryngeal nerve. The ultrasonic scalpel was preferred because the smoke produced by electrocautery rapidly filled the small cavity and obscured the view. The 5-mm clip applier could have been used to ligate the cranial and caudal thyroid vessels. The excised thyroid gland was removed through the trocar site.

Results

THYROIDECTOMY
Thyroidectomy was performed in six dogs by using an external lift device and three ports.[2] The mean operative time for thyroidectomy was 69 minutes (range 58 to 88 minutes). Blood loss was minimal. There were no intraoperative complications. Necropsies 1 week after surgery revealed 2 to 65 mL of serous fluid in the pretracheal space.

PARATHYROIDECTOMY
Parathryoidectomy was completed successfully in five of six dogs.[3] Inadequate exposure was cited as the reason for the failed procedure. The investigators used a balloon dissector and an external lift device to create and maintain the pretracheal space. Bilateral parathyroidectomy was completed in 130 ±6 minutes. There were no intraoperative complications. At necropsy, approximately 20 mL of serous fluid was present in the pretracheal space.

Conclusion

Although the surgical approach and technique proved to be feasible, a minimally invasive thyroidectomy or parathyroidectomy in animals is not recommended. The small optical cavity makes orientation of the surgical field and dissection challenging. The danger of creating pneumomediastinum with insufflation is recognized. Failure to visualize and preserve the recurrent laryngeal nerve can lead to laryngeal paralysis.

REFERENCES
1. Freeman LJ: Unpublished data. 1994.
2. Brunt LM et al: Videoendoscopic thyroidectomy in a canine model. *Minim Invasive Ther* 4(suppl 1):47, 1995 (abstract).
3. Brunt LM et al: Endoscopic parathyroidectomy: an experimental evaluation. *Surg Endosc* 10:225, 1996 (abstract).

CHAPTER 11

MINIMALLY INVASIVE SURGERY OF THE REPRODUCTIVE SYSTEM

Lynetta J. Freeman, Dean A. Hendrickson

Laparoscopy provides superb views of reproductive anatomy with a minimally invasive approach. It is a wonderful way to introduce students to the appropriate use of a Snook ovariectomy hook and what is *really* meant by "strumming" the suspensory ligament. With magnification, the proper ligament of the ovary, oviduct, and gross ovarian and uterine lesions are easily identified. Because of the minimal trauma and excellent view, laparoscopy has been used extensively as a research tool to aid in reproductive studies in pigs, goats, sheep, horses, cattle, dogs, cats, and primates.[1] Investigators studied ovarian morphology and correlated visual changes with hormone levels and sexual behavior.[2] For queens in prolonged estrus, laparoscopy was used to detect and facilitate aspiration of ovarian cysts.[1] Laparoscopy was used to detect changes in appearance of the uterine horns during the reproductive cycle to determine whether ovulation occurred in bitches and queens.[1] By laparoscopically examining the uterus at 21 to 28 days of gestation, segmental swellings were counted to predict the litter size.[1] Laparoscopy also was used to diagnose closed pyometra in queens before clinical signs were apparent.[1]

Until now, laparoscopy of the reproductive system was limited to a single observation port and, occasionally, an accessory working port. Techniques for uterine infusion, insemination, and flushing have been described and used successfully in many species.[3] Sterilization was performed by clipping or cauterizing the oviducts, the uterine horns, or the deferent ducts.[4] Clipping or cauterizing the uterine horn is not recommended because

three of six dogs so treated subsequently developed pyometra. Uterine horns coagulated at the uterotubal junction adjacent to the ovarian bursa in six dogs appeared to be normal when examined 1, 2, and 4 years later.[3] Although conception was prevented, the associated sexual behaviors were not eliminated.

Operative laparoscopic techniques now enable a surgeon to remove the ovaries and uterus and perform advanced operative procedures. The advantages of a minimally invasive approach compared with a conventional ovariohysterectomy include better operative visibility, less adhesion formation,[5] and the opportunity to perform a visual exploration of the entire abdominal cavity.

Minimally invasive approaches are an excellent means of teaching proper surgical technique. Elective ovariohysterectomy, ovariectomy, and cryptorchid orchidectomy laparoscopic procedures enable students to develop hand-eye coordination and the ability to overcome paradoxical movement and work in a small, three-dimensional space while viewing in two dimensions.

Laparoscopy of the Female Reproductive System

Laparoscopy is most applicable for evaluating uterine and ovarian disease, and performing ovariohysterectomy. Diagnostic laparoscopy of the reproductive system should be considered instead of open laparotomy for diagnosis of ovarian and uterine disease. Laparoscopy should also be considered to diagnose ovarian remnants from previous surgery, uterine stump pyometra, fistulous tracts from inflammatory reaction to suture materials, and pregnancy. Depending on the size of the uterus, laparoscopy could also be considered for diagnosis of metritis, subinvolution of placental sites, and pyometra.

INSTRUMENTATION

Standard videoendoscopic instrumentation is listed in Box 11-1 and is described in Chapter 1. Disposable trocars, handheld instruments, clip appliers, and staplers are used. Many of these products are also available as reusable instruments. A 10-mm laparoscope provides the widest field of view. If 5-mm ports are used, have a 5-mm laparoscope available to monitor removal of the uterus from the umbilicus when ovariohysterectomy is performed. Use adjustable stability threads to stabilize the trocar in the body wall and allow the length of the cannula inside the abdomen to be modified. When using 10/12 mm trocars, provide reducing caps to prevent loss of pneumoperitoneum when 5-mm instruments are inserted.

ANESTHESIA AND POSITIONING

Fast the animal for 24 hours and insert an intravenous catheter before administering general anesthetic. Provide assisted ventilation because of increased abdominal pressure and possible hypercapnia from insufflation with carbon dioxide (CO_2).[6,7] Place the animal on a heated, circulating-water blanket to preserve body temperature. Monitor vital signs with an electrocardiogram and oxygen saturation probe if they are available. Express the urinary bladder or insert an indwelling urinary catheter.

Position the animal in dorsal recumbency and prepare the field for sterile abdominal surgery. Tilt the head down (Trendelenburg position), and position the pelvic limbs toward the video monitor (Fig. 11-1). Secure the animal to the table to allow tilting from side to side to enhance ovarian exposure.

INSERTION OF PRIMARY TROCAR

After sterile draping, use one of the techniques described in Chapter 3 to gain access to the abdominal cavity. We prefer the open technique to place a Hasson trocar at the umbilicus. This approach avoids damaging the underlying viscera and reduces lens contamination by fat in the falciform ligament. Insufflate the abdomen and, depending on the animal's size, insert a 5- or 10-mm laparoscope to view the internal anatomy. Placing the animal in Trendelenburg position facilitates movement of the intestines out of the pelvic canal. If extensive adhesions are present, it is usually best to perform a laparotomy.

BOX 11-1

INSTRUMENTS USED IN REPRODUCTIVE SURGERY

0° laparoscope, 5 or 10 mm
Hasson-style trocar
5-mm or 10/12 mm trocars (3)
Reducing caps
Grasping forceps (2)
Curved dissecting forceps
Endoscopic scissors
Bipolar electrocautery forceps
Endoloop sutures
Clip applier
Energy source
Specimen retrieval bag (optional)
Endoscopic needle holders (2)
Endoscopic suture
Irrigation and aspiration device

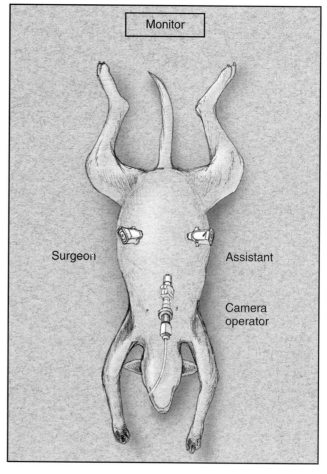

Fig. 11-1   Positioning and port placement for laparoscopic procedures of the reproductive system.

ANATOMY

Laparoscopy provides an opportunity to better understand of the positions of the supporting structures of the uterus and ovaries. The suspensory ligament of the ovary runs from the caudal pole of the kidney to the ovary. In the bitch, it is discrete and lateral to the ovarian pedicle. The round ligament of the uterus is the caudal continuation of the proper ligament of the ovary. It runs to the inguinal canal in the free edge of the broad ligament, which is a double fold of peritoneum containing the uterine horn and uterine artery and veins.

The body of the uterus lies between the rectum and bladder. If the animal has undergone ovariohysterectomy, adhesions may be present between the uterine stump and the bladder or rectum. If the uterus cannot be traced to the ovaries, tilting the table to the right allows the spleen and intestine to gravitate to the right side, exposing the left ovary just caudal to the caudal pole of the left kidney. If positioning changes alone are not sufficient to bring the ovary into view, an additional 5-mm port is inserted to allow retraction of the colon with grasping forceps. Tilting the table to the left and retracting the duodenum exposes the right ovary, caudal to the right kidney.

SECONDARY PORT PLACEMENT

After an initial examination, place one or two secondary 5- or 10/12 mm ports on each side, lateral to the mammary glands and halfway between the umbilicus and pubis (see Fig. 11-1).

UTERINE BIOPSY AND CULTURE

To diagnose uterine disease, uterine biopsy and culture samples can be taken. Use endoscopic scissors to make a 3-mm incision into the uterus. Bleeding from the uterine horn is brisk. Introduce a sterile swab for uterine culture through the trocar cannula and insert it into the uterus. Remove the swab and place it in transport media. Grasp the edge of the incision with grasping forceps. Use the endoscopic scissors to take a small segment of uterus adjacent to the initial incision. Bleeding from the edges of the uterus can be controlled with microbipolar forceps. Place one or two sutures to close the defect. Lavage the abdomen with sterile saline, aspirate the fluid, and inspect the incision to ensure hemostasis before closure.

ENLARGED UTERUS

If the uterus is enlarged, take precautions to avoid trauma during trocar insertion. Remember that the extra weight of the visceral contents applies additional pressure to the diaphragm during positioning. Monitor the animal for signs of respiratory or cardiovascular distress.

Laparoscopy can be used to determine the number of embryos in utero without inducing abortion.[1] Segmental swellings become visible at days 21 to 25 and are distinct by day 28. Grasp the uterine tissue between the swellings with grasping forceps and count the number of swellings in each uterine horn.[1] After day 40 in dogs and cats, the uterus becomes more difficult to manipulate and examine.

Uterine torsion, hydrometra, mucometra, and pyometra often result in an enlarged, friable uterus. The risk of abdominal contamination if the uterus is septic may make removal of a distended uterus safer by laparotomy than by laparoscopy. Distended uterine tissue is often friable and can tear during manipulation. An experienced surgeon may choose to mobilize the ovarian pedicle and suspensory ligaments laparoscopically, then make a small suprapubic incision to remove the uterus and ligate the uterine arteries and uterine body.

ELECTIVE OVARIOHYSTERECTOMY

The steps of a laparoscopic procedure are the same as for open surgery: obtaining access, elevating the uterus, releasing the suspensory ligament, creating a window in the mesovarium, ligating and transecting the ovarian pedicle, taking down the broad ligament, ligating and transecting the uterine body and uterine arteries, removing the genital tract, and closing.[8]

Access

Establish the primary port at the umbilicus and one secondary port in each of the caudal abdominal quadrants as previously described (see Fig. 11-1). Tilt the animal 45° to the right to expose the left ovary. Grasp the uterus with 5-mm grasping forceps and elevate the horn of the uterus to the level of the ovary. One way to mobilize the uterine horn is the "hand-over-hand" technique. The tissue is passed from one grasper to the other in a procedure similar to "running the bowel" in open surgery. The assistant elevates the ovary by applying upward and caudal tension on the proper ovarian ligament.

Suspensory Ligament and Ovarian Pedicle Ligation

The suspensory ligament often contains a small blood vessel. If the ligament is not ligated, the vessel may bleed and obscure visibility. Identify, isolate, ligate, and divide the suspensory ligament of the ovary. Endoscopic ligating clips or an energy source are preferred for this application (Fig. 11-2).

Create a window with dissecting forceps in the broad ligament caudal to the ovarian vessels. Depending on instrument availability and the vascularity, friability, and extent of adipose tissue in the ovarian pedicle, select one of the following techniques to ligate or coagulate the pedicle containing the ovarian vessels:

Bipolar Electrocautery or Ultrasonic Energy

If the pedicle is friable and contains many small vessels, coagulating the vessels with ultrasonic or radiofrequency

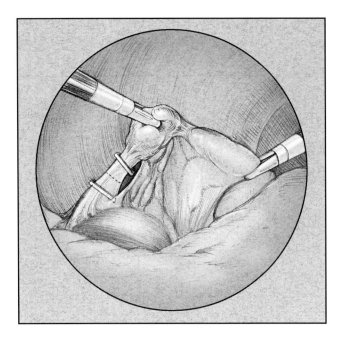

Fig. II-2   Ligation of the suspensory ligament.

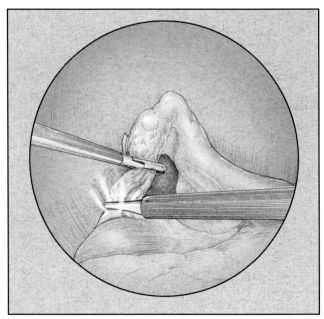

Fig. II-3   Ultrasonic energy can be used for ovarian pedicle occlusion.

energy reduces the risk of damage to adjacent structures. Bipolar forceps and ultrasonic forceps coagulate tissue grasped between their jaws. To use bipolar forceps, set the generator at approximately 20 watts. Isolate the ovarian pedicle and apply the bipolar forceps several times to coagulate a 1 cm-wide section of the pedicle. When coagulation is complete, transect the pedicle with scissors and examine it to ensure hemostasis. Ultrasonic forceps are used with the generator set at level 3. Set the blunt side of the blade against the clamp pad (see Chapter 4). Grasp the tissue in the forceps and apply the energy (Fig. 11-3). As tissue is blanched and coagulated, increase gripping pressure until the tissue has been transected.

Monopolar Electrocautery

Although monopolar electrosurgery is effective when applied properly, its use is discouraged because of excessive lateral spread of the energy and the potential for injury to adjacent bowel. To prevent pathway burns, ensure that current flowing from the activated hand instrument enters a small volume of tissue and leaves the animal's body through extensive contact with a large grounding pad.

Endoscopic Ligating Clips

Endoscopic clips are used if an energy source is not available or if the ovarian artery and vein are larger than 3 mm. Ensure that the clip applier and trocar are of compatible sizes. Most clip appliers are used through a 12-mm trocar, although disposable 5-mm clip appliers are now available. Isolate the ovarian pedicle into smaller sections appropriate for the aperture of the ligating clip. Depending on the width of the ovarian pedicle, two to four sections are isolated. Excessive amounts of fat in the ovarian pedicle can make this procedure difficult to per-

form without causing bleeding. Two clips are applied proximally and one distally (Fig. 11-4). The pedicle is cut between the proximal and distal clips.

Suture Ligation

Sutures are used if the tissue can withstand stretching and the manipulation involved in suture passage and knot tying. Extracorporeal ties make it possible to ligate the ovarian pedicle tightly before the pedicle is transected. Insert a suture through the operative port opposite the ovary and pass it around the ovarian pedicle. Tie half hitches externally and use a knot pusher to tighten them around the pedicle to make a secured square knot. Alternatively, an Endoknot with an extracorporeal Roeder knot or other slipknot can be used. Use the nylon cannula of the Endoknot to push the knot down to secure the ligature around the pedicle. Place two ligatures and cut the pedicle between them.

Vascular Stapler

If the ovarian pedicle is extremely wide and the process of creating windows results in bleeding, a single application of the 35-mm endoscopic linear vascular stapler is used. The stapler places six rows of titanium staples on the ovarian pedicle and simultaneously cuts between the middle rows. After such transection, examine the pedicle for bleeding and use bipolar electrocautery to control bleeding from staple leg penetration through vascular tissue.

Broad Ligament Transection

Elevate the broad ligament and round ligament and transect them with scissors, blunt dissection, or an energy source. Ligating clips or bipolar forceps are occasionally

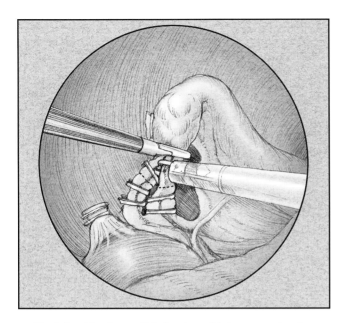

Fig. 11-4   Ovarian pedicle ligation with laparoscopic clips.

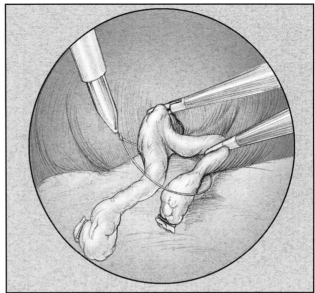

Fig. 11-5   Ligation of the uterine body with Endoloop sutures.

needed for hemostasis of the round ligament. Continue the dissection to the level of the uterine arteries.

To identify the other ovary, tilt the animal to the opposite side. Repeat the entire procedure for the opposite suspensory ligament, ovarian pedicle, broad ligament, and round ligament.

Uterine Body Ligation

To ligate the body of the uterus and the uterine arteries, use an Endoloop or a ligature with an extracorporeal knotting technique. Introduce the Endoloop through a lateral port near the uterine bifurcation. Pass grasping forceps through the suture loop and grasp one of the ovaries. Pull the ovary and uterine horn through the loop (Fig. 11-5). Grasp and pull the other ovary and uterine horn through the same loop. Position the loop cranial to the cervix and tighten it by breaking the nylon cannula near the red band and simultaneously advancing the cannula and pulling the suture attached to the tab (Fig. 11-5). Avoid inadvertent ligation of the bladder or ureters by directly inspecting the ligature site. Apply two ligatures approximately 1 cm apart. Transect the uterine body between the ligatures. As skills are developed, the second ligature to control back bleeding can be eliminated. Ligatures to be tied by extracorporeal knotting can be passed directly around the body of the uterus and uterine arteries.

Tissue Removal

Transfer the telescope from the umbilical port to one of the lateral ports. Pass grasping forceps through the umbilical port and grasp one ovary. Bring the ovary and uterine horn to the base of the trocar cannula. Remove

the cannula, ovaries, uterine horns, and uterine body from the abdominal cavity in a linear fashion. If a cystic ovary is present, bring the ovary to the base of the cannula and drain the cyst percutaneously with a syringe and needle inserted through the port site or directly through the abdominal wall (Fig. 11-6). If the cyst is too large to be passed through an Endoloop, it should be drained before ligating the body of the uterus.

If surgery is performed on an animal with a very large abdominal cavity or if the tissue is malignant or infected, the risks of dropping and losing the tissue during withdrawal may warrant the use of a disposable specimen retrieval bag. Insert the bag through the umbilical port. Place the tissue in the bag and close it. Remove the trocar and bag simultaneously. If necessary, enlarge the incision. The index finger of a surgical glove may be used for a small genital tract if a specimen bag is not available.

Inspection and Closure

Replace the umbilical cannula. To identify venous bleeding, inspect each ligated site with the pressure of insufflation reduced to 4 to 6 mm Hg. Irrigate and examine each site and control any intraoperative oozing with bipolar or monopolar electrocoagulation. It is especially important to obtain *absolute* hemostasis when examining the pedicles under the usual 12 to 14 mm Hg pressure of insufflation. Pedicles thought to be hemostatic at 14 mm Hg may start to ooze when the intraabdominal pressure is reduced to 6 mm Hg. To avoid leaving excessive amounts of irrigation fluids in the abdomen, return the table to the horizontal position during aspiration. Remove the cannulas under direct vision to ensure that there is no evidence of hemorrhage or omental hernia-

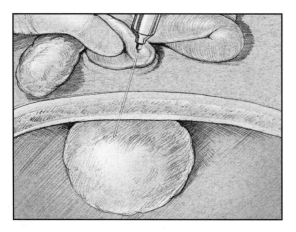

Fig. 11-6   A cystic ovary can be drained with a syringe and long needle percutaneously or through the port site.

tion through the puncture sites. Close the rectal fascia, subcutaneous tissue, and skin. In dogs, ports as small as 5 mm should be sutured to prevent omental herniation through the fascial defect.

Results

Laparoscopic ovariohysterectomy was developed in beagle dogs as a surgical model for preclinical evaluations of endoscopic products. The procedures are performed in pigs and goats to teach endoscopic surgical techniques and evaluate surgical devices in a research setting. Laparoscopic ovariohysterectomy was performed in four lions and a bear at the Audubon Park Zoo and has been used as a learning tool for surgeons or when requested by a client.[9-12] Initial operative times for canine ovariohysterectomy with Endoloops varied from 3 hours, 15 minutes to 1 hour, 15 minutes. Currently, it takes about 1 hour for a canine ovariohysterectomy with extracorporeal knots, 45 minutes for caprine ovariohysterectomy with endoscopic staplers, and about 20 minutes for porcine ovariohysterectomy with an energy source or ligating clips. Animals recover uneventfully and appear clinically normal during the postoperative period.

Postoperative pain and morbidity of laparoscopic and open ovariohysterectomy were compared in dogs.[13] The laparoscopic procedures took longer, and the wound palpation scores 4 hours after surgery in those animals were higher. No differences were noted in blood glucose and plasma cortisol levels at 4, 8, 18, and 24 hours after surgery, nor were differences observed in wound palpation scores at 8, 18, and 24 hours.

Necropsy examinations 7 to 9 days after laparoscopic ovariohysterectomy usually reveal omental adhesions to the ovarian pedicle ligatures and uterine stump. The urinary bladder is occasionally adhered to the uterine stump. Hematomas ranging from 0.5 to 2.5 cm may be present at ligated sites. Omental adhesions to trocar puncture sites also occur.

Potential Complications

Complications encountered during laparoscopic ovariohysterectomy are similar to those in the open procedure. Because of excellent visibility during the operative procedure, the risk of postoperative hemorrhage is reduced.

The most common complication is dropping an ovarian pedicle during ligation. Excessive tension results in tearing of friable vascular and adipose tissue. When using an extracorporeal knotting technique, the suture may saw through the tissue. During Endoloop ligation, the loop may be accidentally positioned around the grasping forceps and become displaced when the forceps are removed.

Locating and controlling a bleeding ovarian pedicle is much easier with laparoscopy than with an open procedure. The technique for locating a dropped pedicle is the same. Ligating clips or an Endoloop suture can be used to ligate the bleeding vessel, or electrocautery can be used.

Accidental ligation of a ureter can occur near the kidney or bladder. Avoid elevating excessive tissue that could include the ureter when ligating the ovarian pedicle (Fig. 11-7). Although the ureter is retroperitoneal, it may be accidentally incorporated into a suture ligature at the caudal pole of the kidney. If the ovarian pedicle is dropped and bleeding, one may unintentionally grasp the ureter while trying to control bleeding from the ovarian pedicle. If electrocautery is used, the ureter may be injured by lateral thermal spread of the cautery.

Take care not to incorporate the ureters or the lateral ligaments of the bladder in tissue ligated near the cervix. Ligatures around the cervix can accidentally incorporate the ureter at the ureterovesical junction if the position of the loop is not controlled during closure. A distended bladder may predispose to including the ureter in the uterine body ligation.[6] If the bladder is distended, it can be drained by cystocentesis under endoscopic guidance. In an animal with considerable fat in the broad ligament, the ureter may be clamped or injured as it crosses the pelvic brim.

Prompt diagnosis and treatment of ureteral injury may allow the ureter to heal uneventfully. Damage to the ureter can also lead to stricture. The animal should be monitored and corrective action taken as indicated. Treatment may include ureteroureterostomy, ureterocystostomy, or nephrectomy, depending on the site of injury.

LAPAROSCOPIC OVARIECTOMY

An alternative to sterilization by ovariohysterectomy is laparoscopic ovariectomy. Veterinary surgeons in Germany have performed laparoscopic ovariectomy in animals since 1992.[14] Although ovariectomy is not practiced in the United States for fear of postoperative pyometra, this complication was not observed in the German series.

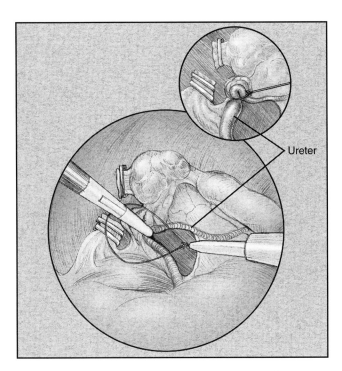

Fig. 11-7 Accidental ureteral ligation when ligating the ovarian pedicle.

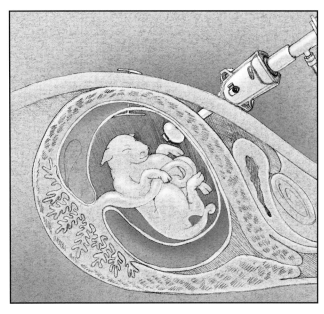

Fig. 11-8 Intrauterine endoscopy. Percutaneous intrauterine access. T-fasteners are used to anchor the amnion to the uterine wall.

An umbilical port is used for the laparoscope. Two 5-mm trocars are placed in the caudal part of the abdomen. One ovary is lifted with grasping forceps. Forceps holding an Ethi-Endo-Ligatur* are used to pierce the peritoneal fold between the suspensory ligament and ovarian vessels. The ligature is passed cranially around the suspensory ligament. The suture is retrieved and removed from the abdomen through the same port. An extracorporeal knotting technique is used, and the ligature is tightened. A window is made in the mesovarium caudal to the ovarian vessels. A second ligature is made around the ovarian pedicle and proper ligament of the ovary. The ovary is freed by cutting the suspensory ligament between the first ligature and the ovary. The ovarian pedicle and proper ovarian ligament are cut between the second ligature and the ovary. The ovary is removed through the cannula or through the abdominal wall after the cannula is removed. The process is repeated on the opposite side. The laparoscopic technique was performed successfully in 60 of 62 dogs.[10]

Ovarian Remnant

Residual ovarian tissue leads to recurrent estrus. Ovarian remnants can be removed by using an Endoloop suture. The technique requires one camera and two operative ports. Use the techniques described previously to locate the ovarian remnant. Introduce the suture loop through

*Ethi-Endo-Ligatur, Ethicon, Inc., Somerville, N.J. 08876.

the ipsilateral port. Pass grasping forceps through the loop to grasp and elevate the ovary. Tighten the suture loop around the ovarian pedicle and transect the pedicle between the ligature and the ovary. If there is concern about dropping the ovary during its removal, use a specimen retrieval bag. Submit the excised tissue for histologic examination.

FETAL SURGERY

Endoscopic fetal surgery in animals is a research tool to evaluate the feasibility of performing minimally invasive surgical procedures in the human fetus. The incidence of preterm labor is very high in women who undergo fetal surgical procedures by hysterotomy. By decreasing uterine trauma, endoscopic fetal surgery may reduce the incidence of preterm labor and facilitate corrective procedures at a much earlier age, when the wounds heal without scars.

Fetoscopy has been performed in pregnant bitches.[1] The feasibility of transabdominal intrauterine endoscopy was tested in a pregnant sow.[15] A sow in midgestation was anesthetized and positioned in dorsal recumbency. Pneumoperitoneum was established with CO_2 at 14 mm Hg, and the primary trocar was inserted at the umbilicus. The gravid uterus was easily seen. The insufflation pressure was reduced to allow the body wall to move closer to the uterus. A 5-mm trocar was inserted through the body wall and into the uterus under direct inspection with the laparoscope (Fig. 11-8). A 3-mm rigid telescope

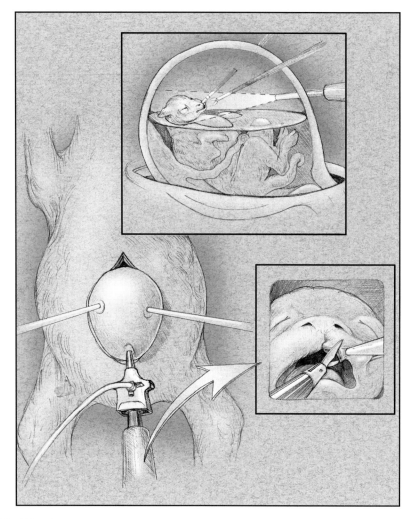

Fig. 11-9   Intrauterine approach to creating and repairing a cleft lip in an ovine fetus.

was inserted into the amnionic sac. Visibility was impaired by the small scope and flecks of material circulating in the amnion. Pneumoamnion was created by attaching the CO_2 tubing to the trocar inside the uterus. Insufflation of the amnion was maintained at 6 to 8 mm Hg pressure. With insufflation, the fetus was easily seen. Two 5-mm ports were inserted into the amnionic sac to allow the introduction of grasping forceps. Trocar cannula positioning was difficult to maintain because there were two points of fixation: (1) the sow's abdominal wall and (2) the wall of the uterus. Amnionic fluid leaked around the cannulas. No therapeutic procedures were performed.

A cleft lip was created and repaired in four fetal lambs.[16] A laparotomy was performed on the ewe, and the uterus was exteriorized (Fig. 11-9). The fetus was stabilized by external means. Carbon dioxide was used to distend the uterus, and the pressure was kept below 3 to 5 cm H_2O. A purse-string suture was placed in the uterine wall and tightened around a trocar cannula. The fe-

tus was examined with a 5-mm scope. A second port was placed, and a cleft lip was created with endoscopic scissors. The defect was repaired with two sutures tied intracorporeally. The uterus was deflated, and the purse-string sutures were tightened and tied. The amnion was distended with warmed lactated Ringer's solution. Two weeks later, the lip wounds were healing with no visible scar.

Two male fetal lambs with surgically induced obstructive uropathy were treated with endoscopically placed wire stents.[17] The urethra was ligated and 7 days later, endoscopic ports were placed in the uterus as described previously. Under endoscopic guidance, a needle was passed from the wall of the uterus into the distended fetal bladder. A J guide wire was passed through the needle, and the needle was removed. The stent was passed over the guide wire into the bladder so urine could leak out of the bladder into the amnion. Seven days later, the stents were patent and showed no evidence of peritoneal urine leakage in the fetus.

Carbon dioxide insufflation at pressures equal to the resting amnionic pressure causes severe fetal hypercapnia and acidosis.[18] Techniques have been modified to use fluid, rather than gas, as the distending medium. Instead of exteriorizing the uterus, percutaneous access has been developed.[19] A needle is inserted through the maternal abdomen and uterus, directly into the amnionic cavity. Warmed saline is used to distend the uterus, and T-fasteners are placed to secure the amnion to the uterine wall (see Fig. 11-8). Trocars are inserted directly into the amnionic cavity. Balloon-tipped trocar cannulas[2] eliminate the need for a purse-string suture at the uterine wall. Low-pressure CO_2 insufflation (3 to 5 cm H_2O) is used.

A comparison of the acute effects of hysterotomy incision and endoscopic access to an ovine fetus showed that hysterotomy was associated with decreased uterine blood flow and uteroplacental oxygen delivery to levels critical for adequate fetal oxygenation.[20] Endoscopic access did not decrease uterine blood flow and oxygen delivery. These results suggest that an endoscopic approach to fetal surgery is less invasive; however, techniques must continue to be validated in animal models before human application. Researchers have been successful in bringing 8 of 10 rhesus monkeys (*Macaca mulatta*) to term after intrauterine fetoscopy at midtrimester.[21]

Laparoscopy of the Male Reproductive System

Veterinary applications for laparoscopy are sterilization of animals by ligating the ductus deferens and removing cryptorchid testicles. Laparoscopy may also be useful in evaluating prostatic disease. Instrumentation, anesthesia, positioning, and access are the same as for the female reproductive system.

ANATOMY

A laparoscopic view of the male genital system includes the ductus deferens and the testicular artery and vein (pampiniform plexus) entering the vaginal ring (Fig. 11-10). The ductus deferens runs in a fold of peritoneum, crossing ventral to the ureter at the lateral ligament of the bladder. Each ductus deferens penetrates the prostate to enter the urethra. The prostate gland is a retroperitoneal structure surrounding the proximal portion of the urethra near the neck of the bladder. A layer of fat covers the ventral surface and must be dissected to provide exposure. As dogs age, the prostate enlarges and moves cranially into the abdominal cavity, and less dissection is required. Varicoceles, which are cystic dilations of the pampiniform plexus, cause infertility in men. The veins can be ligated laparoscopically. To our knowledge, varicoceles have not been reported in animals.

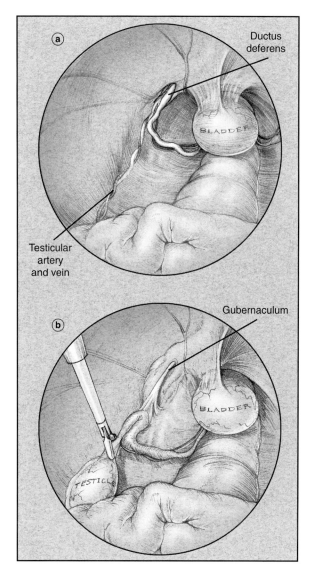

Fig. 11-10 Laparoscopic view of male inguinal ring. Normal inguinal ring (*a*) and cryptorchid testicle (*b*).

LAPAROSCOPIC VASECTOMY

Vasectomy can be performed laparoscopically as an alternative to castration to produce sterility without affecting an animal's behavior, physical characteristics, or hormone production.[22,23] After administering general anesthesia and preparing for aseptic surgery, position the animal in Trendelenburg position. Use a 5-mm laparoscope and two 5-mm working ports. Establish pneumoperitoneum with a Veress needle and maintain the intraabdominal pressure at 12 to 14 mm Hg. Insert a 5-mm port at the umbilicus, avoiding the spleen. Using the transillumination technique, place two 5-mm ports lateral to the rectus abdominis muscle in the caudal abdominal quadrants, midway between the umbilicus and pubis.

With an operating laparoscope and appropriate instrumentation, the procedure could be performed with a

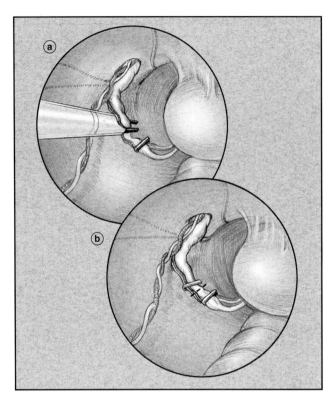

Fig. 11-11 Laparoscopic canine vasectomy. Two clips are applied (*a*), and the ductus deferens is transected between the clips (*b*).

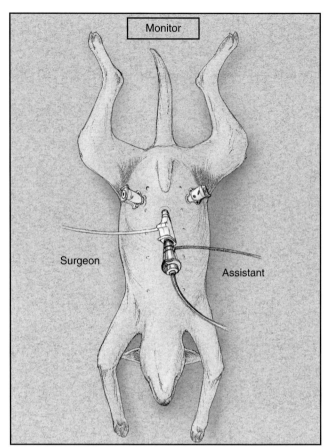

Fig. 11-12 Positioning and port placement for laparoscopic cryptorchidectomy.

single 10/12 mm umbilical trocar. After the laparoscope and working ports are in place, identify the right and left deferent ducts. The ducts can be clipped with a 5-mm clip applier or cauterized with bipolar forceps. If clips are used, place two clips approximately 1 cm apart and cut the tissue between the clips with scissors (Fig. 11-11). To use bipolar coagulation, attach bipolar forceps to an electrosurgical generator set at ~20 watts. Using the forceps, grasp each ductus deferens midway between the prostate and inguinal canal where there is no significant accompanying blood vessel. Apply cautery until 1 to 2 cm of the ductus deferens appears blanched. To prevent recanalization of the ductus, cut the cauterized ductus with scissors. Desufflate the abdomen, remove the trocars, and close the ports routinely. Live spermatozoa may be seen in ejaculate for as long as 21 days after surgery.[24]

The technique was performed safely and quickly in five adult male dogs.[25] The animals had uncomplicated recoveries. Sterilization was confirmed by semen analysis 15 days after surgery.

LAPAROSCOPIC CRYPTORCHIDECTOMY

Testicles that are not palpable in the scrotum may be absent, in the external or internal inguinal canal, or in the abdominal cavity. Laparoscopy offers an excellent means of establishing a definitive diagnosis, as well as a means of therapy, should the testicle be located.

With the animal under general anesthesia and positioned in dorsal recumbency in Trendelenburg position, prepare the abdomen for aseptic surgery. Use an open technique to insert a 10-mm trocar at the umbilicus (Fig. 11-12). Removing the falciform ligament before inserting the trocar helps keep the laparoscope clean during the procedure. Establish pneumoperitoneum and maintain the pressure at 12 to 14 mm Hg. Usually, the right testicle is the retained one. Insert and direct the laparoscope toward the side of the *descended* testicle. Identify the testicular vessels and ductus deferens coursing through the internal ring. Traction on the descended testicle causes the cord structures to move. Examine the inguinal ring to determine whether an inguinal hernia (patent vaginal process) is present.

Direct attention to the side of the *retained* testicle (Fig. 11-13). If spermatic vessels and the ductus deferens are seen entering the internal ring, apply slight pressure to the inguinal canal to express testicles in the inguinal ring back into the abdomen. If the testicle does not appear, inguinal exploration should be conducted because

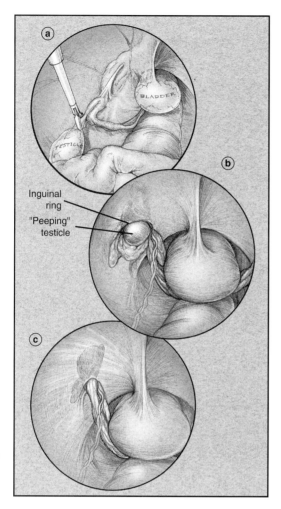

Fig. 11-13 Potential locations of a retained testicle. In the abdomen (*a*), in the inguinal ring (*b*), and in the inguinal canal (*c*).

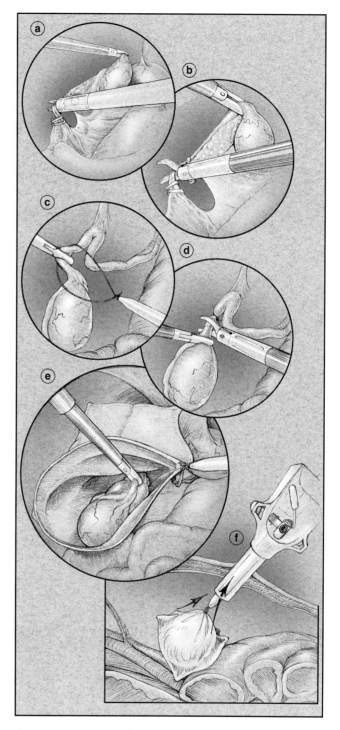

Fig. 11-14 Ligation and transection of the testicular artery and vein (*a* and *b*). Endoloop ligation of the ductus deferens (*c* and *d*). Removal of a retained testicle from the abdomen (*e* and *f*).

of the possibility of remaining "testicular streak tissue."[26] The testicle may be located high in the inguinal canal, or only a gonadal remnant may be present.

Testicles in the abdomen can be located most easily by tracing the ductus deferens to the testicle. An alternative technique is to trace the gubernaculum from the inguinal canal to the testicle. The testicular artery and vein may also be used to locate the testicle. If the vessels and ductus deferens end blindly, with no apparent gonadal tissue, the condition is known as *vanishing gonad* and the tissue at the tip of the vessels is removed.

To perform orchidectomy, two 5-mm trocars, or one 5-mm and one 10-mm trocar, are placed in the left and right lower abdominal quadrants (see Fig. 11-11). Insert the trocars midway between the umbilicus and pubis, lateral to the rectus abdominis muscle. Locate the testicle and create a window between the ductus deferens and the testicular artery and vein. Ligate the testicular artery and vein with two clips and cut between the clips (Fig. 11-14). Introduce an Endoloop

and pass the testicle through the loop. Tighten the loop around the ductus deferens. Cut the ductus deferens between the ligature and testicle. Bring the testicle to the base of the 10-mm trocar and remove it with the trocar, or place it in a specimen retrieval bag and bring it to the body wall (see Fig. 11-14). Occasionally, it is necessary to enlarge the fascial incision to remove the testicle. If a bilateral cryptorchidectomy will be performed on the animal, the trocar is reinserted and the process is repeated for the second testicle. Both inguinal rings are examined for the presence of inguinal hernia. If present, they are addressed as described in Chapter 7.

If one testicle is in the scrotum, perform a routine castration before removing the abdominal trocars. In this way, the transected vascular structures can be examined to ensure hemostasis. Inspect the ligated sites and remove the trocars. Suture the trocar sites and castration incision.

The procedure was performed in six mongrel dogs with unilateral or bilateral cryptorchidism.[27] In all cases, the testicles were removed successfully. Operative time varied from 20 to 45 minutes.

A laparoscopically assisted technique can be used.[28,29] In this procedure, the testicle is identified and mobilized laparoscopically. Grasping forceps are used to hold the ductus deferens and bring the testicle out through an incision in the body wall beside the penis. The vessels are ligated externally. The laparoscopic approach provides better visibility than with a paramedian laparotomy and is less traumatic than a median laparotomy with reflection of the penis and prepuce.

LAPAROSCOPIC ORCHIOPEXY

Although surgeons routinely perform laparoscopic orchiopexy in children,[30,31] orchiopexy is contraindicated in veterinary medicine because of the heritable nature of cryptorchidism.

MINIMALLY INVASIVE PROSTATIC SURGERY

The indications for a minimally invasive approach to the prostate gland in animals have not been established. Laparoscopy can be used to examine the prostate.[32] Biopsy specimens can be obtained if necessary. Potential applications include fine-needle aspiration, percutaneous biopsy, and wedge biopsy under laparoscopic vision.

Laparoscopic prostatectomy was performed in six dogs before the procedure was performed in humans.[33] Five 10/12 mm ports and surgical stapling devices were used to dissect the periprostatic dorsal and lateral venous complexes. The urethral anastomosis was tedious, and suturing required approximately 2.5 hours. An anastomotic leak in one dog necessitated euthanasia the day after surgery. One dog was incontinent. Although the technique was feasible, additional studies are required before this procedure can be performed in clinical cases.

Laparoscopic drainage and marsupialization of prostatic cysts have not been attempted. Only surgeons intimately familiar with open prostate surgery should attempt the laparoscopic approach. Because of the high frequency of prostatic abscesses, surgeons should follow accepted standards for perioperative antibiotic therapy and have a means to control contamination if it occurs during the procedure. Excellent laparoscopic suturing skills are required if surgical therapy is attempted.

REFERENCES

1. Wildt DE: Laparoscopy in the dog and cat. In Harrison RM, Wildt DE, editors: Animal laparoscopy, Baltimore, 1980, Williams & Wilkins.
2. Wildt DE, Levinson CJ, Seager SWJ: Laparoscopic exposure and sequential observation of the ovary of the cycling bitch. *Anat Rec* 189:443-449, 1977.
3. Dukelow WR: Laparoscopy in small animals and ancillary techniques. In Harrison RM, Wildt DE, editors: Animal laparoscopy. Baltimore, 1980, Williams & Wilkins.
4. Wildt DE, Lawler DF: Laparoscopic sterilization of the bitch and queen by uterine horn occlusion. *Am J Vet Res* 46:864-869, 1985.
5. Luciano AA et al: A comparative study of postoperative adhesions following laser surgery by laparoscopy versus laparotomy in the rabbit model. *Obstet Gynecol* 74:220-224, 1989.
6. Leim T, Applebaum H, Hertzberger B: Hemodynamic and ventilatory effects of abdominal CO_2 insufflation at various pressures in the young swine. *J Pediatr Surg* 29:966-969, 1994.
7. Graham AJ et al: Effects of intraabdominal CO_2 insufflation in the piglet. *J Pediatr Surg* 29:1276-1280, 1994.
8. Stone EA, Cantrell CG, Sharp NJ: Ovary and uterus. In Slatter DE, editor: Textbook of small animal surgery, ed 2, Philadelphia, 1993, WB Saunders.
9. Kolata R: Personal communication. 1995.
10. McCarthy T: Personal communication. 1994.
11. Freeman LJ: Unpublished data. 1991.
12. Aguilar RF et al: Endoscopic ovariohysterectomy in two lions (*Panthera leo*). *J Zoo Wildl Med* 28:290-297, 1997.
13. Remedios AM : Laparoscopic versus open ovariohysterectomy in dogs: a comparison of postoperative pain and morbidity. *Vet Surg* 26:425, 1997 (abstract).
14. Thiele S, Kelch G, Gerlach K: Kastration der Hundin durch laparoskopische ovarektomie. *Kleintierpraxis* 38:463-466, 1993.
15. Freeman LJ: Unpublished data. 1991.
16. Estes JM et al: Endoscopic creation and repair of fetal cleft lip. *Plast Reconstr Surg* 90:743-746, 1992.
17. Estes JM et al: Fetoscopic surgery for the treatment of congenital anomalies. *J Pediatr Surg* 27:950-954, 1992.
18. Luks FI et al: Carbon dioxide pneumoamnios causes acidosis in fetal lamb. *Fetal Diagn Ther* 9:105-109, 1994.
19. VanderWall KJ et al: Percutaneous access to the uterus for fetal surgery. *J Laparoendosc Surg* 6S:65-67, 1996.
20. Luks FI et al: The effect of open and endoscopic fetal surgery on uteroplacental oxygen delivery in sheep. *J Pediatr Surg* 31:310-314, 1996.
21. Feitz WF et al: Endoscopic intrauterine fetal therapy: a monkey model. *Urology* 47:118-119, 1996.
22. Wildt DE, Seager SWJ, Bridges CH: Sterilization of the male dog by laparoscopic occlusion of the ductus deferens. *Am J Vet Res* 42:1888-1897, 1981.
23. Moriconi F et al: Sterilizzazione per via laparoscopica nel cane e nel gatto. *Obiettivi Veterinari* 13:13-16, 1989.
24. Pineda MH, Reimers TJ, Faulkner LC: Disappearance of spermatozoa from the ejaculates of vasectomized dogs. *J Am Vet Med Assoc* 168:502-503, 1976.
25. Silva LD et al: Laparoscopic vasectomy in the male dog. *J Reprod Fertil Suppl* 47:399-401, 1993.

26. Brock JW et al: The use of laparoscopy in the management of the nonpalpable testis. *J Laparoendosc Surg* 6S:35-39, 1996.

27. Potter L, Freeman L, Trenka-Benthin S: Laparoscopic castration for canine cryptorchidism. Poster presentation at the annual meeting of the American College of Veterinary Surgeons, 1992, San Francisco, Calif.

28. Gimbo A et al: A new, less invasive, laparoscopic-laparotomic technique for the cryptorchidectomy in the dog. *Arch Ital Urol Androl* 65:277-281, 1993.

29. Van Lue S: Personal communication. 1994.

30. Jordan GH: Management of the abdominal nonpalpable undescended testicle. *Atlas Urol Clin North Am* 1:49-63, 1993.

31. Poppas DP, Lemack GE, Mininberg DT: Laparoscopic orchiopexy: clinical experience and description of technique. *J Urol* 155:708-711, 1996.

32. Jones BD: Laparoscopy. *Vet Clin North Am Small Anim Pract* 20:1243-1263, 1990 (review).

33. Price DT et al: Laparoscopic radical prostatectomy in the canine model. *J Laparoendosc Surg* 6:405-412, 1996.

Minimally Invasive Surgery of the Reproductive System in Large Animals

DEAN A. HENDRICKSON

Cryptorchid Castration

A major benefit of a laparoscopic approach for cryptorchid castration is the ability to see the retained testis if it is within the abdomen, or the spermatic cord entering the vaginal ring if the testis is in the inguinal ring. Standing flank and dorsally recumbent ventral midline laparoscopic approaches have been reported in horses.[1-4] Horses appear to return to normal function more rapidly and with less morbidity with the laparoscopic approaches.

STANDING LAPAROSCOPY

The standing flank approach was developed to reduce the need for general anesthesia in removing abdominal testes. After abdominal insufflation with carbon dioxide (CO_2) and placement of surgical trocars, the abdominal testis is identified and the blood supply is ligated and amputated. Testes can also be exteriorized from the abdomen, and the blood supply ligated and transected with an emasculator.

Surgical Technique

Preparation

Required equipment and sterilization are as described previously. Fast the horse for 24 to 48 hours to decrease the volume of the intestinal contents and thereby improve visibility. Follow accepted standards for administering antibiotics and nonsteroidal antiinflammatory drugs.

Anesthesia

Sedate the horse with xylazine (0.3 to 0.5 mg/kg intravenously [IV]) or detomidine (0.02 to 0.05 mg/kg IV), alone or in combination with butorphanol (0.05 mg/kg).[5-7] The skin and musculature of the flank are infiltrated with 40 to 60 mL of 2% lidocaine or 2% mepivacaine in an inverted L pattern. The spermatic cord can be injected with a local anesthetic agent before ligating and amputating the testis.[1,3] As with any standing procedure, high doses of sedative can cause a horse to collapse during surgery.

To desensitize the caudal part of the abdomen, an epidural anesthetic is administered. If detomidine HCl is the anesthetic agent, intravenous sedation is not required.[8] The epidural space between the first and second coccygeal vertebrae is surgically prepared. Anesthetic protocols are listed in Table 11-1.[9]

Positioning

The horse is placed in "stocks," and its tail is tied to one of its legs or to the stocks to keep it from entering the surgical field. Because of the sedation required, the horse's head is usually supported by suspending it from the top of the stocks. The surgical field is draped to allow access to one or both flanks, as needed. The video monitor is placed behind the animal, and the surgeon and assistant stand on the same side of the animal. Generally there is room only for the surgeon and assistant.

Insufflation

Conventional 120-mm Veress needles and laparoscopic trocars are not long enough to penetrate the flank of most horses. To establish peritoneal insufflation with certainty, insert a trocar catheter* into the peritoneal space or use an open technique to insert a trocar and cannula before insufflating the abdominal cavity.[2,10,11] It is important not to insufflate the retroperitoneal space because that may make the procedure more difficult to per-

---

*12 French Medicut Argyle trocar catheter, Sherwood Medical, St. Louis, Mo.

TABLE 11-1			
Anesthesia Protocols for Caudal Epidural Anesthesia in Horses			
DRUG	DOSE	DILUENT	VOLUME
Xylazine	0.18 mg/kg	2% mepivacaine	5-10 mL
Xylazine	0.18 mg/kg	0.9% sodium chloride	10-15 mL
Detomidine	40-60 μg/kg	0.9% sodium chloride	10-15 mL

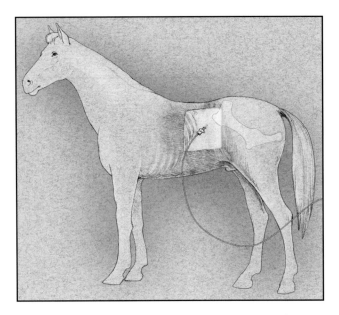

Fig. 11-15   Aseptically prepared left flank of a standing horse with insufflation trocar in place.

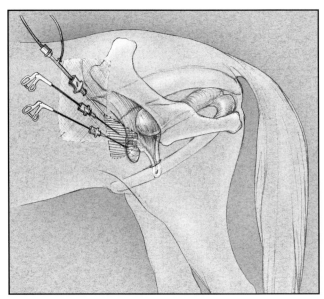

Fig. 11-16   Left flank of a standing horse with instruments and cannulas in position.

form. To insert the catheter, make a 1-cm incision in the skin and external abdominal oblique fascia at the level of the ventral aspect of the tuber coxae, midway between the caudal aspect of the ribs and tuber coxae. In a controlled manner, aggressively insert the trocar catheter through the incision in a slightly downward direction (i.e., toward the opposite stifle). The sound of air entering the abdomen and the loss of negative intraabdominal pressure is confirmation that the tip of the catheter is in the peritoneal space. If air does not enter the abdomen when the trocar catheter is inserted, reinsert the catheter or use a laparoscopic trocar and cannula. Connect the catheter to the insufflator and insufflate the abdomen to 15 to 20 mm Hg (Fig. 11-15).

Port Placement

After the abdomen is distended, insert the primary trocar 5 to 10 cm dorsal to the insufflation catheter. Make a 12-mm skin incision and insert the 10/12 mm trocar and cannula with a slow but constant twisting motion. Remove the trocar, attach the insufflation tubing, and insert the laparoscope. Connect the laparoscope to the light source and video camera. Perform an initial exploration and place the secondary ports. Replace the insufflation catheter with one port and insert another one 5 to 10 cm ventral to the insufflation cannula (Fig. 11-16). If necessary to achieve triangulation, cannulas can be placed to enter the abdominal cavity through the seventeenth intercostal space.

Procedure

Prepare the flank aseptically on the side of the retained testis. If the site of the retained testis cannot be determined before surgery or if both testes are retained, pre-

pare both flanks for aseptic surgery. Because the left testis has a higher incidence of abdominal retention and the spleen is on the right side, approach the left side first to decrease the likelihood of visceral injury.

Using principles of triangulation, identify and grasp the abdominal testis with Babcock or grasping forceps. Verify that the testis, epididymis, and ductus deferens are within the abdomen. If the testis is in the inguinal canal, enlarge the vaginal ring and pull it back into the abdomen. The testis can then be ligated and amputated.

Introduce a loop of size 0 polydioxanone suture* into the abdominal cavity. Release the testis, place the Babcock or grasping forceps through the loop, and regrasp the testis (Fig. 11-17). Position the ligature over the spermatic cord. Tighten the loop and cut the long end of the suture material. For additional security, place another ligature in the same manner. Cut the spermatic cord, leaving the grasping forceps firmly attached to the testis. Observe the castration stump for bleeding. I prefer intracorporeal ligation because it prevents the loss of pneumoperitoneum that occurs when an isolated testis is brought outside the abdomen and an emasculator is used.[1,3] Maintaining pneumoperitoneum is especially helpful in cases of bilateral cryptorchidism.

Retract the small colon and rectum to inspect the opposite inguinal region for an abdominal testis. Use a Babcock or grasping forceps or have an assistant place his or her arm in the rectum to elevate the small colon and rectum. The inguinal area may also be seen by making a window in an avascular region of the mesocolon. If there

---

*Endoloop ligature, Ethicon Endo-Surgery, Cincinnati, Ohio.

is a retained testis on the other side, it may be possible to pull the testis over to the original surgical site. If not, prepare and make a surgical approach from the other paralumbar fossa. Ligate and amputate the testis as previously described. If an undescended testis cannot be returned to the abdomen, the spermatic cord can be cauterized with bipolar cautery, ligated, and divided, leav-ing the testis in situ to undergo avascular necrosis (Fig. 11-18).[12]

Complete the exploration and check the castration stump(s) for bleeding. Enlarge the skin incision for the ventral cannula on the left side to 30 mm (or as large as necessary to remove the testis) and remove the testis from the abdomen. Another option is to place a large cannula* into the surgical site to remove the testis. The large port assists in maintaining pneumoperitoneum if further exploration is necessary, but the port is expensive and is easily dislodged when the horse moves around. Even if bilateral cryptorchid testes require surgical access from both paralumbar regions, both testes can be removed from one side of the abdomen, thereby minimizing trauma to the abdominal musculature. Open the cannulas, release the pneumoperitoneum, and remove the cannulas. Close the small incisions in one layer with simple interrupted sutures of size 2/0 nylon in the skin. Close the extended incision in two layers with size 0 synthetic absorbable suture material in a simple continuous pattern for the external abdominal oblique muscle, and size 2/0 nylon in a simple interrupted pattern for the skin. Allow the animals to return to light exercise the following day, and back to work within a week.

Horses that have one normally descended testis require either a standing castration or a short-acting general anesthetic to remove the descended testis.[13,14]

VENTRAL MIDLINE LAPAROSCOPY
The ventral midline approach enables exploration of the abdomen without moving the small colon. Descended testes can be removed without a second surgical procedure. Insufflation is more easily performed, the animal rarely moves, and there is more room for cannula placement and for the surgeons to stand. General anesthesia is required, and the testis may be more difficult to manipulate because it does not hang from the dorsal body wall as in the standing approach.

Surgical Technique
Preparation
Fast the horse for 24 to 48 hours to decrease the volume of intestinal contents, thereby improving visibility. Follow accepted standards for administering antibiotics and nonsteroidal antiinflammatory drugs.

*Endopath Surgical Trocar, Ethicon Endosurgery, Inc, Cincinnati, Ohio.

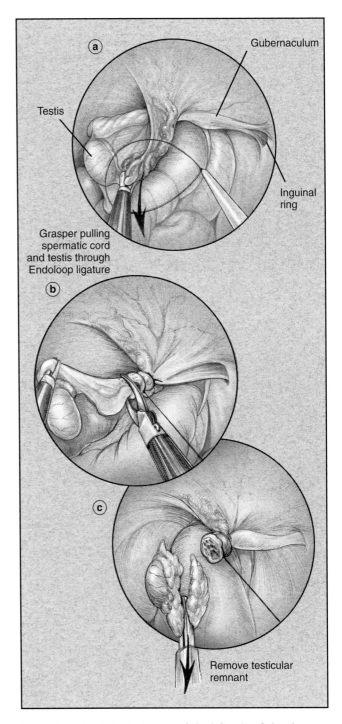

Fig. II-I7 Intraabdominal views of the left side of the abdomen of a standing horse undergoing cryptorchid castration. Grasping forceps hold left abdominal testis while Endoloop is tightened on vasculature, mesorchium, and ductus deferens (*a*). After the loop is tightened, scissors are used to cut ligated structures distal to the ligature (*b*). Ligated stump (*c*).

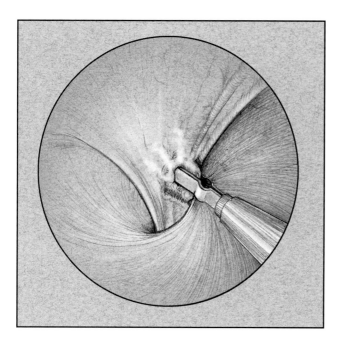

Fig. 11-18 Right inguinal ring in which electrocautery is used to cauterize the vasculature, mesorchium, and ductus deferens.

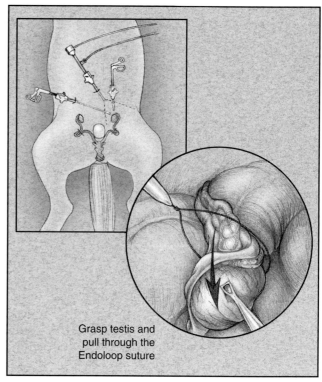

Grasp testis and
pull through the
Endoloop suture

Fig. 11-19 Abdomen of a horse in dorsal recumbency showing instrumentation and cannula placement for ventral abdominal laparoscopy. In this intraabdominal view, the testis is grasped and pulled through the Endoloop suture.

Anesthesia

Anesthetize the horse as for any abdominal procedure. Because of increased abdominal pressure from insufflation and dorsal recumbency, and the potential for peritoneal CO_2 absorption, provide assisted ventilation. Prepare the penis and prepuce aseptically and insert a stallion catheter to drain the bladder.

Positioning

Once the horse is anesthetized, position it in dorsal recumbency, suture the prepuce closed, and prepare the abdomen aseptically. Tie the horse to the table to minimize slippage when the table is tilted. Place surgical drapes at the umbilicus, the folds of the flank, and the inguinal region. Position the video monitor at the foot of the surgery table, or slightly to one side if the hind limbs are between the surgeon and monitor. The surgeon and assistant stand on opposite sides of the abdomen.

Insufflation

Insufflation may be accomplished by the open technique with a Hasson trocar under direct observation, or with a Veress needle or teat cannula (see Chapter 3).

Port Placement

After an initial exploration, tilt the animal so the hind quarters are elevated (Trendelenburg position) to ease

exploration and surgical manipulation in the caudal part of the abdomen. Place secondary ports under direct inspection by using the triangulation principles described previously (Fig. 11-19). Some surgeons prefer to insert a spinal needle to mark the entry points of the additional cannulas to reduce the likelihood of injury to the epigastric vessels. Place one port on each side of midline approximately 10 cm cranial to the cranial aspect of the inguinal rings. For bilateral cryptorchids, place a third instrument port to grasp the testis that is amputated first, so both testes can be removed from the abdomen simultaneously. As an alternative, insert a large trocar and remove each testis as soon as it is amputated.

Procedure

Inspect the inguinal rings and identify the retained testes. I prefer to ligate the spermatic cord within the abdomen. Others prefer to bring the testis outside the abdomen and use an emasculator to crush and divide the spermatic cord.[1,2] Grasp the abdominal testis with Babcock or grasping forceps and manipulate the testis, epididymis, and ductus deferens to ensure that the testis is inside the abdomen. Verify that the testis, epididymis, and ductus deferens are within the abdomen. If the testis

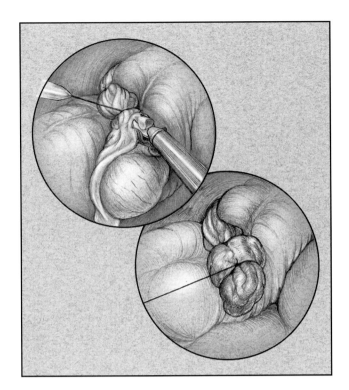

Fig. 11-20 Intraabdominal views of the caudal part of the abdomen of a horse in dorsal recumbency and Trendelenburg position. After the loop is tightened, the spermatic cord is transected with scissors. The vascular stump is examined for bleeding.

is in the inguinal canal, enlarge the vaginal ring and pull the testis back into the abdomen to be ligated and amputated.

Introduce a loop of size 0 polydioxanone suture into the abdominal cavity. Release the testis, place the Babcock or grasping forceps through the loop, and regrasp the testis (Fig. 11-20). Position the ligature over the spermatic cord and tighten the loop. Cut the long end of the suture material. When additional security is required, place another ligature in the same manner. Cut the spermatic cord, leaving the grasping forceps firmly attached to the testis. Observe the castration stump for bleeding.

If both testes are retained, ligate the blood supply and amputate the second testis in the same manner as the first. While the second testis is being ligated, it is helpful to have a third instrument port through which grasping forceps can be passed to secure the first testis. Alternatively, lay the first testis on top of the bowel and remove it after the second testis has been removed. This technique does not require another incision and instrument port, but if the animal moves, the testis may be lost in the abdominal cavity. Both testes are removed from the same incision by enlarging the incision or by using a

large port or a body wall dilator.* Open the cannulas, release or aspirate the pneumoperitoneum, and remove the cannulas. Close the incisions in two layers. Use a cruciate pattern of size 0 synthetic absorbable suture material in the linea alba or external rectus sheath. Close the skin incision with an intradermal or a cruciate pattern of size 2/0 suture material. Recover the horse from anesthesia and institute a postoperative exercise program similar to one for horses having the standing flank approach.

One horse underwent surgery for bilaterally retained testes on a Tuesday and won grand champion halter horse the following Saturday.

Ovariectomy

Standing flank and ventral midline laparoscopic approaches have been described for ovariectomy in mares.[15-17] The main benefit of laparoscopic ovariectomy is the ability to see the ovary and ovarian stump after amputation.

STANDING FLANK OVARIECTOMY

Standing flank ovariectomy is similar to standing cryptorchid castration and can be performed more easily than ovariectomy on an anesthetized mare in dorsal recumbency. Direct inspection of the ovary and ovarian pedicle minimizes the likelihood of visceral trauma and enables the surgeon to ensure complete ligation of the ovarian pedicle. The standing approach is less suitable for removing ovaries enlarged by neoplasia such as a granulosa cell tumor. The approach to the ovarian pedicle is excellent, but it can be difficult to remove an enlarged ovary through the flank incision.

Surgical Technique

Prepare the mare for standing laparoscopy. Approach each ovary from the ipsilateral side. Claw-toothed grasping forceps are mandatory for this procedure, because the ovaries have a very dense covering and can easily slip out of other grasping forceps. Administer nonsteroidal antiinflammatory drugs before and after surgery. Administration of antibiotics is at the discretion of the surgeon.

Administer anesthesia for standing laparoscopic surgery (Table 11-1). Additional anesthesia of the ovarian pedicle has been performed with local infiltration of lidocaine or mepivacaine.[1,16] In my experience, epidural administration of xylazine or detomidine obviates the need for further anesthesia.

Prepare the field aseptically, insufflate the abdomen, and insert the primary port as described for standing

---

*Richard Wolf Medical Instruments Corp, 353 Corporate Woods Parkway, Vernon Hills, Ill.

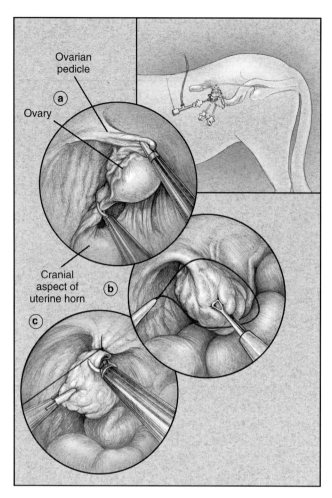

Fig. 11-21 Intraabdominal views of the left side of the abdomen of a standing horse undergoing ovariectomy. Grasping forceps hold the left ovary, while scissors are used to dissect the caudal pole of the ovarian pedicle (*a*). The Endoloop encircles the ovarian pedicle (*b*). After the loop is tightened, the ovarian pedicle is transected between the suture and ovary (*c*).

laparoscopy (see pp. 217-218). Six ports—three on each side—are required to perform this procedure. Begin the procedure on the left side to avoid puncturing the cecum.

Identify the ovary and grasp it with forceps. Using scissors, sharply transect the proper ligament of the ovary between the uterus and ovary (Fig. 11-21). Minimal bleeding is associated with this transection, but it is helpful to have vascular clamps or bipolar cautery available if excess bleeding should be encountered. Introduce a pretied loop ligature, release the ovary, pass the grasping forceps through the loop, and regrasp the ovary. Place the suture loop over the ovary, position it over the ovarian pedicle, and tighten the loop by advancing the nylon cannula. Cut the long end of the suture and place a second ligature in the same manner. Use grasping forceps to hold the ovary securely and use scissors to transect the

ovarian pedicle between the ovary and sutures. Inspect the pedicle for bleeding. Although I prefer to sharply transect the tissue at the caudal pole of the ovary with scissors before ligation, a similar ligation of the ovarian pedicle without dissection was reported with good results.[18] Continue to grasp the ovary while the second ovary is removed.

Place cannulas in the right flank as described for the left side and insert the laparoscope into the abdomen on that side. Identify, dissect, ligate, and amputate the right ovary. Pass the left ovary under the small colon to the right side. Enlarge the ventral incision on the right side so both ovaries can be removed, or extract them through a large trocar. Use claw-toothed grasping forceps during extraction to avoid having the ovary slip out of the forceps and perhaps become lost in the abdominal cavity. In most cases, the ovary simply falls on top of the viscera and can be retrieved, but if the mare moves suddenly, the ovary could be difficult to find. Use Oschner forceps to assist in removing the ovary from the abdominal cavity as it nears the skin incision. Close the incisions and institute the same postoperative treatment as for laparoscopic cryptorchidectomy.

Extracorporeal transection of the ovarian pedicle with an emasculator and intracorporeal transection of the ovarian pedicle with a combination of neodymium:yttrium-aluminum-garnet laser and a laparoscopic stapling device have been described.[1,16] Laparoscopy has also been used to observe ovariectomy performed with a chain écraseur inserted through a colpotomy incision.[10]

VENTRAL ABDOMINAL OVARIECTOMY

The ventral abdominal approach for ovariectomy is similar to that for cryptorchid castration except that the ovaries are near the dorsal body wall and may be more difficult to mobilize. Feed the mare a pelleted ration for a week before surgery and fast her for 48 hours to decrease the volume of intestinal contents and improve visibility of the ovaries. Administer nonsteroidal antiinflammatory drugs before and after surgery. This approach is not convenient for removing ovaries enlarged by neoplasia such as a granulosa cell tumor.

Surgical Technique

Administer general anesthesia with assisted ventilation, position the mare in dorsal recumbency, and prepare the operative table so that the mare's pelvis can be elevated at least 30° and the mare can be rolled slightly to improve exposure of the ovaries.

After aseptic preparation and draping, insufflate the abdominal cavity and insert the primary trocar. Identify the ovaries and place two additional ports, one on each side of the midline. If necessary, place additional ports closer to the mammary gland.

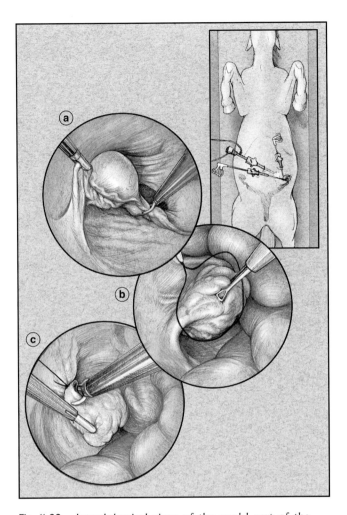

Fig. 11-22 Intraabdominal views of the caudal part of the abdomen of a horse in dorsal recumbency and Trendelenburg position. Grasping forceps hold the ovary while scissors are used to dissect the caudal pole of the ovary (*a*). The ovary is grasped and pulled through the Endoloop suture (*b*). After the loop is tightened, the ovarian pedicle is transected between the suture and ovary (*c*). The ovarian pedicle is then examined for bleeding.

Identify the uterus dorsal to the bladder and follow it craniad until the ovaries are located. Mares with short ovarian pedicles may be rolled to the side opposite the ovary to provide better exposure for ligation and transection. Identify the ovary and hold it with grasping forceps. Using scissors, cut the proper ligament of the ovary between the uterus and ovary (Fig. 11-22). If necessary, control bleeding with vascular clamps or bipolar electrocautery.

Introduce, position, and tighten two pre-tied loop ligatures around the ovarian pedicle as described for the standing ovariectomy. Cut the suture and transect the ovarian pedicle between the sutures and ovary. Inspect the transected pedicle for hemorrhage. Continue to hold

the ovary with the grasping forceps, roll the mare to the opposite side, and ligate and transect the other ovarian artery and veins. Enlarge one of the trocar incisions to remove the ovaries. Alternatively, place a large trocar and remove the ovaries through the cannula.

Just as in the standing procedure, use claw-toothed grasping forceps to keep the ovary and its dense capsule from slipping out of the forceps and becoming lost. As the ovary is pulled out of the body wall, use Oschner forceps to grasp and remove it. Release or aspirate the pneumoperitoneum, remove the cannulas, and close the incisions. The postoperative exercise program is similar to that recommended for the standing flank approach.

STANDING FLANK TUBAL LIGATION
Permanently occluding the oviducts was performed in mares to prove that gamete transfer could be accomplished without risk of fertilizing an egg from the ovary of the recipient mare. The standing flank laparoscopic approach allowed direct inspection during ligation and transection of each oviduct. The effectiveness of ligating only one oviduct was examined in six mares. All became pregnant when they ovulated on the undisturbed side. None became pregnant when they ovulated from the side on which the oviducts had been ligated and transected.[19]

Surgical Technique
Prepare both flanks aseptically to allow exposure to both oviducts. An endoscopic clip applier and scissors are required. Six cannulas—three on each side—are required for this procedure (see Fig. 11-16).

Insufflate the abdomen and place the trocars as described. Use triangulation to locate and identify one ovary and oviduct. Move the endoscopic clip applier into position (Fig. 11-23) and place two clips on the oviduct, leaving enough room between the clips to transect the oviduct with scissors. Repeat the procedure on the opposite side. Release the pneumoperitoneum, remove the cannulas, and close the incisions.

STANDING FLANK OVIDUCTAL INSEMINATION
A standing flank laparoscopic approach is being developed to provide a reliable technique for repetitive oviductal fertilization. Because of the time required for the incisions to heal, the open flank approach used currently cannot be performed more than once during a single breeding season. The laparoscopic approach allows injection of semen under direct inspection of the oviduct and fimbriae. The most difficult step is advancing the small tubing into the oviduct, but the technique is not otherwise technically demanding. Trauma to the oviduct and fimbriae may cause fibrosis and subsequent infertility.

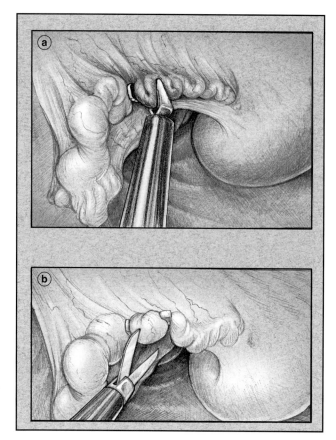

Fig. 11-23   Intraabdominal views of the left side of the abdomen of a standing horse undergoing tubal ligation. A clip applier is used to place ligation clips over the oviduct (*a*). A second clip is applied approximately 1 cm closer to the ovary, and the oviduct is transected between the two clips (*b*).

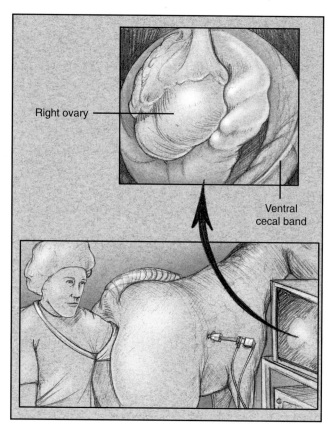

Fig. 11-24   Standing horse showing port placement and video monitor setup for laparoscopically guided palpation of the abdomen per rectum.

Surgical Technique

Only the flank associated with the follicle that is near ovulation is approached. Required equipment includes atraumatic grasping forceps, a small-diameter cannula, and polyvinyl chloride tubing that will fit inside the cannula.

Anesthesia, positioning, insufflation, and port placement are performed as for other standing laparoscopic procedures. Identify the selected ovary and oviduct and grasp the ovary with atraumatic grasping forceps. Manipulate the ovary until the fimbriae in the ovulation fossa are identified. Pass a small-diameter cannula into the trocar and position it at the ovary. Pass the polyvinyl chloride tubing into the cannula until its tip exits the cannula. Advance the tip of the tubing into the fimbriae and up the oviduct as far as possible without causing undue trauma. Inject the semen through the tubing and then remove the tubing. Release the pneumoperitoneum, remove the cannulas, and close the incisions. Postoperative care is the same as for standing laparoscopic cryptorchid castration.

LAPAROSCOPICALLY GUIDED RECTAL EXAMINATION

Laparoscopy enables students to see what they are palpating while learning to perform rectal examinations on standing horses. The procedure is not technically demanding and is very rewarding to the students. Two laparoscopes, two cameras, and two video monitors allow students to view both sides of the abdomen at the same time or, alternatively, a single laparoscope can be moved from side to side.

Surgical Technique

Anesthesia, positioning, insufflation, and port placement are performed as for other standing laparoscopic procedures. Prepare both flanks so that they are accessible for aseptic surgery. Place the video monitor on one side of the thorax so students can see the monitor as they perform rectal palpation (Fig. 11-24).

Place one port for the laparoscope on each side of the horse. After the laparoscope is in the abdomen, a student begins a rectal examination (see Fig. 11-24). The camera operator follows the student's hand while the ipsilateral side of the abdomen is palpated. When the student has finished palpating one side of the abdomen, move the telescope to the opposite side and repeat the process. At the end of the procedure, release the pneumoperitoneum, remove the cannulas, and close the incisions. Postoperative care is the same as for other standing laparoscopy procedures. No complications have been noted.

LAPAROSCOPICALLY GUIDED OPEN CRYPTORCHID CASTRATION

Laparoscopy enables students to observe the internal anatomy while performing a limited open approach such as a parainguinal or inguinal cryptorchidectomy. The procedure requires placement of one port at the umbilicus and a standard operating pack.

Surgical Technique

Perform anesthesia, positioning, insufflation, draping, and primary port placement as for the ventral abdominal laparoscopic cryptorchidectomy. Place the video monitor to the side of the horse and allow the student surgeon to work between the legs. The student may need to stand on a stool while the horse is placed in Trendelenburg position. Place the laparoscope inside the abdomen and perform an exploratory laparoscopy. Allow the student to perform a standard parainguinal[20] or inguinal[14] approach for castration as he or she observes the surgical anatomy and the actions of their fingers with the laparoscope. Following the castration, close the incisions routinely, release the pneumoperitoneum, remove the trocar cannula, and close the port site as previously described.

REFERENCES

1. Fisher AT Jr: Standing laparoscopic surgery. *Vet Clin North Am Equine Pract* 7:641-647, 1991.
2. Fisher AT Sr et al: Diagnostic laparoscopy in the horse. *J Am Vet Med Assoc* 189:289-292, 1986.
3. Fisher AT Jr, Vachon AM: Laparoscopic cryptorchidectomy in horses. *J Am Vet Med Assoc* 201:1705-1708, 1992.
4. Wilson DG: Laparoscopy as an aid in the surgical management of the equine hemicastrate. Proceedings of the Thirty-fifth Annual Conference of the American Association of Equine Practitioners, 1989.
5. Hendrickson DA, Wilson DG: Laparoscopic cryptorchid castration in standing horse. *Vet Surg* 26:335-339, 1997.
6. Galuppo LD, Snyder JR, Pascoe JR: Laparoscopic anatomy of the equine abdomen. *Am J Vet Res* 56:518-531, 1995.
7. LeBlanc PH: Chemical restraint for surgery in the standing horse. *Vet Clinic North Am Equine Pract* 7:521-533, 1991.
8. Skarda RT: Antagonist effects of atipamezole on epidurally administered detomidine-induced sedation, analgesia, and cardiopulmonary depression in horses. *J Vet Anesth Special Supplement* 79-81, 1991.
9. Gaynor JS, Hubbell JAE: Perineural and spinal anesthesia. *Vet Clin North Am Equine Pract* 7:501-519, 1991.
10. Embertson RM, Bramlage LR: Clinical uses of the laparoscope in general equine practice. Proceedings of the Thirty-eighth Annual Conference of the American Association of Equine Practitioners, 1992.
11. Witherspoon DM, Kraemer DC, Seager SWJ: Laparoscopy in the horse. In Harrison RM, Wildt DE, editors: Animal laparoscopy, Baltimore, 1980, Williams & Wilkins.
12. Wilson DG et al: Laparoscopic alternatives to scrotal castration. *Vet Surg* 24:444, 1995 (abstract).
13. Beard W: Standing urogenital surgery. *Vet Clin North Am Equine Pract* 7:669-684, 1991 (review).
14. Trotter GW: Normal and cryptorchid castration. *Vet Clin North Am Equine Pract* 4:493-513, 1988 (review).
15. Hendrickson DA: Standing laparoscopic surgery in the horse. *J Am Vet Med Assoc* 209:383, 1996 (abstract).
16. Palmer SE: Standing laparoscopic laser technique for ovariectomy in five mares. *J Am Vet Med Assoc* 203:279-283, 1993.
17. Ragle CA, Schneider RK: Ventral abdominal approach for laparoscopic ovariectomy in horses. *Vet Surg* 24:492-497, 1995.
18. Boure L, Marcoux M, Laverty S: Laparoscopic ovariectomy in mares using Endoloop ligatures. *Vet Surg* 24:422, 1995 (abstract).
19. Hendrickson DA: Unpublished data. 1996.
20. Wilson DG, Reinertson EL: A modified parainguinal approach for cryptorchidectomy in horses: an evaluation in 107 horses. *Vet Surg* 16:1-4, 1987.

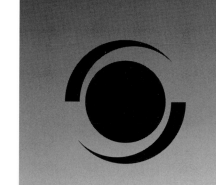

CHAPTER 12

MINIMALLY INVASIVE SURGERY OF THE URINARY SYSTEM

Ray G. Rudd, Dean A. Hendrickson

Minimally invasive access to the kidneys and urinary bladder is less traumatic than the conventional surgical approach. Adhesion formation to the wound site is substantially reduced.[1] Enhanced visibility and magnification of the operative field are additional benefits. Urologists routinely perform a laparoscopic approach in humans for nephrectomy, bladder neck suspension, pelvic lymph node dissection, ligation of varicoceles of the spermatic cord, and management of an undescended testicle. Veterinarians use a cystoscope to evaluate the urethra and urinary bladder, and they perform renal biopsy under laparoscopic guidance. The feasibility of performing advanced surgical procedures is limited only by the size of the animal and one's laparoscopic surgical skill. Included in this chapter are techniques for cystoscopy, placing peritoneal dialysis catheters, renal biopsy, nephrectomy, and cystotomy closure.

Anatomy

The kidneys and ureters are retroperitoneal structures. In dogs and cats, they are in nearly the same sagittal plane as the umbilicus. The cranial pole of the right kidney lies in a fossa of the caudate lobe of the liver. The caudal vena cava is very near the medial surface of the right kidney. Each adrenal gland is adjacent to the cranial pole of the corresponding kidney. The left kidney is more caudal than the right kidney and often has direct contact with the spleen and descending colon. The ureter and the renal artery and vein arise from the medial

renal hilus. Anatomic variations are often seen. The left renal artery is frequently paired in dogs, and multiple renal veins are often seen in cats.[2] The left gonadal vein empties into the left renal vein rather than into the vena cava.

The ureters extend to the bladder in the retroperitoneal space. The right ureter is near the caudal vena cava and 1 to 2 cm lateral to the aorta. The left ureter is 1 to 2 cm to the left of the aorta. The ureters cross the deep circumflex iliac and external iliac arteries and veins at the pelvic brim. They then become enveloped between the two layers of peritoneum that create the lateral ligaments of the bladder.[3] From their positions in the lateral ligaments of the bladder, the ureters enter the bladder on its dorsolateral surface and perforate the bladder wall obliquely.

The urinary bladder is also retroperitoneal and, when empty, lies in the pelvic cavity between the colon and uterus in females or the ductus deferens in males.[3] The bladder moves into the abdominal cavity as it fills with urine. The urinary bladder wall has three layers of muscle that may be difficult to distinguish. The muscle is very thin, even in a nondistended bladder. Chronic infection or inflammation causes thickening of the bladder wall. The medial iliac lymph nodes lie ventral to the deep circumflex iliac arteries and veins. Middle and lateral sacral lymph nodes and deep inguinal lymph nodes are located medial to the internal iliac arteries and veins. Sympathetic (hypogastric nerve) and parasympathetic (pelvic nerve) innervation to the urinary bladder passes through the lateral ligaments of the bladder near the caudal vesical arteries.

Indications and Contraindications

Most surgical procedures that can be performed by celiotomy can also be performed by laparoscopy. They include biopsy, nephrectomy, live donor nephrectomy, partial nephrectomy, cystotomy, cystectomy, and bladder wall closure. Disorders of the ureterovesical junction can be managed laparoscopically if the surgeon is skilled in endoscopic suturing. Contraindications to the laparoscopic approach include large neoplastic disorders. Dissection and removal are difficult, increasing the probability of tumor seeding. Large masses cannot be removed from the abdomen without enlarging a port or morcellating the mass. Waterproof morcellating bags are not uniformly reliable.[4] Morcellating the tissue can interfere with the pathologist's evaluation. Extremely obese animals should be evaluated critically because excessive amounts of adipose tissue add substantially to the difficulty of dissection and may contribute to postoperative morbidity.[5]

Anesthesia

The anesthetic protocol is no different than that used for laparotomy. Renal insufficiency and metabolic acidosis are common, and coagulation disorders occur occasionally in animals that require surgery of the urinary system. The acid-base status should be stabilized, and appropriate crystalloids infused intravenously. An orogastric tube should be passed to decompress the stomach. An indwelling urinary catheter (Foley when possible) is inserted to monitor urinary output intraoperatively and postoperatively. Barbiturate anesthesia should be avoided to reduce the possibility of splenic engorgement. For short procedures, such as cystoscopy, laparoscopic peritoneal dialysis catheter placement, and laparoscopic renal biopsy, sedation and local anesthesia may be all that is required.

Instrumentation

Cystoscopy is performed with rigid or flexible endoscopes varying from 1.9 to 6 mm in diameter. Rigid scopes provide the best view for cystoscopy in female dogs and cats, male cats, and male dogs with a perineal urethrostomy. Flexible endoscopes are used for cystoscopy in male dogs. Biopsy forceps, grasping forceps, basket forceps, and cytology brushes are used to obtain biopsy specimens.

Five- or 10-mm trocars are used for laparoscopic procedures, depending on the animal's size. A 30° laparoscope provides optimal visibility of the surgical site. The

BOX 12-1

INSTRUMENTATION FOR LAPAROSCOPIC UROLOGIC PROCEDURES

4 or 5 trocars (either 5 or 10 mm, depending on the size of the animal)
Endoscopic dissecting forceps
Endoscopic grasping forceps
Endoscopic curved scissors
Endoscopic Kelly and right-angled forceps
Endoscopic Babcock forceps
Endoscopic DeBakey forceps
Organ retractor
Suction/irrigation/cautery cannula and probe
Endoscopic clip appliers
Endoloop pre-tied loop ligature
Endopouch disposable specimen retrieval bag
2 needle holders
Lapra-Ty suture clip applier
Lapra-Ty suture clips
UltraCision harmonic scalpel and accessories
Bipolar forceps

surgeon should always be prepared for conversion to an open laparotomy by having a sterile laparotomy pack available. Basic instrumentation for performing laparoscopic urologic procedures is listed in Box 12-1.

Cystoscopy

Cystoscopy provides a means to diagnose and treat diseases of the lower urinary tract.[6] Usually, a transurethral approach is used to examine the urethra and bladder.[7] Occasionally, percutaneous cystoscopy or video-assisted percutaneous cystoscopy is used to gain access to the bladder or proximal urethra when they are not accessible by the transurethral approach.[8,9]

TECHNIQUE
Place the animal in dorsal, ventral, or lateral recumbency at the end of the surgical table. Create an optical cavity by distending the urethra and bladder with warmed irrigation fluids such as saline or lactated Ringer's solution. Attach the fluids to the port on the cystoscope cannula and establish an egress path with an intravenous extension set attached to an opposite port.

Although most cystoscopes are equipped with an obturator that can be used to advance the cystoscope cannula blindly, most veterinarians prefer to use an endoscope and advance the cystoscope while viewing the

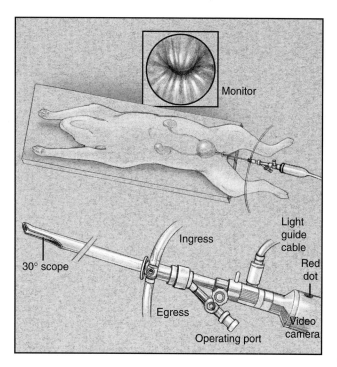

Fig. 12-1   Rigid cystoscopy can be performed in male dogs with a perineal urethrostomy. The dog is placed in the ventral lithotomy position. The video camera, 30° scope, and cysto-scope sheath are aligned.

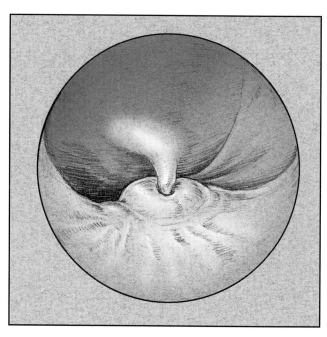

Fig. 12-2   Right ureteral orifice during urine ejection in a male rabbit.

vagina or urethra. Attach the light guide cable to the endoscope and, for optimal viewing, attach the video camera to the eyepiece of the scope. Insert the scope into the cystoscope cannula and extension bridge. Ensure that all fittings are locked together. When looking "down" with a 30° telescope, be sure that the light guide cable is "up" and the video camera is properly oriented so the monitor image correctly reflects the anatomic position (Fig. 12-1).

Lubricate the tip of the cystoscope with water-soluble gel. Begin the fluid flow and insert the tip of the cystoscope into the vagina or urethra. Allow the fluid to distend the structure and carefully pass the cystoscope while examining the walls of the vagina or urethra. To prevent fluid backflow, it may be helpful to hold the labia or the tip of the penis gently around the cystoscope.

In females the urethral tubercle identifies the external orifice of the urethra. It is common to see vaginal bands and the openings of Gartner's ducts in the cranial portion of the vagina. The urethral wall is smooth, and the wall of the vagina cranial to the urethral tubercle has longitudinal folds that flatten as the vagina is distended.

In males the urethra is smooth, with longitudinal folds that flatten with distention. In the middle part of the prostatic urethra, the seminal hillock (colliculus sem-inalis) protrudes into the lumen. Numerous prostatic ducts and the deferent ducts open around the colliculus seminalis.

Continue to advance the cystoscope while the urethra is being distended until the neck of the bladder is identified. Palpate the bladder to ensure that it is not being overly distended. If it is, open the egress port and drain the urine until a clear view is obtained. If the bladder is distended too much, it will be difficult to see the cranial aspect of the bladder wall. Rotate the cystoscope so that all of the bladder wall and trigone area are inspected. Identify the ureteral orifices and observe urine flow into the bladder (Fig. 12-2). To view the caudal aspect of the bladder wall adequately, a 70° scope is preferred.

Take biopsy specimens, passing the forceps or brush through the operating channel of the cystoscope. If a cystoscope with an operating channel is not available, forceps or needles can be passed percutaneously to obtain a biopsy specimen under direct inspection. Alternatively, biopsy forceps can be passed alongside the cystoscope into the bladder.

After the procedure, drain the fluid from the bladder. In animals with questionable bladder wall integrity, consider leaving an indwelling urinary catheter in place for 24 to 48 hours.

Omentectomy and Catheter Placement for Peritoneal Dialysis

Laparoscopic techniques have been used to insert and correct malfunctioning peritoneal dialysis catheters in humans. The correction overcomes subcutaneous leakage of dialysate and allows patients to resume treatment much sooner than with open surgery. The primary port is placed lateral to the edge of the rectus abdominis muscle at the level of the umbilicus.[10] The laparoscope is inserted and used to monitor entry of the second port. Excising the omentum may decrease the incidence of catheter obstruction. If omental resection is planned, a third port is inserted and omentum is removed caudal to the gastroepiploic vessels on the greater curvature of the stomach. Hemostasis is achieved with Endoloop sutures, monopolar electrocautery, bipolar cautery, or the ultrasonic dissector. The excised omentum is removed through one of the ports.

To introduce the catheter, make a 1-cm skin incision at the desired exit point. Use a 7/8 mm trocar to tunnel into the subcutaneous space for a distance of 4 to 5 cm before inserting the trocar into the abdominal cavity. Introduce the catheter through the trocar cannula and position the tip of the catheter cranial to the pubis. Remove the trocar cannula and secure the Dacron cuff on the catheter inside the peritoneal cavity with sutures or staples.

An alternative technique involves placing a 5-mm trocar for the laparoscope and using a system of dilators and sheaths to introduce the catheter (Fig. 12-3).[11] Required instrumentation includes a Veress needle, 8 French sheath, 8 French flexible stylet, and 18 French dilator and sheath. After the abdomen has been insufflated, place the primary trocar away from the umbilicus to minimize fluid leakage. Identify and mark the abdominal entry site on the skin. Place the catheter on the abdominal wall and mark sites for penetration of the internal and external rectus sheaths. Make a skin incision cranial to these sites to allow the cuff to be placed in the subcutaneous tissue.

Trim the 8 French sheath to fit over the outside of the Veress needle, leaving the tip of the needle exposed. Introduce the Veress needle and sheath through the skin incision, tunnel into the subcutaneous space, pop through the external fascia, tunnel into the rectus abdominis muscle, pop through the internal fascia, and tunnel into the retroperitoneal space before entering the abdomen (see Fig. 12-3). The long retroperitoneal tunnel prevents fluid leakage. Remove the Veress needle, leaving the sheath in place. Insert the flexible 8 French stylet and remove the sheath. Pass the 18 French dilator and sheath over the outside of the flexible stylet. Remove the dilator, leaving the sheath in place. Pneumoperi-

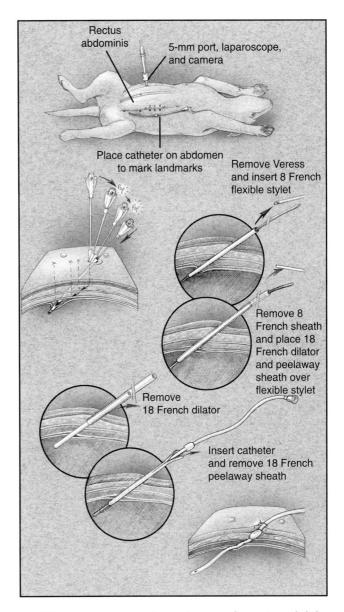

Fig. 12-3 Laparoscopic catheter placement for peritoneal dialysis. The Veress needle and sheath are tunneled obliquely. The needle is replaced with an obturator, and the tract is dilated. The catheter is advanced, and the peelaway sheath is removed.

toneum will be lost. Insert the catheter into the sheath and allow pneumoperitoneum to be reestablished. Remove the peelaway sheath and secure the cuff of the catheter in the subcutaneous space. Confirm that the catheter is in the correct location and functioning properly. Remove the laparoscope and trocar cannula. Close the port site and skin incision.

The most common causes of catheter obstruction are omental wrapping and catheter sequestration.[12] Usually, such problems can be corrected laparoscopically by lysing adhesions and freeing the catheter. If dense adhesions are present, laparotomy is indicated.

Kidney

Laparoscopic procedures involving the kidney include renal biopsy, nephrectomy, and partial nephrectomy. Although all procedures have been performed successfully in animals, nephrectomy and partial nephrectomy require advanced laparoscopic skills.

POSITIONING AND PORT PLACEMENT

Position the animal in reverse Trendelenburg (head-up) position, leaning 30° to 60° to the right for access to the left kidney or 30° to 60° to the left for access to the right kidney. Insert a blunt-tipped 10/12 mm port at the umbilicus and stabilize it appropriately. To provide the largest field of view, the cannula should not extend more than a few millimeters past the peritoneum. In small animals the laparoscope may be too close to the operative site, and the camera port must be moved 2 to 4 cm caudal to the umbilicus. Insert a 12-mm trocar near the fold of each flank. If necessary, insert a 5-mm trocar over the kidney, lateral and slightly cranial to the umbilical port (Fig. 12-4).

Renal Biopsy

Laparoscopy provides an opportunity to obtain a renal biopsy under direct inspection and magnification.[13] Fine-needle aspiration or Tru-Cut biopsy specimens can be obtained easily without biopsy artifact.[14] The diagnostic yield is similar to or better than that obtained with a keyhole approach.[15]

Technique

For renal biopsy only, laparoscopy in small animals can be performed with sedation and local anesthesia or with general anesthesia. Dogs and cats are placed in left lateral recumbency, and a right midabdominal approach is used because the right kidney is less mobile during the biopsy procedure.[7] Small animals are placed in dorsal recumbency under general anesthesia if it is necessary to take a biopsy specimen from both kidneys. In large animals, a standing approach can be used.

Establish pneumoperitoneum and place the primary port at the umbilicus or in the right flank approximately 5 cm caudal to the last rib and 5 cm ventral to the lumbar muscles (see Fig. 12-4). Unless additional ports are needed to retract tissue, no other ports are necessary for a biopsy. One should consider placing an additional 5-mm port if it becomes necessary to apply pressure to control bleeding. Insert a biopsy needle perpendicularly through the abdominal wall directly above the kidney or lesion of interest. Under direct vision, insert the needle at a shallow angle to the renal capsule, directing it away from the hilus (Fig. 12-5). Advance the needle to obtain the specimen or, if using fine-needle biopsy, aspirate the syringe. Control the depth of penetration so the biopsy

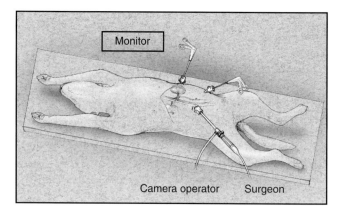

Fig. 12-4   Port placement for laparoscopic approach to the left kidney.

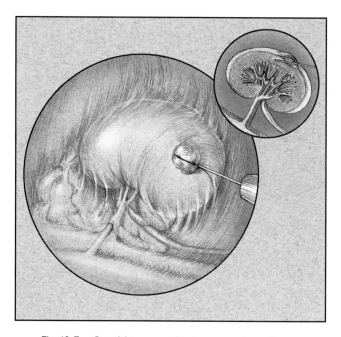

Fig. 12-5   Renal biopsy under laparoscopic guidance.

needle does not injure the renal vasculature. Remove the needle and apply pressure to the renal surface with a cautery probe or grasping forceps. Take additional biopsy specimens as needed. Use cautery or topical hemostatic agents if necessary to ensure hemostasis. As with other approaches, postoperative hematuria may occur.

Nephrectomy

Laparoscopic nephrectomy is performed after irreparable traumatic injury; for diagnosis or treatment of benign, nonfunctioning symptomatic disease; and to harvest kidneys for renal transplantation.[16] Early studies have shown that human kidney donors have less blood loss, less pain, shorter hospitalization, and a faster return to work with a laparoscopic approach than with open procedures.[17]

Technique

Perform insufflation and port placement as described previously. To identify the left kidney, retract the bowel medially and the spleen cranially with 10-mm Babcock retractors from the lower ports. To expose the right kidney, retract the duodenum medially. Grasp the peritoneum with Babcock forceps and create tension between the kidney and abdominal wall. Incise the peritoneum lateral to the kidney from its caudal to its cranial pole, by using an energy source (Fig. 12-6). Use the Babcock forceps with the tips closed as a blunt dissector to free the kidney completely from the surrounding tissue and peritoneum. Control hemorrhage with monopolar or bipolar forceps. Completely free the body wall attachments and allow the kidney to fall medially. Dissect and isolate the ureter. Apply traction on the ureter to tense the renal hilus (Fig. 12-7). Tension aids in dissecting the renal artery and vein. Carefully dissect and isolate the renal blood supply. Clip each artery, leaving two clips on the host side and one clip on the specimen side (Fig. 12-8). Transect the vessels. Place two clips on the ureter and transect between them.

Titanium clips are as secure as size 2/0 or size 0 silk ligatures for occluding the renal artery; however, care should be taken not to dislodge the clips during further dissection.[18] Triple staggered lines of vascular staples are not as secure as are clips or silk sutures. Arteriovenous fistulas may develop when the renal pedicle is ligated with en masse stapled occlusion.[18]

Place the kidney in a disposable specimen retrieval bag of an appropriate size. Pull the bag through a slightly enlarged umbilical port. If the kidney is not neoplastic, it can be crushed inside the bag to allow it to be removed through a smaller incision. At the conclusion of the procedure, irrigate and aspirate the surgical site before removing the trocars. Close the fascia with absorbable sutures and the skin with staples or sutures.

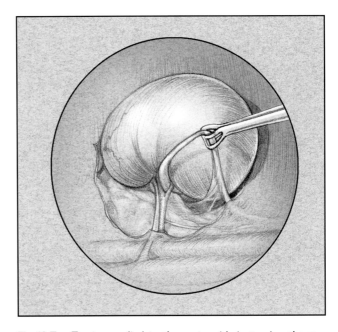

Fig. 12-7   Tension applied to the ureter aids in tensing the renal artery and vein.

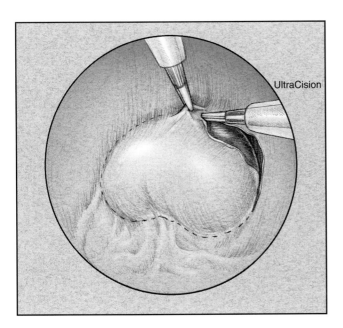

Fig. 12-6   Peritoneal incision for performing nephrectomy.

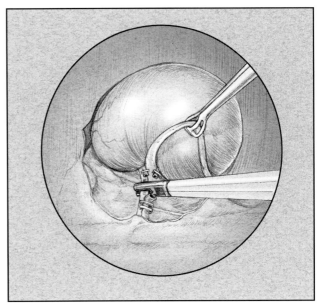

Fig. 12-8   Clipping the renal artery. Two clips are placed on the patient side, and one clip is placed on the specimen side. The vessel is transected between the clips.

Instead of using specimen retrieval bags or morcellators, some surgeons prefer to make a 5- to 7-cm incision to allow a hand to be introduced inside the abdominal cavity. Loss of peritoneum is prevented by sealing the fascia with a purse-string suture or a special device called a Dexterity Pneumo Sleeve* that attaches to the body wall (Fig. 12-9).[19] With laparoscopic guidance and magnification, the surgeon inserts his or her nondominant hand into the abdomen to retract, grasp, and bluntly dissect tissue while the dominant hand uses laparoscopic instruments to cut, clip, or staple tissue. Hand-assisted laparoscopic nephrectomies in pigs required less operative time than when the procedure was performed with entirely laparoscopic techniques.[20] The surgeon's tactile sense is retained, and the animal benefits from a slightly smaller incision.

Partial Nephrectomy

Partial nephrectomy is indicated when an animal needs a nephron-sparing operation. Trauma confined to one pole of the kidney is an ideal indication. Controlling bleeding from the renal parenchyma is a primary concern in performing this procedure. Partial nephrectomy is performed by isolating the blood supply to the portion of kidney to be removed. The renal artery and vein are occluded with an atraumatic vascular clamp. The procedure has been performed experimentally in pigs by using a plastic cable tie to provide ischemia and an argon beam coagulator* to fulgurate the transected surface.[21] The nephrotomy can also be made with a laser or monopolar needle-pointed cautery tip (Fig. 12-10). The intraabdominal pressure must be monitored carefully when using an argon beam coagulator because high argon gas flows can result in dangerously high intraabdominal pressures. Topical hemostatic agents can be used in combination with an argon beam coagulator.

Smaller sections of a kidney can be ablated selectively with lasers or cryosurgery.[22] The neodymium:yttrium-aluminum-garnet (Nd:YAG) laser has been used for coagulation and necrosis of small lesions of the kidney. At energies of 480 J, coagulation necrosis of the renal parenchyma predominantly occurs. At 720 J, pronounced tissue vaporization surrounded by a zone of coagulation necrosis results. The holmium:YAG laser provides more

---

*Pilling Weck, Inc, Research Triangle Park, N.C. 27709.

*Argon Beam Coagulation System, ConMed Corp, Utica, N.Y. 10351.

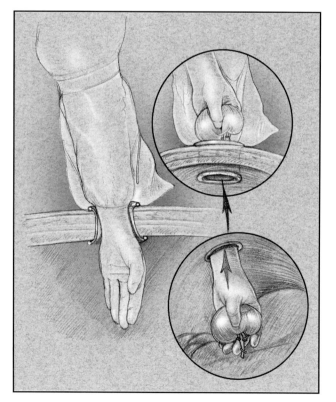

Fig. 12-9 A pneumo sleeve prevents loss of pneumoperitoneum during insertion of a hand into the abdomen. The sleeve attaches to a wound protector in the incision and to the surgeon's arm.

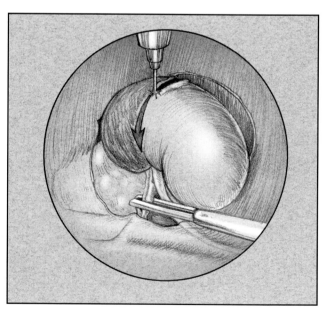

Fig. 12-10 Laser incision for partial nephrectomy.

precise cutting with a more superficial zone of coagulative necrosis than the Nd:YAG laser and, when combined with electrocautery, provides adequate hemostasis.[23] When the laser is used, minimal manipulation is required.

RESULTS

Laparoscopic nephrectomy has been reported in numerous human clinical cases and is used at some centers for liver-donor nephrectomy. Most procedures are completed laparoscopically, but the extent of adhesions, pathology of the kidney, and experience of the surgeon influence the outcomes. Five centers reported results from a 4-year study of 185 patients.[24] Complications occurred in 30 patients (16%). The rate was higher in patients with renal cancer. Intraoperative complications included vessel injury, splenic injury, and pneumothorax.

Swine have been used as a training model for laparoscopic nephrectomy in humans. Several studies have been performed in pigs and goats to refine the port placement and technique for human surgery.[25-28] The procedure was performed successfully with minimal bleeding. Laparoscopic nephrectomy has been performed in rats.[29] With increasing experience and access to instrumentation, the technical feasibility of these procedures will be proven in veterinary surgery.

Urinary Bladder

The development of minimally invasive procedures involving the urinary bladder has focused mainly on correction of vesicoureteral reflux because of the high incidence of this disease in children. In veterinary medicine, trauma, urinary calculi, and removal of mass lesions are more likely to be encountered.

CORRECTION OF VESICOURETERAL REFLUX

The clinical significance of vesicoureteral reflux has not been fully assessed in dogs and cats. Ureteral reflux does not ordinarily occur because the oblique insertion of the ureter into the bladder causes the ureter to collapse when the bladder fills. If reflux is associated with a persistent renal infection, hydronephrosis, or renal calculi, permanent renal damage could occur and the condition would require correction. When vesicoureteral reflux occurs in adults, the surgical correction involves creating a submural tunnel five times longer than the diameter of the ureter. Laparoscopic reflux repair has been shown to be a viable alternative to standard open surgical repair.[30-32]

Studies have shown that this procedure is technically possible and effective in normal pigs with surgically induced ureteral reflux. Surgical time was approximately 2 hours, and the animals were able to eat the day after surgery. Urinary tract infections or other difficulties were not encountered.

CYSTOTOMY CLOSURE

Closure of the bladder may be necessary after trauma, surgical errors, or cystotomy incisions for removal of calculi or resection of mural lesions. Bladder incisions can be closed with laparoscopic suturing and knot tying, suturing and endoscopic knot clips, or a laparoscopic stapling device.[33,34] Care should be taken when using the stapling device. When the edges are inverted with a linear stapling device, calculi can develop on the staple line. Everted staple lines do not appear to result in calculi formation.

Technique

Anesthesia, positioning, and port placement are the same for cystotomy as for other pelvic surgery (see Fig. 11-1). Place the camera port at the umbilicus and additional ports in the caudal abdominal quadrants. If necessary, resect an affected area of the bladder with endoscopic Metzenbaum scissors attached to monopolar electrocautery or another energy source such as ultrasound. The incision can be closed with a simple continuous pattern of size 3/0 Vicryl (polyglactin 910) or a suture secured with suture clips (Fig. 12-11). As with an open cystotomy closure, an inverting suture pattern with sutures that do not penetrate the mucosa is ideal. Place a second row of

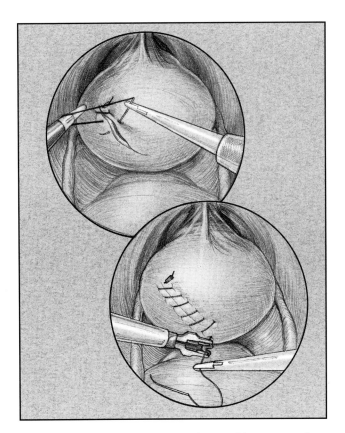

Fig. 12-11 Laparoscopic cystotomy closure with sutures and Lapra-Ty clips.

sutures if necessary. Surgeons proficient with intracorporeal suturing may prefer size 3/0 PDS (polydiaxanone) suture because of smooth tissue passage. Polydiaxanone sutures should not be used with suture clips, because the monofilament suture may place additional stress on the hinge of the clip and cause premature opening.

Bladder closure has also been achieved with an endoscopic linear stapling device applied across the bladder wall. An everted staple line with three rows of titanium staples is the result. Each application of staples extends 3 cm, and additional firings may be required. Similar techniques can be used to close a traumatic bladder rupture.

At the conclusion of the surgical procedure, place the animal in head-up position and irrigate and aspirate the surgical site. If an infectious process is involved, administer antibiotics as appropriate. The bladder may be drained by an indwelling urinary catheter for 24 to 48 hours. The animal should be encouraged to void frequently during the recovery period.

Results

Laparoscopic stapled bladder closure was performed successfully in eight pigs.[35] Calculi did not form at the staple site in short-term studies in pigs; however, calculi were detected 6 months after cystotomy closure with staples in a foal.[36] Laparoscopic cystotomy closure was performed in four healthy beagle dogs to evaluate the function of absorbable suture clips.[37] The ventral aspect of the bladder was incised for approximately 2 cm. Laparoscopic suturing techniques were used to place a continuous vertical mattress suture line. The sutures were placed approximately 3 mm apart and did not penetrate the mucosa of the bladder. Each end of the suture was secured with a laparoscopic suture clip. The procedures required approximately 45 minutes to perform. When the sites were examined approximately 2 weeks later, there was no evidence of leakage, adhesions, or calculi formation in any of the dogs. Although the feasibility of these techniques has been demonstrated, advanced laparoscopic skills are essential for a good result.

REFERENCES

1. Moore RG et al: Adhesion formation after transperitoneal nephrectomy: laparoscopic vs. open approach. *J Endourol* 9:277-280, 1995.
2. Christie BA, Bjorling DE: Kidneys. In Slatter DE, editor: Textbook of small animal surgery, ed 2, Philadelphia, 1993, WB Saunders.
3. Evans HE, Christensen GC: The urogenital system. In Evans HE, editor: Miller's anatomy of the dog, ed 3, Philadelphia, 1993, WB Saunders.
4. Ordorica RC, Moran ME: Vital dye sham intrarenal lesions: assessment of risk of intra-abdominal tumor spread during laparoscopic nephrectomy and morcellation. *Minim Invasive Ther* 3:105-109, 1994.
5. Mendoza D et al: Laparoscopic complications in markedly obese urologic patients (a multi-institutional review). *Urology* 48:562-567, 1996.
6. McCarthy TC, McDermaid SL: Cystoscopy. *Vet Clin North Am Small Anim Pract* 20:1315-1339, 1990.
7. Jones BD: The role of cystoscopy in the diagnosis of lower urinary tract disease. Seminar notes from the Fourth International Course in Small Animal Rigid Endoscopy, March 21-22, 1997, Colorado State University.
8. McCarthy TC, McDermaid SL: Prepubic percutaneous cystoscopy in the dog and cat. *J Am Anim Hosp Assn* 22:213-219, 1986.
9. Van Lue SJ, Cowles RS III, Rawlings CA: Video-assisted percutaneous cystoscopy of the bladder and prostatic urethra in the dog: new approach for visual laser ablation of the prostate. *J Endourol* 9:503-507, 1995.
10. Thompson SE: Unpublished data. 1994.
11. Stevenson R, Freeman LJ: Unpublished data. 1995.
12. Amerling R et al: Laparoscopic salvage of malfunctioning peritoneal catheters. *Surg Endosc* 11:249-252, 1997.
13. Grauer GF, Twedt DC, Mero KN: Evaluation of laparoscopy for obtaining renal biopsy specimens from dogs and cats. *J Am Vet Med Assoc* 183:677-679, 1983.
14. Grauer GF: Laparoscopy of the urinary tract. In Tams TR, editor: Small animal endoscopy. St. Louis, 1990, Mosby.
15. Wise LA, Allen TA, Cartwright M: Comparison of renal biopsy techniques in dogs. *J Am Vet Med Assoc* 195:935-939, 1989.
16. Fornara P, Doehn C, Fricke L: Laparoscopic bilateral nephrectomy: results in 11 renal transplant patients. *J Urol* 157:445-449, 1997.
17. Ratner LE et al: Laparoscopic assisted live donor nephrectomy: a comparison with the open approach. *Transplantation* 63:229-233, 1997.
18. Kerbl K et al: Ligation of the renal pedicle during laparoscopic nephrectomy: a comparison of staples, clips, and sutures. *J Laparoendosc Surg* 3:9-12, 1993.
19. Bemelman WA et al: Laparoscopic-assisted colectomy with the Dexterity pneumo sleeve. *Dis Colon Rectum* 39:S59-S61, 1996.
20. Bannenberg JJG et al: Hand-assisted laparoscopic nephrectomy in the pig: initial report. *Minim Invasive Ther Allied Technol* 5:483-487, 1996.
21. McDougall EM et al: Laparoscopic partial nephrectomy in the pig model. *J Urol* 149:1633-1636, 1993.
22. Lofti MA, McCue P, Gomella LG: Laparoscopic interstitial contact laser ablation of renal lesions: an experimental model. *J Endourol* 8:153-156, 1994.
23. Johnson DE, Cromeens DM, Price RE: Use of the holmium: YAG laser in urology. *Lasers Surg Med* 12:353-363, 1992.
24. Gill IS et al: Complications of laparoscopic nephrectomy in 185 patients: a multi-institutional review. *J Urol* 154:479-483, 1995.
25. Higashihara E et al: Laparoscopic nephrectomy: animal experiment and clinical application. *Nippon Hinyokika Gakkai Zasshi* 83:395-400, 1992.
26. Kerbl K et al: Retroperitoneal laparoscopic nephrectomy: laboratory and clinical experience. *J Endourol* 7:23-26, 1993.
27. Gill IS et al: Laparoscopic live-donor nephrectomy. *J Endourol* 8:143-148, 1994.
28. Guillonneau B et al: Retroperitoneal laparoscopic nephrectomy: animal and human anatomic studies. *J Endourol* 9:487-490, 1995.
29. Giuffrida MC et al: Laparoscopic splenectomy and nephrectomy in a rat model: description of a new technique. *Surg Endosc* 11:491-494, 1997.
30. Schimberg W et al: Laparoscopic correction of vesicoureteral reflux in the pig. *J Urol* 151:1664-1667, 1994.

31. Atala A et al: Laparoscopic correction of vesicoureteral reflux. *J Urol* 150:748-751, 1993.
32. McDougall EM et al: Laparoscopic repair of vesicoureteral reflux utilizing the Lich-Gregoir technique in the pig model. *J Urol* 153:497-500, 1995.
33. Adams JB et al: New laparoscopic suturing device: initial clinical experience. *Urology* 46:242-245, 1995.
34. Anderson KR et al: Laparoscopic assisted continent urinary diversion in the pig. *J Urol* 154:1934-1938, 1995.
35. Kerbl K et al: Laparoscopic stapled bladder closure: laboratory and clinical experience. *J Urol* 149:1437-1440, 1993.
36. Edwards RB, Ducharme NG, Hackett RP: Laparoscopic repair of a bladder rupture in a foal. *Vet Surg* 24:60-63, 1995.
37. Freeman LJ: Unpublished data. 1991.

Repair of a Ruptured Bladder

DEAN A. HENDRICKSON

Overview

Laparoscopic repair of a bladder rupture in a foal has been described.[1] The bladder rupture was diagnosed by laparoscopy and repaired with a laparoscopic stapling device. The foal subsequently developed a urinary calculus 10 months later. The use of nonabsorbable staples in the bladder is questioned.

Surgical Technique

PREPARATION

Foals with ruptured urinary bladders are generally presented for emergency repair. Fasting before surgery therefore typically is not feasible. Because most are just a few days old and consuming milk only, fasting is not considered necessary. Use of nonsteroidal antiinflammatory drugs and antibiotics is variable and depends on the surgeon's preference.

ANESTHESIA

Anesthetic protocol for laparoscopy is similar to that used for open surgery for a foal with a ruptured bladder. Electrolyte abnormalities are common in foals with uroperitoneum. The surgeon and anesthesiologist should work together to ensure that the foal is stable before it receives anesthesia. Assisted ventilation is indicated because of increased abdominal pressure secondary to insufflation, positioning of the foal, and the potential for peritoneal carbon dioxide (CO_2) absorption.

POSITIONING

Once anesthetized, the foal is placed in dorsal recumbency. The ventral abdomen is aseptically prepared for surgery. Secure the foal to the surgical table to minimize slippage when the table is tilted. Drapes are placed at the umbilicus, the lateral flank folds, and over the inguinal region. After the abdomen is insufflated and the laparoscope inserted, the animal is tilted head down (Trendelenburg position). The video monitor is positioned directly at the rear of the animal, or slightly to one side if the hind legs are between the surgeon and monitor. The surgeon and assistant stand on either side of the abdomen.

PROCEDURE

Insufflation

One of two techniques may be used to gain access to and insufflate the abdomen.

Open Technique

The open technique is performed by making an incision through the skin and linea alba at the level of the umbilicus, and placing the trocar cannula under direct visualization. The abdomen is then insufflated with CO_2 to a constant pressure of 15 to 20 mm Hg. One advantage of this technique is that iatrogenic damage to the underlying viscera is avoided. One disadvantage is that if the incision is slightly too large, CO_2 may escape around the cannula, making pneumoperitoneum difficult to maintain.

Insufflation With a Veress Needle or Teat Cannula

A Veress needle or teat cannula is inserted into the peritoneal space through a small stab incision at the umbilicus. The needle is connected to a CO_2 insufflator to distend the abdomen to 15 to 20 mm Hg pressure. Once the abdomen is distended, the Veress needle or teat cannula is removed and the skin incision increased to accommodate the telescope cannula. The trocar is placed through the body wall with a slow, but constant, twisting motion. The insufflation tubing, telescope, and video camera are then connected.

Placement of Secondary Ports

After initial exploration, the animal is placed in Trendelenburg position to ease further exploration and surgical manipulation in the caudal part of the abdomen. Secondary ports are placed under direct visualization using the same principles described previously. Some surgeons prefer to preplace a spinal needle to determine the exact entry point of the additional cannulas. Two

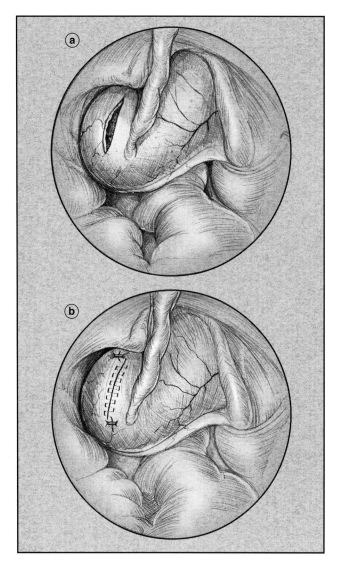

Fig. 12-12 Intraabdominal views of the caudal ventral abdomen of a dorsally recumbent horse, showing repair of a ruptured urinary bladder. View of the ventral aspect of the bladder, showing the tear (*a*). Same view with intracorporeal suturing of the bladder, using absorbable clips to replace knots (*b*).

secondary ports generally are placed. A trocar is placed on each side of midline, approximately 10 cm cranial to the cranial aspect of the inguinal rings. It may be necessary to aspirate some of the abdominal fluid to improve visualization of the operative site.

Staple Technique

For the staple technique the bladder is grasped with an atraumatic grasping forceps, and the tear in the bladder wall is identified. (Fig. 12-12). The edges of the tear should be freshened and then apposed. Sutures, a hernia stapler, or a linear stapling instrument may be used. A linear stapling instrument was used in the report, and a urolith was noted after 10 months. The urolith may have formed secondary to the use of nonabsorbable staples or nonabsorbable suture material. Alternatively, the tear can be closed with intracorporeal suturing, either by tying intracorporeal knots or by using absorbable clips at the ends of the suture lines (see Fig. 12-12, *b*).

At the end of the procedure, the cannulas are opened, the pneumoperitoneum released or actively suctioned, and the cannulas removed. The incisions are closed in two layers. A cruciate pattern of a size 0 synthetic, absorbable suture material is used in the linea alba or external rectus sheath. For skin closure, either an intradermal pattern with a size 00 synthetic absorbable suture material or a cruciate pattern using a size 00 synthetic nonabsorbable suture material is used. The horse is recovered from anesthesia and allowed to resume normal exercise.

Complications of Bladder Repair

Complications of bladder repair include urolith formation secondary to the use of nonabsorbable suture material.

POTENTIAL COMPLICATIONS
Anesthetic complications are as described previously but need to be specifically addressed in foals with severe electrolyte disturbances. Laparoscopic complications are as described previously.

Conclusion

Bladder repair using laparoscopic techniques can be performed, but I recommend that stapling equipment not be used. It is more technically demanding to place intracorporeal sutures, but the risks of subsequent urolith formation can be reduced with absorbable suture material.

REFERENCE
1. Edwards RB, Ducharme NG, Hackett RP: Laparoscopic repair of a bladder rupture in a foal. *Vet Surg* 24:60-63, 1995.

CHAPTER 13

ARTHROSCOPY

Timothy C. McCarthy

Veterinarians are beginning to adopt arthroscopy techniques for use in small animals. Tissues are traumatized less with arthroscopy than with arthrotomy, producing shortened recovery times.[1] Arthroscopy facilitates inspection of intraarticular soft tissue and cartilage not apparent on radiographs, and the visibility of most structures is better than with arthrotomy.[2-5] Direct examination of joint surfaces with magnification and optimal lighting improves diagnostic accuracy. With proficiency, operative time, anesthesia time, and the potential for complications from anesthesia are reduced.

Three factors make arthroscopy the most difficult rigid endoscopic technique to master: (1) small optical cavities with rigid, bony confinement; (2) the complexity of some joints; and (3) the fragility of the instruments, which must be handled carefully. During the learning phase, arthroscopic procedures take longer to perform than do open surgical procedures. It has been suggested that the learning curve for performing arthroscopy of the shoulder joint in dogs encompasses approximately 30 cases.[6] I have experience in 250 arthroscopic procedures and am approaching proficiency. Practice, patience, and persistence are required to master the appropriate skills and obtain good results.[7] This chapter provides a foundation for continued learning.

Indications

DIAGNOSIS

Diagnostic arthroscopy may be indicated when joint disease is suspected from clinical or radiographic findings. Clinical signs of joint disease include lameness, pain, joint capsule distention, periarticular soft-tissue swelling, crepitus, laxity, and thickening or enlargement of a joint by fibrosis or osteophytosis. Radiographic indications for arthroscopy include evidence of increased joint fluid, joint capsule thickening, periarticular soft-tissue swelling, osteophyte formation, sclerosis, joint space narrowing, cartilaginous or osseous deformities or defects, bone chips or fragments, and joint laxity or subluxation. Arthroscopy provides direct examination of joint cartilage, synovial membranes, menisci, and ligaments.

Conditions that have been diagnosed arthroscopically include osteochondritis dissecans (OCD) of the shoulder, stifle, elbow, and hock joints; meniscal injuries; partial and complete cruciate ligament ruptures; fragmentation of the medial coronoid process; degenerative joint disease; intraarticular fractures; synovitis; bicipital tendinitis; bicipital tendon rupture; and neoplasia. Cartilage lesions can be detected before the onset of degenerative joint disease. Obtaining biopsy specimens of synovial membrane from more than one joint with a minimally invasive technique is particularly helpful in the diagnosis of immune-mediated arthropathies. For long-term research studies, serial samples to evaluate pathologic changes can be obtained.

THERAPY

Arthroscopy is used for definitive surgical treatment of selected conditions. Treatment of OCD of the shoulder, elbow, stifle, and hock joints has been described. The articular cartilage flap is removed, and the subchondral bone is curetted. Internal stabilization of the stifle joint after rupture of the cranial cruciate ligament was per-

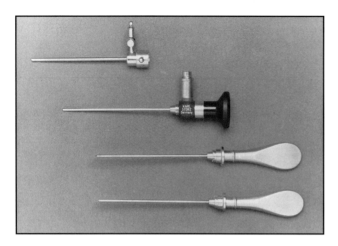

Fig. 13-1 Cannula, 2.4-mm, 30° arthroscope, sharp trocar, and blunt obturator. (Courtesy Karl Storz Veterinary Endoscopy America.)

formed successfully in dogs; however, carbon fiber implants failed and the instability returned.[8] Coronoid process fragment removal with debridement of the defect has been successful. As technical expertise grows and equipment is made available, new therapies will be developed.

Instrumentation and Equipment

Rigid telescopes used for arthroscopy are 1.9 to 5.0 mm in diameter. The sizes used most frequently in small animals are 1.9, 2.4, and 2.7 mm. The 2.4- or 2.7-mm arthroscopes appear to be appropriate for the majority of procedures. In animals that weigh less than 20 kg and in small joints, a 1.9-mm scope may be more useful. A 25° or 30° viewing angle greatly facilitates examination of joints by increasing the field of view. By rotating the telescope, regions of the joint not in direct alignment with the arthroscope can be seen.

Trocar cannulas are selected to correspond in size with the arthroscope and instruments to be used. Each cannula is equipped with a blunt obturator and a sharp trocar. The cannula houses a stopcock to control the flow of fluid into the joint (Fig. 13-1).

Small light sources are adequate for direct inspection during diagnostic procedures. Video instrumentation, which is essential for operative arthroscopy, requires at least a 250 W xenon light source. Video equipment enables the entire operating team to see the procedure and work together. Use of video equipment helps in maintaining sterile technique for operative procedures and facilitates conversion from diagnostic arthroscopy to open surgery. With the direct inspection technique, conversion to arthrotomy requires that the surgical site, team, and instruments be prepared again for sterile surgery.

The optical space is established and maintained by distention with a fluid. Appropriate fluids include normal saline and lactated Ringer's solution. In one study, proteoglycans were depleted when saline was used.[9] In another, there were no significant differences between normal saline, lactated Ringer's solution, and sterile water.[10] Lactated Ringer's solution has no disadvantages; I have used it with no adverse clinical effects.

Fluid flow is maintained in several ways. An intravenous set connected to a 1-L bag provides gravity flow. If necessary, a syringe and three-way stopcock, a manual pressure bag, or an infusion pump can be added. Gravity flow is easy to set up and is effective for all diagnostic and many operative procedures. Ingress fluids are attached to the arthroscopic cannula and help maintain a clear view. Continuous drainage is provided by an egress needle or cannula. Overzealous fluid infusion can result in subcutaneous fluid collection, which compresses the joint capsule and interferes with the examination.

A single telescope port and egress cannula can be used for diagnostic arthroscopy. Two or more cannulas are used for therapeutic procedures. Instruments for cartilage, bone, and synovial tissue removal are inserted through the second port. A variety of hand- and power-driven equipment is available. Specific requirements for instrumentation in dogs have not been completely elucidated. Many procedures appear to be feasible with a limited number of hand instruments. Grasping forceps, a graduated probe, basket forceps, a curette, and an arthroscopic knife are essential instruments for small-animal arthroscopy (Fig. 13-2). Power instruments, including small joint and maxillofacial cartilage shavers, are being evaluated for application in small-animal practice. A cartilage shaver for human maxillofacial applications uses shavers, bits, and burrs similar to small arthroscopy units. The maxillofacial cartilage shaver's handpiece is shorter and weighs less than the arthroscopy units, making it much easier to use in small joints.

Preparation

Arthroscopy requires general anesthesia and aseptic technique. The animal is prepared and draped as for an arthrotomy, using impervious drape materials. Endoscopes and other instruments are sterilized with glutaraldehyde or ethylene oxide, or by autoclaving. Manufacturers recommendations for sterilization of specific instruments should be followed.

The limb is positioned and stabilized by an assistant, or it can be immobilized in a holding device. Basic principles of endoscopic operating room setup are followed. The patient and video monitor are arranged so the telescope is pointed toward the monitor for most of the procedure (Fig. 13-3). This concept is essential to effective

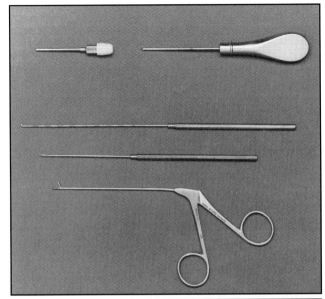

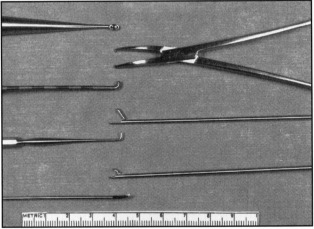

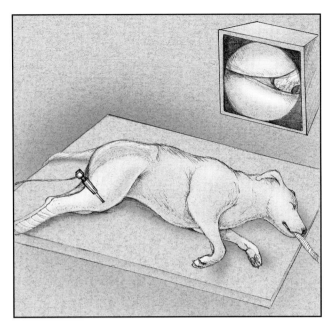

Fig. 13-3 Operative setup for stifle arthroscopy. The animal is positioned and prepared for sterile surgery as would be done for an arthrotomy. The monitor is positioned so the scope faces the monitor for most of the procedure.

Fig. 13-2 **A,** Instruments used for arthroscopy. *Top to bottom:* Operative instrument port with blunt obturator, graduated probe, curved knife, grasping forceps. (Courtesy Karl Storz Veterinary Endoscopy America.) **B,** *Left, top to bottom:* 0000 curette, hook probe with graduations, hook/right-angle probe, curved arthroscopy knife. *Right, top to bottom:* Mosquito hemostatic forceps, 2.0-mm arthroscopic grasping forceps, and 2.0-mm arthroscopic rongeur.

arthroscopy. The techniques are difficult enough to learn and master without adding the problem of disorientation caused by improper monitor placement. Having a radiograph in the operating room of the joint being examined helps maintain orientation.

Basic Operative Technique

Prepare the limb aseptically as for an open arthrotomy. Effective arthroscopy requires that the joint be freely movable, and draping must allow a full range of flexion, extension, and rotation of the joint. To achieve this mobility, suspend the limb and drape it with a stockinette and waterproof barrier drape.

Insert a 1- to 2-inch, 20-gauge hypodermic needle into the joint (Fig. 13-4). Withdraw synovial fluid to ensure intraarticular placement. If desired, save the fluid sample and submit it for analysis. Distend the joint capsule with sterile lactated Ringer's solution. Make an incision in the skin with a No. 15 blade at the site selected for joint entry, just large enough to insert the initial cannula. The arthroscope cannula with a blunt obturator is inserted into the joint (Fig. 13-5). Although more force is required to enter the joint with a blunt obturator than with a sharp trocar, the risk of damage to the articular cartilage is dramatically reduced. When the cannula has been properly positioned, remove the obturator and insert the arthroscope. Ensure that the telescope locks into position on the cannula (Fig. 13-6).

Attach an intravenous administration set and 1-L container of sterile lactated Ringer's solution to the endoscope cannula injection port. Maintain continuous irrigation of the joint with lactated Ringer's solution to provide a clear view and maintain joint distention. The fluids can be allowed to flow from the joint through the hypodermic needle used for the initial joint distention, a hypodermic needle placed at a secondary location, or a specially designed egress cannula.

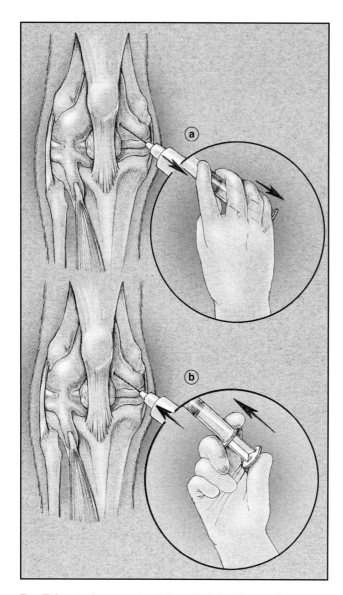

Fig. 13-4 Arthrocentesis of the stifle joint. The needle is inserted above the fat pad either medial or lateral to the patellar tendon. A sample of synovial fluid is withdrawn for analysis and to confirm the intraarticular needle placement (*a*). Saline is injected to distend the joint capsule until it is firm, but not hard (*b*).

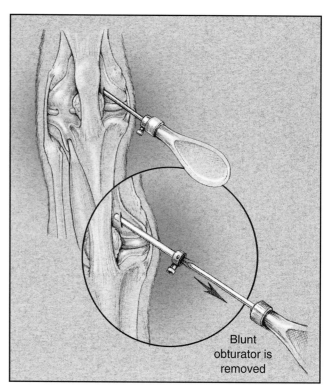

Fig. 13-5 The arthroscope cannula is inserted through a skin incision. A blunt obturator reduces the risk of articular cartilage damage. The cannula is placed either medial or lateral to the patellar tendon proximal to the fat pad.

Although distention of the joint capsule is necessary for examination, constant flow to provide a clear visual field is more important than pressure for joint distention. Dogs are especially susceptible to fluid extravasation into subcutaneous tissues. Pressures higher than 50 mm Hg should be avoided.[11] Wise port placement, minimal joint movement, and avoidance of excessive distention help minimize fluid extravasation. If fluid begins to accumulate in the subcutaneous or periarticular tissues, the superficial tissue incision is enlarged to create a tapered channel and allow fluid to escape.

High-flow, low-pressure systems facilitate examination by providing a clear visual field without excessive fluid extravasation. Power instruments require a very high flow system because aspiration through the hollow shaver blade removes debris created by the shaving procedure. Negative pressure created by the aspiration causes air to be pulled into the joint, interfering with visibility. To overcome this, fluid inflow is increased and aspiration is carefully controlled. With power equipment, the shaver tip becomes the egress port and fluid inflow can be increased by using a large, multiport egress cannula for fluid inflow. Specialized high-flow, low-pressure pumps are available.

If needed, additional instrument and telescope portals can be created. Follow the principle of triangulation for additional port placements so the telescope does not interfere with the operative procedure (Fig. 13-7). The arthroscope and operative instrument form two sides of the triangle, with the apex of the triangle located at the lesion. The angle of convergence of the two sides of the triangle is critical. Too narrow an angle makes orientation and manipulation of the instruments difficult and it increases interference by the telescope. The tip of the instrument and the optical field of the telescope must meet at the desired point within the joint. The anatomy of the

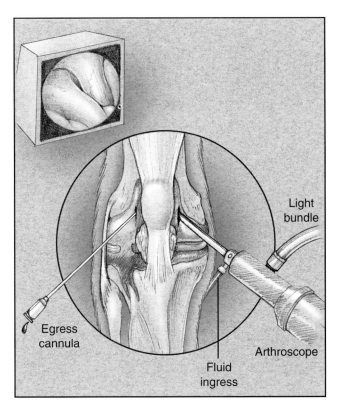

Fig. 13-6 The arthroscope is inserted and locked onto the cannula. The image appears on the video monitor. Fluids are attached to the ingress port on the arthroscope cannula. With the telescope portal medial to the patellar tendon, a secondary portal is initially placed laterally for egress of fluids. The egress portal is converted to an operative portal if indicated.

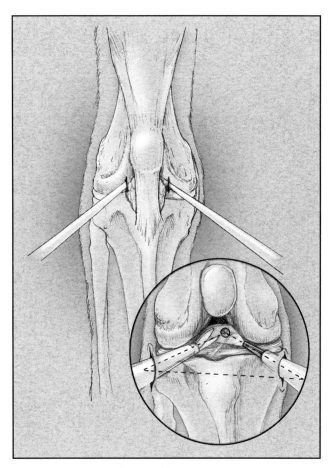

Fig. 13-7 Principles of triangulation. The arthroscope and operative instrument form two sides of the triangle. The desired point within the joint at which the instruments meet forms the apex of the triangle. The angle between the operative instrument and arthroscope is known as the *angle of convergence.*

joint must be considered when selecting the point and angle of insertion, to avoid interference by the surrounding bony structures. Care must be taken to avoid damage to articular cartilage and instrumentation. Encroachment of a black edge into the circular view on the monitor indicates that the scope is being bent.

To use the principle of triangulation, insert a 20-gauge, 1- to 2-inch hypodermic needle at the intended site. While viewing the surgical site and needle inside the joint, withdraw and reposition the needle until the optimal point of insertion and the correct angle are achieved. Remove the needle, incise the skin, and insert the operative cannula or instrument. Frequently, it is easier to insert instruments directly into the joint through a stab incision in the skin without using a cannula. Practitioners disagree about the use of instrument cannulas vs. the free-passage technique. Both techniques have applications. Debriding joints with hand instruments requires many passes, and a cannula is useful. A cannula may also be useful to pass instruments through thick muscle, such as the caudal operating port in shoulder arthroscopy. In tight joint spaces, the pressure of a cannula interferes with instrument manipulation. Removing large bone or cartilage fragments requires free passage. Frequently, both techniques are used in the same joint.

At the end of the procedure, instill a local anesthetic if desired, remove the instruments and allow excess fluid to drain from the joint. If needed, apply compression to ensure that fluid is completely drained. Place a single skin suture at each puncture site.

Surgical Approach

Arthroscopic ports have been established in dogs for the stifle, shoulder, elbow, hock, and hip joints. The locations of instrument ports and egress cannula sites for each joint have been tentatively defined.

SHOULDER JOINT

Arthroscopy can be used to examine or diagnose OCD of the humeral head, instability of the shoulder joint, tenosynovitis of the biceps brachii tendon, rupture of the biceps brachii tendon, articular fractures, and traumatic lesions. Arthroscopic techniques can be used to obtain synovial biopsy specimens in suspected inflammatory or immune-mediated arthropathies. In OCD of the humeral head, osteochondral flaps can be removed and the subchondral defects debrided. The bicipital tendon can be transected to facilitate screw fixation to the humerus.

Position the animal in lateral recumbency with the affected limb up so traction can be applied by an assistant or with a leg-holding device. After aseptic preparation, palpate the acromion. The preferred telescope port site is distal to the tip of the acromion process, directly over the joint space. This site has been described in the literature as 1 to 2 cm caudal and 1 cm distal to the tip of the acromion process.[6] This is an accurate description when studying an anatomic drawing or specimen. Clinically, on palpation the acromion process with the attached tendon of origin of the deltoid muscle is more blunt, and the insertion point is more directly distal than caudodistal. An alternative site for arthroscope placement is on the cranial aspect of the joint, dorsolateral to the greater tubercle of the humerus.[7] I determined recently that a site between these two ports may be better. Move cranially from the lateral port site until the cranial margin of the deltoid muscle can be palpated (Fig. 13-8). A space is present between the deltoid muscle and greater tubercle in which no muscles overlay the joint. This site allows examination of the most common OCD location on the humeral head and the bicipital tendon and bursa, and it provides a better site for triangulation of the instrument port site for removal of the humeral head OCD lesions.

For needle insertion, apply traction while abducting the scapula and adducting the distal end of the limb to produce varus angulation and distraction of the shoulder joint. Pass the needle medially, perpendicular to the skin surface, directly into the joint space between the scapula and the head of the humerus. Make a skin incision and, with the joint distended, insert the telescope cannula. After the arthroscope is inserted and fluid flow is established, place an egress portal dorsomedial to the greater tubercle. Placement of the egress portal is facilitated by observing a needle placement from inside the joint. The needle is inserted dorsomedial to the greater tubercle into the joint lateral to the bicipital tendon. Accurate placement to miss the bicipital tendon can be ensured by arthroscopic examination. A needle is an adequate egress portal for diagnostic arthroscopy and for most operative

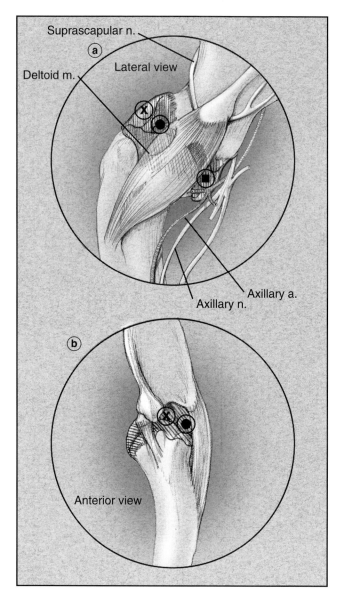

Fig. 13-8 Arthroscopy port sites for the left shoulder joint for OCD lesion removal. Lateral view showing placement of the telescope portal (●), operative portal (■), and the egress cannula or needle (x) relative to the axillary artery and nerve and the suprascapular nerve (a). Anteroposterior view showing placement of the arthroscope portal (●) and the egress needle or cannula (x) (b).

procedures. If drainage is inadequate, replace the needle with an egress cannula.

Begin a systematic examination. Structures of interest in the shoulder are the origin of the bicipital tendon, the caudal aspect of the humeral head, and the caudal cul-de-sac of the joint. A meniscus-like structure is identifiable in the medial joint space between the humeral head and glenoid joint surfaces. The bicipital tendon is seen best by directing the telescope cranially (Fig. 13-9) and

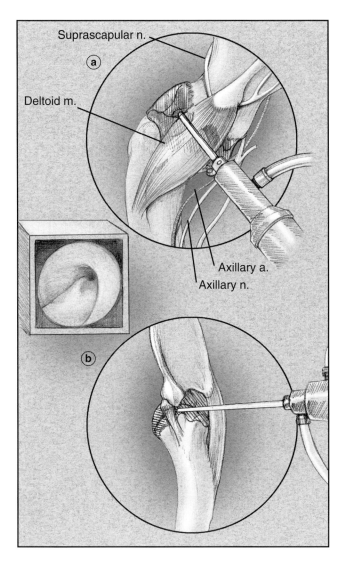

Fig. 13-9   Lateral (a) and anteroposterior (b) views of the left shoulder joint showing placement of the arthroscope for viewing the bicipital tendon and bursa.

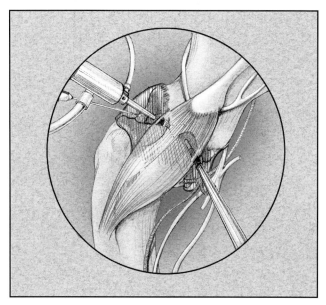

Fig. 13-10   Lateral view of the left shoulder joint showing placement of arthroscope, instruments, and egress needle for treatment of humeral head OCD lesions.

extending the shoulder with internal or external rotation as needed. Examine the bicipital tendon from its origin, progressing distally into the bicipital groove. The tendon and bicipital extension of the joint capsule can be followed a variable distance, depending on individual anatomy and the exact placement of the arthroscope. The caudal aspect of the humeral head and the caudal cul-de-sac are seen best by directing the telescope caudally (Fig. 13-10) and manipulating the joint through flexion, extension, external rotation, and internal rotation. Internal and external rotation of the joint—varus, neutral, and valgus angulation—with flexion and extension are necessary to examine the joint thoroughly.

For therapeutic procedures, establish one or more operative ports after the lesions have been accurately de-

fined. For removal of a humeral head OCD lesion, the instrument port is 2 to 4 cm caudal to and 1 to 2 cm distal to the telescope port.[3] Take care to avoid the axillary artery, vein, and nerve (see Fig. 13-8, *a*). Confirm the correct location of the instrument port by inserting a needle and applying the principles of triangulation.[12] Initial manipulation of the OCD lesion can usually be performed with this needle.

Incise the skin and insert an instrument through a cannula or by free passage without a cannula. Extraction of the OCD flap is most easily accomplished through a tissue tract created by instrument passage without a cannula because a cannula will not permit removal of large, intact cartilage fragments. If a cannula was placed, remove it, enlarge the tissue tract, and pull the cartilage flap through the tissue tract. If a cannula was not placed, create a tissue tract at the operative port site large enough to permit instrument passage and fragment removal. If an operative cannula was not used or was removed for cartilage flap extraction, one may be placed for the debridement phase of the procedure. Curettage of the subchondral bone with hand instruments is more easily performed through a cannula because repeated instrument insertions are required. The shaving blade of power cartilage shavers is passed through the tissue tract or through a cannula.

Transection of the bicipital tendon for treatment of bicipital synovitis or partial tears of the bicipital tendon is performed through a port dorsal or dorsomedial to the greater tubercle at the site of the egress portal (see

Fig. 13-9). Insert a curved or hooked arthroscopy knife and transect the tendon under direct inspection.

ELBOW JOINT

Evaluation of the medial coronoid process of the ulna and medial condyle of the humerus can be performed through either a medial or lateral approach.

Medial Approach

The medial approach is preferred because joint entry and placement of operative instruments is easier and visibility of the humeral condyle and other medial joint structures is better.[13] This approach also eliminates the need for repositioning the animal when converting to open surgery. With the animal in dorsal recumbency, both elbows can be examined without repositioning. For unilateral procedures, position the animal in lateral recumbency, with the elbow to be examined placed downward and the upper limb retracted caudally. Place the elbow joint over a sandbag or pad at the edge of the table to allow the limb to be abducted.

The arthroscope port is distal to the prominence of the medial epicondyle and caudal to the medial collateral ligament (Fig. 13-11). For the initial arthrocentesis, insert the needle into the caudolateral or anconeal fossa region of the joint. Position the needle caudal to the caudal margin of the lateral supracondylar ridge and proximal to the proximal margin of the olecranon. Direct the needle axially and slightly distally into the anconeal fossa. After confirmation of joint penetration and distention, leave the needle in place as an egress port. After the joint is distended, open the medial aspect of the joint space by rotating the limb internally and abducting the antebrachium to produce valgus angulation of the elbow. Locate the joint space and the exact point for the telescope portal by inserting a hypodermic needle approximately 1 cm distal and 0.5 cm caudal to the medial epicondyle of the humerus (see Fig. 13-11). Insert the arthroscopic cannula, attach fluids, and use the arthrocentesis needle as the egress port.

Direct the telescope cranially to examine the medial coronoid process, medial collateral ligament, and craniomedial synovium. Move the arthroscope caudally, laterally, and proximally until the anconeal process and other structures come into view (Box 13-1).

To remove coronoid process fragments and medial humeral condyle OCD lesions, insert an instrument port approximately 1 cm cranial to the arthroscope, immediately caudal to the medial collateral ligament (Fig. 13-12; also see Fig. 13-11). The puncture sites should be located to avoid damage to the neurovascular structures on the craniomedial aspect of the elbow joint. Instruments are inserted through a cannula or by free passage.

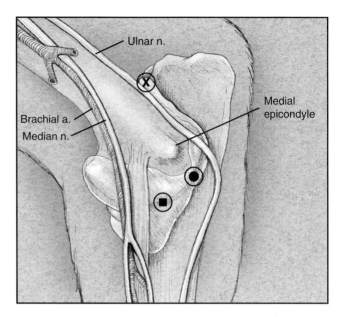

Fig. 13-11   Right elbow joint, medial view, showing positions of the arthroscope portal (●), operative portal (■), and egress cannula or needle (x) relative to the ulnar and median nerves and brachial artery.

BOX 13-1

ARTHROSCOPIC ELBOW EXAMINATION

Medial humeral condyle
Medial collateral ligament
Medial coronoid process of the ulna
Middle and caudal parts of the radial head
Medial aspect of the lateral humeral condyle
Lateral coronoid process of the ulna
Ulnar semilunar notch
Anconeal process
Joint capsule

Lateral Approach

The lateral approach to the elbow is used when several joints in the same forelimb are to be examined for polyarthritic conditions or when the involved joint cannot be identified with a less invasive technique. Rapid examination of the shoulder, elbow, and carpus is feasible and multiple synovial biopsies can be obtained without repositioning the animal.

Make the initial joint puncture into the anconeal fossa. Insert the needle between the caudal aspect of the medial supracondylar ridge and the most proximal part of the olecranon and direct it axially and slightly distally. The arthroscope port is cranial and slightly distal to the

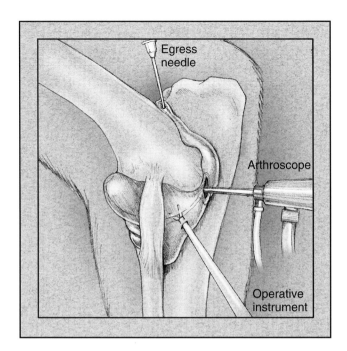

Fig. 13-12 Right elbow joint, medial view, showing placement of the arthroscope, operative instrument, and egress needle for removal of fragmented coronoid process and medial humeral condyle OCD lesions.

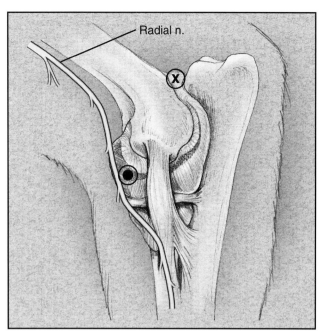

Fig. 13-13 Left elbow joint, lateral view, showing the location of the arthroscope portal (●) and the egress cannula (x) relative to the radial nerve.

prominence of the lateral epicondyle. Insert the arthroscope cannula with a blunt obturator where the joint capsule is distended cranial to the articulation of the radial head and the lateral humeral condyle (Fig. 13-13). Remove the obturator, insert the arthroscope, and attach the fluid inflow line (Fig. 13-14).

Examine the joint by passing the telescope across the cranial aspect of the humeral articular surface until the craniomedial area of the joint is visible (Fig. 13-15). The structures of primary interest are the coronoid process of the ulna and the medial condyle of the humerus. The articular surface of the radial head, the intercondylar region of the humerus, and the lateral humeral condyle can also be examined. The coronoid process is readily examined from the lateral approach with the distal part of the limb rotated externally. Moving the joint through the full range of flexion and extension facilitates examination of the coronoid process and establishes the optimum position for visibility. To evaluate the humeral condyle for OCD, extend the joint and rotate the limb internally. Take the limb through various positions to find the one that is best. Examination of the humeral condyle is somewhat limited with the lateral approach.

Arthroscopic removal of fragmented coronoid processes can be performed using the lateral approach. Place the instrument port directly cranial or craniomedial to the coronoid process. Determine the site by exploratory

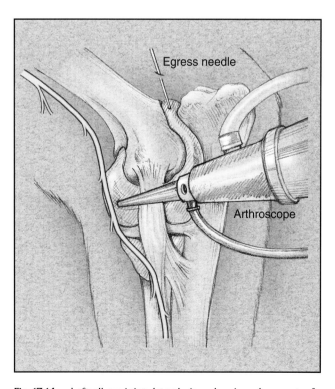

Fig. 13-14 Left elbow joint, lateral view, showing placement of the arthroscope for viewing the medial coronoid process of the ulna and the medial condyle of the humerus from the lateral approach.

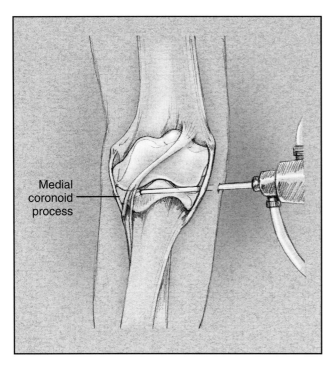

Fig. I3-I5 Left elbow joint, cranial view, showing the telescope position for viewing the medial coronoid process (MCP) of the ulna and the medial humeral condyle from the lateral approach.

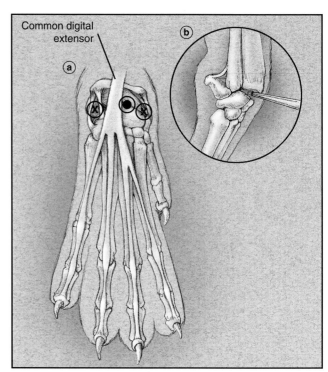

Fig. I3-I6 Right carpus, dorsal view, showing positions for the arthroscope portal (●) medial to the common digital extensor tendon and two potential sites for the egress cannula or an operative port (x) (*a*). Lateral view demonstrating flexion of the carpus (*b*).

needle placement. Carefully dissect and pass instruments to avoid the craniomedial neurovascular bundle (see Fig. 13-13).

RADIOCARPAL JOINT

Arthroscopy of the carpal joint is indicated for taking synovial biopsy specimens and for assessing radial carpal bone fractures.

Position the animal in lateral recumbency with the carpus to be examined placed upward and the leg rotated externally, or in dorsal recumbency with the limb pulled caudally. Prepare the field aseptically. Flex the carpal joint and insert a hypodermic needle medial to the common digital extensor tendon with the needle directed caudally (Fig. 13-16). Aspirate joint fluid to confirm entry. Distend the joint. Incise the skin and insert the arthroscope cannula. Place the egress needle lateral to the common digital extensor tendon (see Fig. 13-16). The integrity of the radial carpal bone and condition of the articular cartilage are evaluated. The joint is also examined for signs of synovial inflammation.

HIP JOINT

Arthroscopy of the hip joint has been used to examine the weight-bearing surfaces of the acetabulum and femoral head in young, dysplastic dogs before performing a pelvic osteotomy. Because of joint laxity, dysplastic hips in young dogs are easily accessed for arthroscopy. The procedure is difficult in normal hips and has not been attempted in older, dysplastic dogs.

Position the dog in lateral recumbency and prepare the hip region aseptically. Arthroscopy has been performed through a port dorsal to the greater trochanter (Fig. 13-17).[14] Traction is applied to the limb at approximately 90° to the long axis of the body without abduction or adduction and without lateral displacement of the proximal end of the femur. This opens the joint space and facilitates infusion of the joint. Insert a 2- to 3-inch spinal needle dorsal to the greater trochanter and direct it medially into the joint space (see Fig. 13-17). After distention of the joint, incise the skin and insert the cannula for the arthroscope. Entry can be difficult if the joint capsule is thickened in response to hip dysplasia. If needed, a sharp trocar can be used but with caution. Entry can also be facilitated by separating the gluteal muscles with hemostatic forceps to create a passage for insertion of the trocar cannula. After the cannula and arthroscope have been inserted, establish fluid flow. Insert an egress needle 1 to 2 cm cranial to or caudal to the telescope portal. If the needle is inserted caudally, take care to avoid the sciatic nerve and caudal gluteal artery. Maintain traction on the limb during the examination to provide the largest

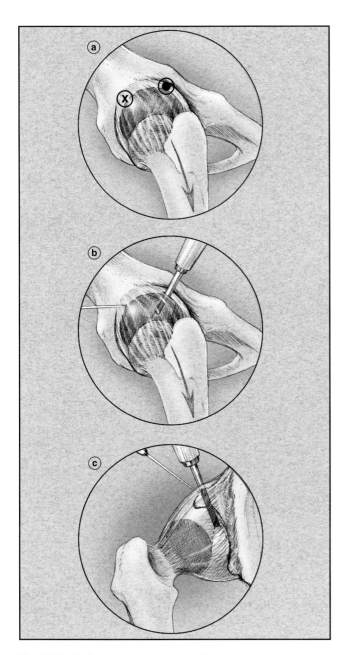

Fig. 13-17   Left hip joint subluxated for arthroscopic examination. Lateral view showing the arthroscope portal (●) and a cranial egress cannula or needle site (x) (*a*). Lateral view showing placement of the telescope and egress cannula or needle (*b*). Anteroposterior view of the pelvis showing telescope placement (*c*).

optical cavity. Flex and extend the hip and abduct, adduct, and rotate the limb internally and externally to bring as much of the articular surface of the femoral head as possible into view. Direct the arthroscope cranially and caudally to examine the acetabular joint surface, acetabular rim, dorsal aspect of the joint capsule, and teres ligament. The condition of the weight-bearing surfaces of the acetabulum and femoral head are of primary interest in evaluating candidates for pelvic osteotomy.

BOX 13-2

INDICATIONS FOR STIFLE ARTHROSCOPY

Hind limb lameness without an obvious cause
Stifle joint capsule distention
Stifle joint thickening or swelling
Crepitus
Radiographic evidence of increased joint fluid
Radiographic evidence of degenerative joint disease
Radiographic evidence of flattening or distortion of the femoral condyle
Drawer instability

STIFLE JOINT

Indications for arthroscopy include hind limb lameness coupled with physical findings suggesting stifle involvement or radiographic evidence of increased joint fluid or degenerative joint disease (Box 13-2). OCD lesions of the femoral condyle can be treated surgically.[15] Stifles with ruptured cranial cruciate ligaments have been stabilized with arthroscopically placed carbon fibers; however, the implants broke and the repairs failed.[8]

To access the stifle joint, position the dog in lateral recumbency with the limb rotated externally. I prefer to position dogs in lateral recumbency and use video equipment because many cases are partial or complete cranial cruciate ligament ruptures that are immediately converted to open procedures. If both stifles are being evaluated, the dog may be positioned in dorsal recumbency with the limbs extended.

Place the arthroscope into the cranial aspect of the joint, either medial or lateral to the patellar ligament. The most common port site for stifle arthroscopy is immediately lateral to the patellar ligament, approximately midway between the distal end of the patella and the point of insertion of the patellar ligament on the tibial crest (Fig. 13-18). Placing the telescope laterally facilitates inspection of the cranial cruciate ligament and medial meniscus. The scope should enter the joint just above the proximal margin of the fat pad. Selecting the proper site is made easier by examining lateral radiographs of the stifle and palpating the joint capsule after the joint has been distended.

Insert the infusion needle on the side opposite the intended arthroscope port. When significant joint lesions with increased joint fluid are present, additional distention may not be required and this step is omitted. Placing the needle into normal joints or those with a minimal increase in joint fluid can be difficult. An alternative technique can be used to facilitate needle placement. With the stifle hyperextended, place the needle into the joint space between the patella and the trochlear

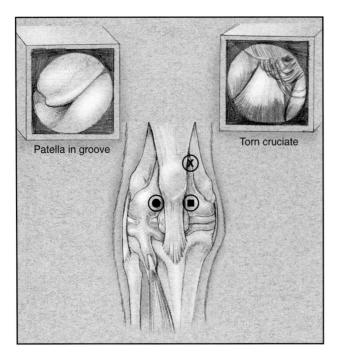

Patella in groove

Torn cruciate

Fig. 13-18   Port placements for stifle arthroscopy demonstrating the locations for the arthroscope (●), operative instrumentation (■), and an egress cannula (x). The arthroscope and instrument portals can be interchanged.

TABLE 13-1	
Arthroscopic Stifle Examination—Dorsolateral Port	
STRUCTURE	LEG POSITION
Suprapatellar cul-de-sac	Hyperextended
Trochlear groove	Hyperextended
Articular surface of patella	Hyperextended
Lateral joint capsule	Standing position
Medial joint capsule	Standing position with lateral rotation
Trochlear ridges	Hyperextension
Medial meniscus	Valgus stress, standing position to flexion
Medial femoral condyle	Valgus stress, flexion
Lateral meniscus	Varus stress, standing position to flexion
Lateral femoral condyle	Varus stress, flexion
Cranial cruciate ligament	Standing position to flexion
Caudal cruciate ligament	Standing position to flexion
Origin of long digital extensor tendon	Standing position to flexion

groove. The joint can then be distended and the arthroscopic port placed as outlined previously.

Direct the cannula from the port site into either the suprapatellar pouch parallel to the trochlear groove or into the intercondylar area. If resistance from a thickened joint capsule is encountered, the skin incision can be deepened to include the retinaculum and joint capsule. Access to the suprapatellar pouch is gained by hyperextending the stifle to elevate the patella from the trochlear groove and placing the cannula between the patella and the trochlear groove. The intercondylar area is approached by placing the joint at a standing angle and directing the cannula caudally. The intercondylar approach can be associated with a higher risk of iatrogenic cruciate ligament damage.

After the arthroscope is inserted, attach the inflow fluid line and establish an egress port. Place the egress cannula on the opposite side of the patellar ligament or into the suprapatellar pouch. Examine all areas of the joint systematically (Table 13-1). A partially ruptured cruciate ligament may appear as wavy cross striations. To complete the examination, extend, flex, and rotate the joint internally and externally. Apply varus stress to open the lateral joint space and valgus stress to open the medial joint space. To view OCD lesions of the lateral femoral condyle, insert the arthroscope through the medial port and instruments through the lateral port.[11]

HOCK JOINT

The hock joint can be entered through dorsomedial, dorsolateral, and plantarolateral portals.[3] OCD, which is a common indication for arthroscopy of the hock, usually affects the plantar part of the medial trochlear ridge. Lesions may also affect the proximal part of the lateral trochlear ridge.

Dorsomedial and Dorsolateral Approaches

The dorsal approaches provide access to the dorsal part of the trochlear ridges of the tibial tarsal bone and the distal edge of the articular surface of the tibia (Fig. 13-19). The dorsomedial approach is used to visualize the lateral joint structures, specifically, OCD lesions on the dorsal part of the lateral trochlear ridge. Instrument port insertion for the dorsomedial arthroscope position is dorsolateral. The telescope and instrument ports are reversed for the dorsolateral approach.

Position the dog in dorsal recumbency and extend the hind limb. After aseptic preparation and draping, palpate the long digital extensor tendon and the tendon of the cranial tibial muscle as they cross over the dorsal (anterior) aspect of the joint (see Fig. 13-19). Insert a needle lateral to the extensor tendons to distend the joint. Insert the arthroscope cannula medial to the extensor tendon at the point of maximal joint capsule distention. Allow the initial centesis needle to function as an egress cannula. Extend the joint to see the dorsal portion of the trochlear ridges. The egress needle site is used for operative instrument placement if arthroscopic examination determines that it is appropriately located. A cannula is not usually required for removal of OCD lesions and debridement of the cartilage defect.

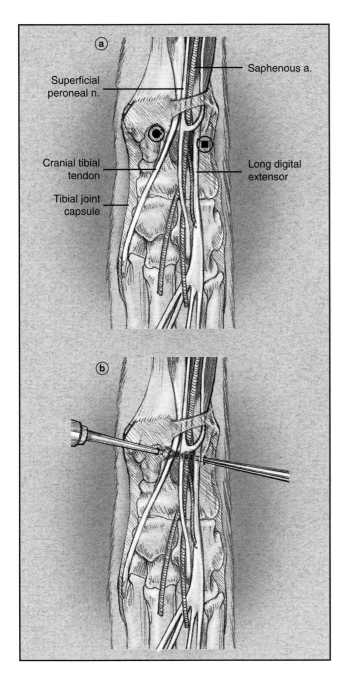

Fig. 13-19 Left hock, dorsal view, showing dorsomedial arthroscope portal (●) and dorsolateral instrument portal sites (■) (*a*) and instrument positioning for dorsolateral talar ridge OCD lesion removal (*b*). Port sites are shown relative to the superficial peroneal nerve, saphenous artery, long digital extensor tendon, and tendon of the tibialis cranialis muscle.

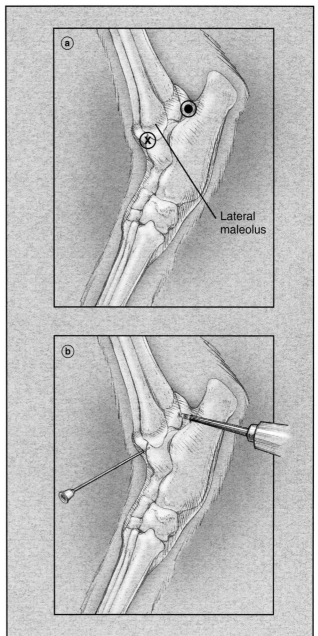

Fig. 13-20 Left hock, lateral view, showing the plantaromedial telescope portal (●) and dorsomedial egress portal (x) (*a*), and instrument positioning for plantaromedial talar ridge OCD lesion evaluation (*b*).

Plantarolateral Approach

The plantarolateral approach provides good visibility of the plantar part of the medial trochlear ridge, distal part of the tibia, and deep flexor tendon. Position the dog in lateral recumbency with the affected limb up. Palpate the lateral malleolus, the caudolateral extent of the tibia, and

the plantarolateral trochlear ridge. Insert an infusion needle caudal to the malleolus at the intersection of the caudal tibial articular margin and lateral trochlear ridge, and direct it medially (Fig. 13-20). If joint capsule thickening makes entry at this location difficult, the dorsolateral portal site can be used. When the joint has been distended, incise the skin and insert the arthroscope cannula caudal to the malleolus at the point of the initial needle insertion. Insert the arthroscope, attach the fluid lines, and establish the egress cannula.

Exposure of the trochlear ridges is enhanced by flexing the joint. Osteochondritic lesions on the plantar portion of the medial trochlear ridge of the tibiotarsal bone can be seen easily. These lesions are generally large and difficult to remove. Occasionally the free OCD flap will fragment, facilitating arthroscopic removal.

Combined Approach

For examination of the dorsal and plantar aspects of the tarsocrural joint, the dorsal and plantarolateral approaches can be combined. If cannulas are maintained in both portals, escape of infusion fluid is minimized. This is an important factor because excessive periarticular fluid compresses the joint capsule, increasing the difficulty of the procedure.

Complications

When techniques are applied carefully, few significant complications of arthroscopy result. Most of the problems are technical ones, and their incidence decreases with experience. Such complications include failure to establish or maintain an optical cavity, iatrogenic damage to underlying structures, difficulty in triangulation, and equipment failure or breakage. Infection, neurovascular damage, injury to articular cartilage and joint structures, and postoperative swelling have been reported.[16]

Establishing the initial joint capsule distention may be difficult in heavily muscled animals because palpable landmarks are obscured. This may be especially true in arthroscopy of the shoulder. It may be difficult to penetrate a thickened joint capsule or a joint space that is too small. Maintaining the optical cavity is difficult if fluid leaks through multiple holes in the joint capsule and accumulates in the subcutaneous space. Periarticular fluid interferes with the examination by compressing the optical cavity, but it is not detrimental to the animal and it is absorbed without treatment. In chronic cases, significant synovial proliferation may obscure visibility, making joint examination difficult if not impossible.

Iatrogenic damage to articular cartilage with trocars and instruments is common in the early phase of the learning curve. Damage to neurovascular bundles may occur during approaches to the medial aspect of the elbow or the caudal approach to the shoulder. The cranial cruciate ligament may be injured if the intercondylar approach to cannula placement is used. The biceps brachii tendon, long digital extensor tendon, and common digital extensor tendon should be avoided when approaching the shoulder, hock, and radiocarpal joints. Forceful manipulation of instruments or using them as levers may cause them to break within the joint. Fragments of broken instruments usually can be removed arthroscopically.

Locating instrument ports and mastering triangulation may require practice. Using pilot needle punctures helps develop the correct three-dimensional view. It is difficult or impossible to extract specimens through a cannula or tissue path that is too small. Failure of the light source, video camera, or other equipment, and inability to complete the operative portion of a procedure may be reasons for conversion to open arthrotomy.

Editor's note: The editor and illustrator sincerely appreciate the assistance of Tori Guy with the illustrative layout and rough sketches for this chapter.

REFERENCES

1. Person MW: Arthroscopic treatment of osteochondritis dissecans in the canine shoulder. *Vet Surg* 18:175-189, 1989.
2. van Bree H, Van Ryssen B, Desmidt M: Osteochondrosis lesions of the canine shoulder: correlation of positive arthrography and arthroscopy. *Vet Radiol Ultrasound* 33:342-347, 1992.
3. vanGestel MA: Diagnostic accuracy of stifle arthroscopy in the dog. *J Am Anim Hosp Assoc* 21:757-763, 1985.
4. Miller CW, Presnell KR: Examination of the canine stifle: arthroscopy versus arthrotomy. *J Am Anim Hosp Assoc* 21:623-629, 1985.
5. van Bree H, Van Ryssen B: Imaging the canine elbow: radiology, computed tomography, and arthroscopy. The Veterinary Annual, 35th issue, pp 118-129.
6. Van Ryssen B, van Bree H, Vyt P: Arthroscopy of the shoulder joint in the dog. *J Am Anim Hosp Assoc* 29:101-105, 1993.
7. Siemering GH: Arthroscopy of dogs. *J Am Vet Med Assoc* 172:575-577, 1978.
8. Person MW: Prosthetic replacement of the cranial cruciate ligament under arthroscopic guidance: a pilot project. *Vet Surg* 16:37-43, 1987.
9. Reagen BF et al: Irrigating solutions for arthroscopy. *J Bone Joint Surg* 65A:629-631, 1983.
10. Arciero RA et al: Irrigating solutions used in arthroscopy and their effect on articular cartilage: an in vivo study. *Orthopedics* 9:1511-1515, 1986.
11. Taylor RA: Proceedings of the first national canine arthroscopy seminar. Colorado State University, May 21, 1994.
12. Van Ryssen B, van Bree H, Missinne S: Successful arthroscopic treatment of shoulder osteochondrosis in the dog. *J Small Anim Pract* 34:521-528, 1993.
13. Van Ryssen B, van Bree H, Simoens P: Elbow arthroscopy in clinically normal dogs. *Am J Vet Res* 54:191-198, 1993.
14. Person MW: Arthroscopy of the canine coxofemoral joint. *Comp Cont Ed Pract Vet* 11:930-936, 1989.
15. McLaughlin RM, Hurtig MB, Fries CL: Operative arthroscopy in the treatment of bilateral stifle osteochondritis dissecans in a dog. *Vet Comp Orthop Traumatol* 4:158-161, 1989.
16. Person MW: Arthroscopy of the canine shoulder joint. *Comp Cont Ed Pract Vet* 8:537-546, 1986.

CHAPTER 14

MINIMALLY INVASIVE SURGERY IN NONDOMESTIC ANIMALS

Robert A. Cook

Laparoscopy has been a valuable research tool in zoologic medicine for the past 20 years. Applications of this technology are continually expanding. Initially, laparoscopy was used to observe the reproductive organs. Later, sequential biopsy and observation of organs, such as the liver, kidney, and spleen, were performed. With training and experience, progress is being made in performing more complex surgical procedures.

Improved optics and light sources now provide better visibility of small spaces. Manufacturers have been willing to provide customized instrumentation to facilitate minimally invasive procedures in both small and large animals. As technical proficiency improves, minimally invasive surgery is being more widely practiced.

Benefits

Clinical diagnosis of illness in wild animals is a continual challenge. Because many nondomestic species mask overt signs of clinical disease to prevent attraction of predators, improved methods for making clinical diagnoses are needed. Many animals must be immobilized or anesthetized before they can be examined and have blood and laboratory samples or radiographs taken. Minimally invasive surgery can be performed at the same time or as a subsequent diagnostic procedure. Minimally invasive surgical techniques can be used to diagnose disease in many physiologic systems, including the cardiovascular, auditory, respiratory, digestive, renal, and reproductive systems. Surgeons should consider performing minimally invasive diagnostic procedures because earlier diagnosis and definitive therapy improve the animal's prognosis.

Wild animals do not adapt well to lengthy environmental or activity restrictions required for proper healing after many conventional surgical procedures. Minimally invasive surgery reduces tissue trauma and may provide additional benefits of shorter recovery, decreased postoperative care, and fewer complications. As with any surgical procedure, the value of the diagnosis and therapy must outweigh the risks of anesthesia and surgical manipulation. Minimally invasive surgery is considered when it is likely to reduce postoperative morbidity and improve the potential for rapid recovery so the animal can return to its normal habitat quickly. One advantage of minimally invasive surgery over conventional procedures is that much less human intervention may be required during the recovery and healing phases. Magnification provided by the telescope allows one to see structural detail better than with conventional surgical procedures. Minimally invasive surgery in zoo animals should be used whenever visual inspection of an organ or structure may provide additional diagnostic information.

Considerations

One of the assumptions for advancing from diagnostic to therapeutic procedures is that the surgeon should always be prepared to convert to an open procedure. Therefore,

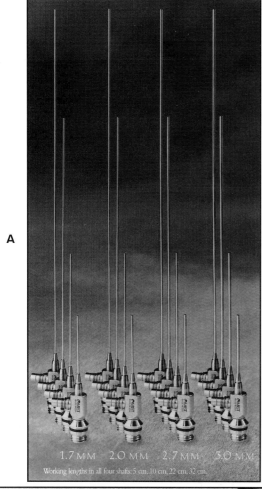

A

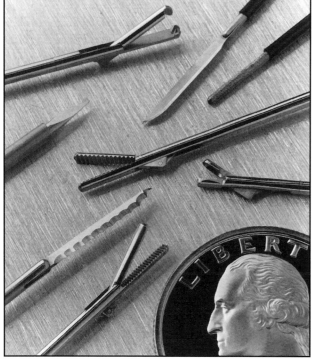

B

Fig. 14-1   1.7-mm telescopes (A) and instrumentation (B).

beginning laparoscopists should not attempt minimally invasive surgery if the risks of open surgery are great.

Advances in anesthetic techniques have made it safer to immobilize and recover zoo animals. Nevertheless, the surgical team must be able to work rapidly. The physiologic effects of insufflation and position on each species are relatively unknown. Anatomic variations must be anticipated. Equipment and instrumentation necessary to accomplish the procedure must be readily available. Relative contraindications, such as pregnancy, obesity, and previous abdominal surgery, are similar to those for domestic animals.

An animal's size may restrict the use of minimally invasive surgery in some species. The megavertebrates (e.g., elephant, rhinoceros) have massive, heavy, internal organs that are difficult to manipulate. The vast intraabdominal space may preclude viewing of distant abdominal structures with current light sources and laparoscopes. Conversely, conventional instruments are too large to maneuver in animals weighing less than 100 g. However, 1.7-mm scopes and instruments can be used to perform basic procedures in animals with a small optical cavity (Fig. 14-1).

A veterinarian who treats nondomestic animals is challenged by the diversity of species in six major classes. This chapter will cover the use of minimally invasive surgical techniques in four of those classes: amphibians, reptiles, birds, and mammals. Anatomic differences among the classes require that different approaches be used. It is beyond the scope of this chapter to detail all variations; however, important differences are noted. Suggested readings listed at the end of the chapter give more detailed descriptions of the taxonomy, anatomy, anesthesia, imaging modalities, and diseases of nondomestic species.

Instrumentation

Because veterinarians examine animals varying in size from the smallest fishes or amphibians to whales and elephants, they must be prepared with several sizes of surgical telescopes and instruments (Box 14-1). Guidelines for selecting a telescope diameter based on the animal's weight are provided in Table 14-1. The largest diameter appropriate for the size of the animal provides the best illumination and the largest field of view. Telescopes vary in length from 5 to 54 cm. Shorter telescopes weigh less and are easier to manipulate in animals with a small optical cavity. Longer telescopes are necessary for examining large optical cavities and structures distant from the insertion site. An angled scope facilitates examination of small optical cavities.

The internal diameter of a trocar cannula should match the outside diameter of the telescope and instruments. The 120-mm shaft of conventional trocar cannu-

Surgery Set (for incision and closure)

- Microsurgery or ophthalmic surgical instruments for small patients
- Traditional surgery set for larger patients
- Skin stapler or appropriately sized skin sutures

Surgical Telescopes

- 1.7, 2.4, 5.0, 7.0, 10.0 mm diameter
- 0°, 30°, 45°, 70° angle (Note: For the beginner a 0° angle may be easier.)
- Lengths as short as 5 cm

Trocars, Cannulas, and Insufflation

- To match the telescope
- Cannulas (sheaths) with insufflation ports preferred
- Lightweight cannulas for small telescopes
- Veress needle

Exploratory and Biopsy Procedures

- Cautery (monopolar or bipolar electrosurgical generator)
- Endosurgical cautery instrument adaptor
- Double spoon flexible biopsy instruments
- Double spoon rigid biopsy instruments with monopolar cautery capabilities
- Grasping forceps (with monopolar cautery adaptors)
- Dissectors

Advanced Diagnostic and Therapeutic Procedures

- Scissors
- Ligating clip appliers
- Pre-tied loop ligatures
- Cherry dissectors
- Clamps
- Laparoscopic sutures and needle holders
- Stapling devices (cut and staple or staple alone)

TABLE 14-1

Guidelines for Selecting Telescopes for Use in Nondomestic Animals

ANIMAL WEIGHT	PREFERRED SCOPE DIAMETER
30-500 g	1.7-2.4 mm
500 g-5 kg	3.0-4.0 mm
5-25 kg	5.0 or 10 mm
>25 kg	10 mm
Megavertebrates	Custom made

---

las may be too short in an animal with a thick abdominal wall or too long for an animal with a thin abdominal wall. Trocars with variable shaft lengths are available. Metal trocars and sleeves are not used routinely in very small animals because the body wall is not thick enough to support the weight of the cannula. Plastic trocar cannulas weigh less and may provide an advantage. A 3-mm plastic sleeve with a carbon dioxide (CO_2) port is light and allows insufflation. A 14-gauge sleeve is used with 1.7-mm telescopes and instruments (see Fig. 14-1). Unless insufflation is needed to expand the optical cavity, trocar cannulas do not require an internal seal to prevent loss of pneumoperitoneum.

Creating an Optical Cavity

Amphibians, reptiles, and birds have a coelomic cavity with no true diaphragmatic separation that houses all of the internal organs. Insufflating the coelomic cavity provides an adequate optical cavity for inspection of the visceral structures in amphibians and reptiles. Because of its air sac system, the avian coelomic cavity does not require insufflation to expand the field of view. Mammals have a diaphragm that separates the thoracic and abdominal cavities. In mammals, the abdominal cavity is insufflated to create an optical cavity. An optical cavity in the thorax is provided by creating pneumothorax through insufflation or by using open ports with one-lung ventilation.

Insufflation flow rates are based on the animal's size. For small animals, the initial flow rate is 1.4 L/min; for medium-sized animals, it is 2.4 L/min; and for large animals, it is 9 L/min. Loss of pneumoperitoneum through the operative ports may require that the flow rates be increased. For megavertebrates, several cannulas and insufflators running simultaneously may be required.

In addition to monitoring insufflation pressure, the thickness and distensibility of the overlying coelomic or abdominal musculature and skin should also be evaluated. A pressure is chosen to allow optimum visibility without drum-tight stretching of the skin over the body cavity. The lowest pressure that provides adequate exposure without impairing cardiovascular or respiratory functions is used. Continuous monitoring of coelomic or abdominal wall distention is necessary to prevent tissue damage or vascular compromise. Although it is relatively well established that pressures of 12 to 14 mm Hg are safe in mammals, safe insufflation pressures and the effects of CO_2 absorption for other animals are not known.

Amphibians

Amphibians, such as frogs, toads, newts, and salamanders, have adapted to various environments and bridge the gap between aquatic and terrestrial existence. Amphibians have paired fat bodies that in frogs and toads appear as large, fingerlike projections within the coelomic cavities. Many amphibians that inhabit terrestrial environments have a large urinary bladder; aquatic amphibians lack this organ completely. Reproductive organs in amphibians vary considerably. In some male frogs and toads, such as the common toad, the Bidder's organ is an ovary-like structure that is present in addition to the testes. In the genus *Rana*, older females may shift to the production of sperm. Reproduction is sexual, and both internal and external fertilization occurs. Although most amphibians lay eggs, a few species bear live young. In males, the testes are ventral to the head of the kidneys and adrenal glands and distal to the paired fat bodies. In females, the oviducts are lateral and distal to the kidneys; the egg-laden ovaries are ventral to the oviducts and kidneys. The oviduct is the major reproductive organ in the female. In gravid females, half of the coelomic cavity may be distended with eggs.

ANESTHESIA

As in reptiles and birds, an amphibian's respiratory inspiration does not depend on negative pressure in the thorax. Respiration is by one or a combination of gills, lungs, the tissues of the oropharyngeal cavity, or the skin of the body and appendages. Because of its respiratory function, the skin in many amphibians is relatively thin and absorptive. This can be used to advantage by the anesthetist, who can provide an anesthetic agent, such as tricaine methanesulfonate, in a shallow pan of water or by applying it with a soaked sponge. Anesthetic gels can be applied to skin, injectable agents can be administered into muscle, and gas can be provided by chamber, mask, or endotracheal intubation, or bubbled into the aquatic environment.[1]

SURGICAL PREPARATION

To decrease the risks of anesthesia, assess the animal's health status before surgery and take corrective action as indicated. In terrestrial species, loose skin or dry mucous membranes may indicate dehydration. Malnutrition may appear as malaligned long bones or weight loss. Skin infections in frogs appear as a generalized reddening of the ventral body surface.

Preoperative antibiotic or antifungal therapy is not routinely administered unless specifically indicated. Depending on the species, drugs may be given by mouth, parenterally, or in the aquatic environment. Because amphibians have a high metabolic rate and feed intermittently, large meals should be avoided but food is usually not withheld before surgical procedures. Standard disinfectants and their application may be irritating and toxic.

Sterile, waterproof dressings* or waterproof, plastic drapes† are preferred. To facilitate recovery, appropriate body temperatures should be maintained during and after the procedure.

SURGICAL TECHNIQUE

With the amphibian positioned in dorsal recumbency, a single port in the coelomic cavity allows examination of the heart, lungs, liver, gallbladder, gastrointestinal tract, urinary bladder, and reproductive organs (Fig. 14-2). Use a 1.7- or 2.4-mm surgical telescope. Make a paramedian approach to avoid the large ventral abdominal

---

*Tegaderm, 3M Medical-Surgical Division, St. Paul, Minn. 55144-1000.
†SteriDrape, 3M Health Care, St. Paul, Minn. 55144-1000.

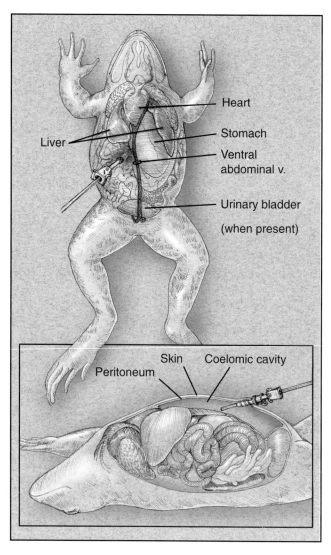

Fig. 14-2   Port placement and anatomy of frogs and toads.

vein coursing down the ventral midline. Because the skin is thin and the coelomic cavity is distended with contents, use the Hasson approach for open trocar placement. Incise the skin to create an opening slightly smaller than the diameter of the primary trocar cannula. The shorter incision allows the skin to stretch around the cannula during placement. If the incision is too long and a tight seal around the telescope sheath is not obtained, place a purse-string suture of size 4/0 or 5/0 around the cannula. It is easy to mistake the space between the skin and peritoneum for the coelomic cavity. To avoid insufflation injury, ensure that the trocar fully penetrates the peritoneum.

Set the insufflation at 1.4 L/min and begin insufflating through the primary trocar. Avoid rapid overfilling of the small cavity to prevent skin and organ damage. Place secondary ports if required and if the animal is large enough. Species such as marine toads *(Bufo marinus)* are large enough that one can easily manipulate instruments and perform procedures with more than one port. Transilluminate the thin body wall to reveal vessels that should be avoided in secondary port placement. Minimize incision lengths to avoid leakage of the insufflation gas. Place secondary ports under direct vision. In smaller species, use a single port for the telescope. To obtain a biopsy specimen, use a 2.7-mm telescope with an integral instrument channel or introduce the biopsy needle percutaneously.

RECOVERY

After the procedure, remove the ports and close the incisions. When the environment is aquatic, seal the incisions with a waterproof, nontoxic protectant. One example is a paste used in human dental procedures* to facilitate healing and prevent the entry of aquatic-borne pathogens such as *Aeromonas* and *Pseudomonas* species.[2] Provide a warm, clean environment for recovery. Amphibians recover quickly from anesthesia once they have been removed from contact with the agent. To decrease postoperative stress, return the animal to its normal environment rapidly.

Reptiles

The three most commonly encountered groups of reptiles in nondomestic practice belong to the orders Testudinata (turtles, tortoises, terrapins, and sea turtles), Squamata (snakes and lizards), and Crocodilia (crocodiles, alligators, caimans, and gavials). Like amphibians, reptiles (except for crocodilians) have a coelomic cavity

with no true diaphragmatic separation. Respiratory inspiration does not depend on negative pressure. Reptiles are poikilothermic (cold-blooded). Because reptiles can hold their breath and have a slow metabolic rate, reaching a surgical plane of anesthesia can take a long time. The natural stoicism of a restrained reptile can make it difficult to ascertain when surgical anesthesia has been achieved.

TESTUDINATA

A turtle shell consists of a bony carapace and plastron, which present a formidable barrier to traditional surgical procedures. Minimally invasive exploration and biopsy are performed by gaining access to the coelomic cavity between the hind limb and shell (Fig. 14-3).

Anesthesia

Turtles are perhaps the most challenging reptile to anesthetize because of their ability to draw their head and limbs into the shell, making masked gas anesthesia and even injections difficult. Injectable anesthetic agents, inhalation anesthesia administered by chamber, or a

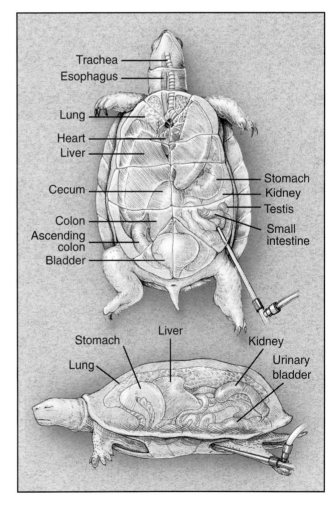

Fig. 14-3 Port placement and anatomy of the turtle.

---

*Orabase, Colgate Oral Pharmaceuticals, Colgate-Palmolive, Canton, Mass. 02021.

combination of injectable and inhalation anesthetics have been used successfully. For prolonged procedures, intubation and inhalation anesthesia are preferred.

Surgical Technique

Depending on the animal's size and the space available between the hind limb and shell, select the largest telescope that can be inserted and manipulated easily. Position the turtle in right lateral recumbency and extend the left hind limb caudally (see Fig. 14-3). Tent the skin proximal to the left hind limb and make a shallow stab incision. To avoid lacerating a full urinary bladder, use the Hasson technique to place the initial port. Place the cannula, using a purse-string suture if necessary, to secure the port in place. Although the coelom is surrounded by a nondistensible shell, one can use low levels of insufflation to distend the soft tissues and expand the field of view. Remember that the shell restricts the ability of the tissues to expand. To improve visibility, express the urinary bladder by applying gentle pressure with the laparoscope or another blunt instrument. If this fails, perform abdominocentesis with a laparoscopically guided 2½ -inch, 18-gauge spinal needle without a stylet* or a 14-gauge, needle-tipped trocar† introduced through the skin adjacent and parallel to the primary port. Connect the needle or trocar to a syringe or suction apparatus and drain the bladder.

After the primary puncture and urinary bladder drainage (if indicated), position the turtle in dorsal recumbency. Examine the liver and intestinal structures. The right liver lobe is usually larger than the left lobe. Tilt the animal in several oblique postures to move the intestine and liver out of the field and examine the gonads lying ventral to the kidney and spleen. With further distraction of liver and intestine to the animal's right side, observe the heart and lungs and the gallbladder on the left dorsal aspect of the liver.

To obtain a biopsy specimen, introduce forceps through the ancillary channel of an operating telescope or insert a second port proximal and parallel to the primary one. It takes practice to guide biopsy forceps on a plane parallel to the telescope, but once beyond the distal end of the scope, biopsy specimens can be retrieved easily. Consider using monopolar biopsy forceps to minimize bleeding. After the procedure, remove the ports and close the incision sites with size 3/0 to 4/0 absorbable suture on a cutting needle. Seal the incisions with cyanoacrylate, especially in aquatic species.

Recovery

Provide a clean, warm environment for postoperative recovery. Because of the slow nature of anesthetic metab-

*Becton Dickinson Co, Franklin Lakes, N.J. 07417.
†MIST, Inc, Smithfield, N.C. 27577.

olism, recovery may take from several minutes to several hours, depending on the animal's physiologic status and the duration of anesthesia. Maintain aquatic species in a dry environment until normal head or limb withdrawal reflexes are evident. One can extend the time out of water by maintaining the animal in a moist environment with warm, damp towels.

SQUAMATA
Snakes

Although a snake's unique anatomy compromises simultaneous examination of all abdominal structures, minimally invasive surgery allows one to examine several sites without an extensive laparotomy. Once it is determined where the problem exists, minimally invasive surgery or a laparotomy can be used. Identifying the problem site before major surgical intervention reduces the risk of postoperative complications.

Surgical Preparation

Snakes characteristically feed on large food items at extended intervals. Because of the increased risk of regurgitation, avoid handling snakes after a feeding. Snakes undergo intermittent molting when the external skin becomes devitalized and is shed. Handling during this period is contraindicated because the new outer skin is very easily damaged.

Antimicrobial therapies are not routinely given to surgical candidates. Every effort should be made to address nutrition and hydration. Malnourished snakes have loose skin and appear wasted. Signs of dehydration are sunken eyes and lack of skin turgor. Fluids can be administered either subcutaneously or intracoelomically when indicated.

Anesthesia

Injectable anesthetics or an inhalation anesthetic delivered in a chamber environment are the most common induction agents. In some species, combining injectable and inhalation anesthetics can avoid the long induction times experienced with gas anesthesia alone. After induction, insert an endotracheal tube and maintain inhalation anesthesia.

Surgical preparation of the snake can also be a challenge. Using tape, one may choose to secure the snake to a long, narrow piece of flat wood or plastic. Because snakes live in warm environments that stimulate the growth of microorganisms and their ventral surfaces are in constant contact with the substrate, thoroughly disinfect the surgical site. Use a sterile, transparent adhesive drape to be able to view the animal and maintain a sterile field.

Surgical Technique

An extensive skeletal system, which can consist of more than 300 vertebrae and ribs, creates a relatively nondistensible cavity. This, along with the snake's long, narrow body, leaves little potential space within the coelomic cavity. Because of these restrictions, it is a challenge to extend the telescope from the site of entry for any distance into the coelomic cavity. Therefore, use radiography or ultrasonography to determine proper trocar placement for access to the organ of surgical interest. Several entries may be required to view an entire single organ.

With the snake in dorsal recumbency, make a stab incision between scutes lateral to the ventral midline. Use a paramedian approach distal to the apex of a rib or midway between the distal point of the rib and the ventral midline to avoid the ventral abdominal vein coursing along the midline (Fig. 14-4). Use the Hasson technique for primary port placement because the internal organs are close to the skin surface. Tent the ventral scutes and make a superficial stab incision with a small blade between the scutes. It is easier to penetrate between scutes initially and easier to suture there after the procedure.

After the trocar cannula is secured in the coelomic cavity, introduce the laparoscope. The weight range guidelines for the size of a laparoscope are not applicable to snakes. A smaller scope generally is used. Insufflation

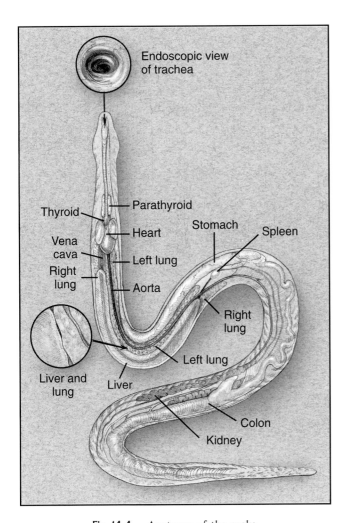

Fig. 14-4 Anatomy of the snake.

is of limited value because the cavity is constrained by the ribs. Because of the small optical cavity, additional ports may be difficult to establish within the field of view. Use a telescope sheath with an integral instrument channel to obtain biopsy specimens. Move to other sites as necessary to complete the examination.

Recovery
Remove the ports and close the incisions. It is preferable to appose the scales during wound closure to facilitate wound healing. Because the snake's ventrum is in contact with the substrate, protect the incision by applying cyanoacrylate over the incision line. Allow the snake to recover from anesthesia in a clean, warm environment.

Lizards
Lizards are the most widely distributed reptiles and have adapted to various environments. Their skin may be so thin as to be traumatized during gentle handling or so thick and spiny as to cause injury to the handler.

Anesthesia
Injectable anesthetic agents, inhalation anesthesia delivered by mask or chamber, and combination anesthetic protocols are used. After induction, intubate and maintain the lizard on inhalation anesthesia. Determine optimal temperature before beginning the procedure and maintain it during and after the procedure.

Surgical Technique
Position the lizard in dorsal recumbency and use a paramedian approach to avoid the ventral abdominal vein coursing along the midline (Fig. 14-5). Use an open method of primary trocar placement to avoid penetrating the internal organs close to the skin surface. Tent the skin and make a superficial stab incision with a small blade between the scales. This location is easier to penetrate initially, and it facilitates suturing after the procedure. After the primary trocar has been placed, insufflate the coelomic cavity.

For diagnostic procedures in most species, direct the telescope caudad to examine the urinary bladder. The kidneys, located dorsal to the bladder deep within the pelvic canal, may be difficult to see. Tilt the lizard in several oblique postures to facilitate movement of structures into and out of the field of view. If necessary, insert a second port to introduce instruments to manipulate the bladder and intestinal structures and to gain access to the kidneys, gonads, and adrenal glands. Direct the telescope craniad to examine the liver and gallbladder. The gallbladder is on the ventral surface of the right liver lobe and can be seen when the left liver lobe is lifted. The heart is cranial to the liver, and the lungs are dorsal and lateral to the heart. Remove the ports and close the incisions.

Recovery
Because a lizard's ventrum contacts the ground, take care to prevent wound contamination. Apply cyanoacry-

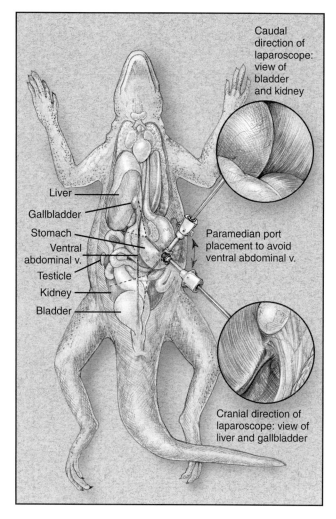

Fig. 14-5   Port placement and anatomy of the lizard.

[labels in figure]
Caudal direction of laparoscope: view of bladder and kidney

Liver
Gallbladder
Stomach
Ventral abdominal v.
Testicle
Kidney
Bladder

Paramedian port placement to avoid ventral abdominal v.

Cranial direction of laparoscope: view of liver and gallbladder

late or a waterproof dressing* over the suture line to protect the incision. Lizards tend to recover slowly from the effects of anesthesia. A clean and warm postoperative environment is essential because hypothermia will delay recovery from anesthesia.

Crocodilia

Crocodilians possess a body form similar to that of lizards and therefore the approach is similar. They have a diaphragm different from higher vetebrates in that it functions to separate the heart and lungs from the remaining abdominal organs. A crocodilian's size and organ structure make it a good candidate for minimally invasive procedures.

Anesthesia

Injectable anesthetics are essential for the large crocodilians. Competitive and noncompetitive neuromuscular

*Tegaderm, 3M Medical-Surgical Division, St. Paul, Minn. 55144-1000.

blocking agents, with or without centrally acting muscle relaxants, have been used in larger animals. Neuromuscular blocking agents alone do not provide analgesia or anesthesia. If invasive procedures are planned, humane protocols dictate using anesthetic agents or neuromuscular blocking agents in combination with anesthetic agents. Injectable anesthetics alone, gas anesthetics alone, and injectable anesthetics for induction followed by intubation and delivery of gas anesthetics have been used in smaller crocodilians, which are more easily handled.

Surgical Technique

Although a crocodilian is often larger and the ventral skin is much thicker and more fibrous than a typical lizard, the approach to the coelomic cavity is similar. With the animal in dorsal recumbency, make a paramedian incision between the scales where the skin is more pliable, taking care to avoid the ventral abdominal vein. Use the open technique to insert the primary trocar and begin insufflation with CO_2. Alternatively, tent the skin to allow inspection of more distant structures. Tilt larger animals from side to side to facilitate examination of organs farther from the primary port. Place secondary ports as necessary, making the incisions between the scutes.

Organ landmarks in crocodilians are similar to those in lizards, with paired lobulated kidneys, liver lobes, gonads, and lungs. Depending on the animal's size, one can retract the liver to see the lungs and heart. Remove the ports and close the incisions so the scales are apposed to facilitate wound healing. Use a large cutting needle to penetrate the skin if necessary. Seal the incisions with cyanoacrylate.

Recovery

Provide warm temperatures appropriate to the species to promote recovery from anesthesia. Because of a slower metabolic rate, impaired physiologic status, or lowered body temperature, anesthetic recovery can be prolonged. Crocodilians that require repeated handling for wound care, medication, or intravenous fluid therapy can be maintained out of water in moist environments for extended periods.

Birds

The class Aves is divided into two superorders, palaeognathous and neognathous, and 34 orders. The palaeognathous include tinamous and ratites. Tinamous are partridgelike birds. Ratites include flightless birds such as the ostrich, rhea, cassowary, and emu. The neognathous include 12 orders that comprise all other bird forms, including Psittaciformes (e.g., parrots), Falconiformes (birds of prey), Sphenisciformes (penguins), Galliformes (pheasants and chickens), and Passeriformes (song birds).

Birds were the first nondomestic animals to undergo routine laparoscopy. Many avian species have no external indicators of sexual dimorphism. In psittacines, especially those popular in the pet trade, sex was determined by rapid anesthetic induction and laparoscopic examination of internal reproductive organs. Laparoscopic determination of gender (surgical sexing) has now been superseded in many psittacines and other species by the use of restriction fragment length polymorphism (RFLP).* Laparoscopy is still used for less common species for which RFLP may not yet be available, when rapid results are required for large numbers of birds, and when simultaneous examination of other internal structures is desired.

ANATOMY

Birds are excellent candidates for minimally invasive surgery because they lack a diaphragm, and they have a unique respiratory system that provides a large space within the coelomic cavity without insufflation. Air sac morphology varies between species. In general, there are eight air sacs: one cervical, one clavicular, two cranial thoracic, two caudal thoracic, and two abdominal (Fig. 14-6).

The peritoneal cavity is divided into five distinct parts: left and right ventral hepatic peritoneal, left and right dorsal hepatic peritoneal, and intestinal peritoneal. Knowledge of the location of the air sacs and their association with subdivided peritoneal cavities and coelomic viscera is key to successful laparoscopy.[3,4] Specific endoscopic approaches to examine visceral structures, based on their anatomic location, are described.

PREOPERATIVE CONSIDERATIONS

After a comprehensive medical examination and evaluation, prepare the bird for surgery by correcting any fluid or electrolyte abnormalities. Hypoglycemia is a concern in birds that weigh less than 500 g, so they are usually only fasted for 2 to 3 hours before surgery. To prevent regurgitation during anesthesia, fast larger birds long enough to allow emptying of the crop. Raptors consume large boluses of whole food and may require fasting for up to 36 hours.

Large stores of intraabdominal adipose tissue make endoscopic examination difficult. Fat is stored on the air sac membranes, and it can be difficult to see through them to examine other structures. This is especially true in captive raptors. If possible, consider delaying the examination for 6 to 8 weeks and instituting an improved diet to reduce the fat stores.

ANESTHESIA

Use anesthesia to minimize surgical stress and avoid trauma if the bird should move while the laparoscope is being inserted. The approach to anesthesia depends on

*RFLP Zoogen, Inc, Davis, Calif. 95616.

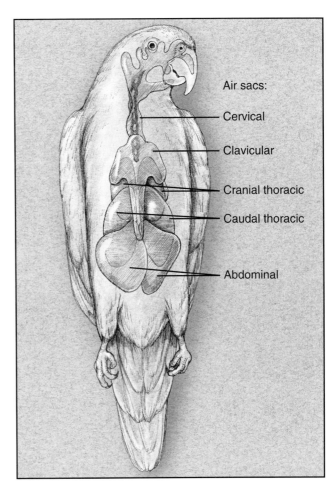

Fig. 14-6 Air sac anatomy of birds.

Air sacs:
- Cervical
- Clavicular
- Cranial thoracic
- Caudal thoracic
- Abdominal

the bird's disposition, size, and jaw strength, and on the anticipated length of the procedure. The larger ratites pose a particular set of challenges in restraint and anesthesia because of their great size and strength. An adult ostrich may grow to a height of 3 m and weigh more than 150 kg.[5] With adult ratites, administer an injectable anesthetic agent for induction and follow it with intubation and delivery of gas anesthetics.

For most endoscopic procedures, use isoflurane. If the procedure will last more than 15 minutes, intubate the bird before beginning. For smaller species that tolerate manual restraint, induce anesthesia with mask inhalation followed by intubation. A darkened anesthetic chamber lowers the risk of self-trauma and stress-induced physiologic abnormalities in fragile species.

EQUIPMENT AND INSTRUMENTATION

Assess the bird's size to determine the optimal telescope size. Use a 1.7-mm telescope in the smallest birds. Use a 2.7- or 4-mm arthroscope in larger birds to provide an acceptable field of view. In ratites, using the 5- and 10-mm telescopes and multiple instrument ports provide the best fields of view and the greatest variety of instruments for diagnosis and therapy.

SURGICAL PREPARATION

Pluck the feathers and prepare the surgical sites as for any avian surgery. Air sac and peritoneal granulomas may occur if skin contaminates the endoscope tip. Use sterile, transparent adhesive drapes to maintain the surgical field and allow anesthetic monitoring during the procedure.

Place the bird in dorsal, left lateral, or right lateral recumbency according to the organs of interest and the adjoining air sacs. The positions of the laparoscope and secondary ports also vary with the structures of interest.

TROCAR INSERTION

Closed or open approaches can be used for primary port placement in larger birds. To make a closed approach, introduce the pointed trocar and cannula through a small incision in the skin. Before incising the skin, distract it proximally or distally so the external incision will be offset from that of the deeper layers. When the incision is closed, this misalignment helps ensure a tight seal of the body layers and helps avoid subcutaneous emphysema caused by air escaping from the coelomic air sacs.

Direct the trocar cranially and parallel to the vertebral column. When the coelomic wall is penetrated, a characteristic "pop" may be sensed. With the trocar cannula inside the body cavity, remove the trocar from the cannula and replace it with the telescope. Control hemorrhage during port placement because even small volumes of blood can obstruct the view within the air sacs.

Use an open approach for birds that weigh 30 to 500 g or if there is doubt about using the closed approach in larger birds. Make a small incision and dissect through fascia and muscle into the coelomic cavity. Insert the cannula and telescope through the incision. Because of the air sac system, insufflation and a tight seal around the telescope sheath are not necessary.

SURGICAL APPROACHES

Endoscopic approaches to the bird were first described by Bush[6] and followed with an expanded treatise by Taylor.[7] Five approaches will be described: ventrolateral thoracic, lateral, postpubic, ventral, and intercostal. The left lateral approach is used most commonly for reproductive examinations.

Ventrolateral Thoracic

In the ventrolateral thoracic approach, the telescope is inserted at a depression in the V notch between the sternum and last rib (Fig. 14-7) and enters the cranial thoracic air sac. The approach is usually performed on the left side and is used to examine the heart and pericardial sac, liver, and lungs. By directing the scope caudally and

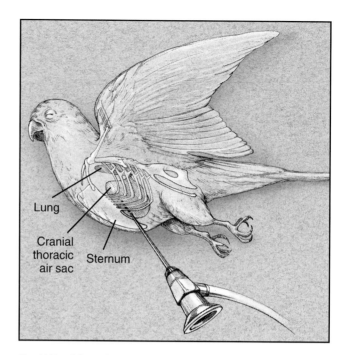

Fig. 14-7 Ventrolateral thoracic approach to the cranial thoracic air sac.

penetrating the posterior air sac membrane, the adrenal glands, gonads, kidneys, and intestines can be examined.

Position the bird in lateral recumbency with the wings reflected dorsally. Expose the sternal notch, where the last rib joins the sternum, by moving the leg cranially or caudally. Pluck feathers from the sternal notch region and prepare the site aseptically.

Make a 3- to 5-mm skin incision, depending on the size of the laparoscope. Holding the trocar parallel to the vertebral column, direct the trocar craniad and use controlled pressure to insert it through the abdominal wall. A loss of resistance signals complete penetration of the abdominal wall. Hold the cannula in place, remove the obturator, and insert the laparoscope. From the anterior thoracic air sac, examine the liver, heart, lungs, and bronchi.

Although the liver can be approached from the anterior thoracic air sac (ventrolateral approach), this approach is not recommended in birds with ascites because fluid could drain into the air sac and be aspirated. In the lateral approach, the confluent walls of the caudal thoracic air sac and ventral hepatic peritoneal cavity are breached by grasping and tearing a small window with endoscopically guided forceps or by bluntly penetrating the air sac with the telescope. The lateral approach avoids the fat pad.

Direct the laparoscope caudad to observe the posterior wall of the air sac. If it is transparent, observe the kidneys and gonads. If the air sac is opaque due to fat infiltration or air sacculitis, penetrate the posterior wall and enter the left abdominal air sac. From the left abdominal air sac, observe the kidneys, spleen, gonads, adrenal glands, stomach, and intestines.

Lateral

The left lateral approach is preferred for examining the gonads. Most female birds have only a left ovary; males have paired testes. A left lateral approach ensures that the gonads of either sex can be seen.

In the lateral approach, the flank is entered caudal to the last rib. Depending on the species, the telescope is inserted directly into the abdominal air sac, or it enters the caudal thoracic air sac first and then passes into the abdominal air sac through a tear in the posterior wall of the caudal thoracic air sac. The upper limb is moved cranially or caudally to provide the best access to the telescope insertion site.

The intestinal peritoneal cavity is a potential space extending caudally from the kidneys to the vent. Within the intestinal peritoneal cavity are the proventriculus, intestines, gonads, and supporting structures. The intestinal peritoneal cavity is entered by extending the lateral approach through the abdominal air sacs. The left coelomic structures of a hen near the time of ovulation should not be examined because the ova and oviduct enlarges so much that it fills the intestinal peritoneal cavity.

Cranial Position of Upper Leg

Place the bird in right lateral recumbency with the wings extended dorsally. The wing extension facilitates a true lateral position. Direct the upper limb cranially in birds with heavily muscled thighs (e.g., many members of the order Psittaciformes). Make the skin incision and surgical approach in the upper part of the triangle formed by the proximal end of the femur, the last rib, and the cranial edge of the pubis (Fig. 14-8), or where the semimembranosus muscle crosses the last rib. Separate the semimembranosus muscle (flexor cruris medialis) from the body wall and reflect the muscle dorsally. Insert the trocar just caudal to the last rib, beneath the reflected muscle, into the caudal thoracic air sac.

Caudal Position of Upper Leg

In birds without heavily muscled thighs, the caudal position of the upper leg facilitates a lateral approach to access the caudal thoracic air sac. Extend and hold the upper leg caudally. Palpate the point of trocar insertion by identifying the triangle cranial to the muscle mass of the femur, ventral to the synsacrum, and caudal to the last rib (Fig. 14-9). Species variability may dictate that the trocar should be placed more dorsally or cranially. In Psittaciformes, the entry site is in the seventh intercostal space (in front of the last rib).

Whether the leg is held cranially or caudally, the endoscope enters the caudal thoracic air sac. Direct the

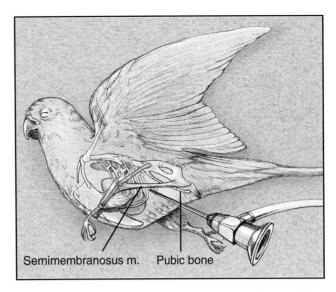

Fig. 14-8 Left lateral approach with the hind limb extended cranially in the bird. The landmarks for primary trocar insertion are the proximal femur, last rib, and pubis.

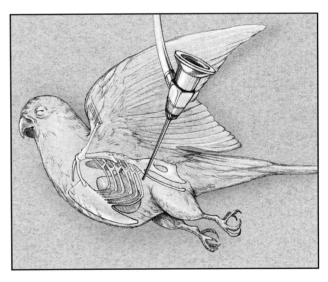

Fig. 14-9 Left lateral approach with the hind limb extended caudally in the bird. The landmarks for primary trocar insertion are the femoral muscles, synsacrum, and last rib.

telescope craniodorsad to view the pericardial sac, heart, lobe of the liver, proventriculus, and caudal region of the lungs. Redirect the laparoscope caudad to observe the abdominal air sac membrane. Using the telescope, create a rent in the posterior wall of the caudal thoracic air sac to enter the abdominal air sac. Carefully advance the laparoscope so its distal tip penetrates the air sac at a point devoid of vessels and fat and removed from underlying organs. Retract the telescope to view the slit and then advance the telescope through it. Direct the telescope into the abdominal air sac to observe the proventriculus, the edge of the liver, and the kidneys, adrenal glands, spleen, intestines, and gonads.

Examine the ovary or testes, kidneys, adrenal glands, stomach, spleen, and intestines. The gonad is located at the cranial aspect of the left kidney and may vary in size depending on seasonal hormonal influences. Testes appear in pairs as smooth, cylindrical, or elliptical structures with blood vessels over their surface. A single ovary appears flatter and more granular and lacks vascularity on the surface. An active ovary may appear as a cluster of yellow to white grapes during breeding season, while an inactive ovary is often a dull cream color with many tiny bumps on the surface. Testes and ovaries may be pigmented. The ductus deferens is smaller than the ureter, and the oviduct is two to four times larger than the ureter.[7]

Postpubic

The postpubic approach, first described by Lumeij,[8] enters the intestinal peritoneal cavity through the caudal body wall. Palpate the pubis and ischium and make a small skin incision. Introduce the laparoscope dorsal to the pubic bone and caudal to the ischium to enter the intestinal peritoneal cavity (Fig. 14-10). Penetrate the thin membrane between the intestinal peritoneal cavity and the abdominal air sac to observe the kidneys, adrenal glands, gonads, spleen, proventriculus, ventriculus, and intestines. This approach should not be performed in hens near the time of ovulation because it may damage the oviduct or egg.[7]

Ventral

The ventral approach is best for examining and sampling both lobes of the liver (Fig. 14 11). The paired ventral hepatic peritoneal cavities are accessed by incising the skin on the midline, just caudal to the sternum. Incise the linea alba and bluntly penetrate the ventral hepatic peritoneal cavity.[7] Insert the telescope. A fat pad overlying the ventral hepatic peritoneal cavity may be encountered. This is the approach of choice in birds with ascites because it avoids drainage of fluids into the air sacs, as would result from the ventrolateral thoracic approach.

Intercostal

To obtain lung biopsy specimens, make an approach through the third or fourth intercostal space, just ventral to the scapula (Fig. 14-12). Make a small skin incision and bluntly dissect the intercostal muscles to the level of the pleura. Avoid penetrating too deeply, which could injure the lung parenchyma. Insert the cannula and telescope to observe the lung surface. Use biopsy forceps to obtain a sample of lung tissue.

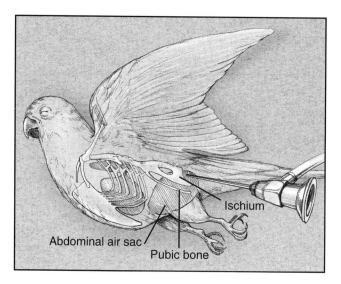

Fig. 14-10   Postpubic approach to access the intestinal peritoneal cavity in birds.

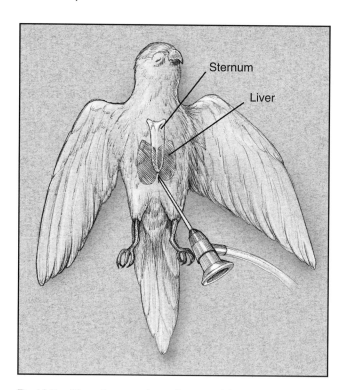

Fig. 14-11   Ventral approach to the ventral hepatic peritoneal cavity in birds.

BIOPSY TECHNIQUES

Examine organs and air sacs for gross alterations in appearance. Take biopsy specimens, cultures, fluid samples, or swabs for cytology. Using a telescope with an integral instrument port facilitates biopsy of selected organs. A specialized sleeve to accommodate biopsy forceps is available for use with 2.7-mm telescopes. Several flexible

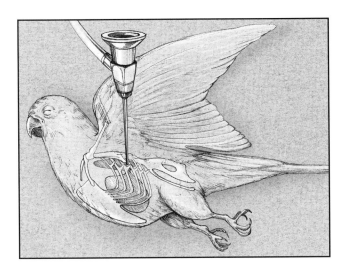

Fig. 14-12   Intercostal approach to the lung in birds.

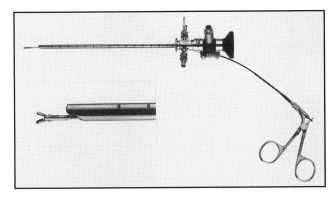

Fig. 14-13   Biopsy instruments useful in zoo and small animals. (Courtesy Karl Storz Veterinary Endoscopy.)

instruments are available for biopsy of selected organs (Fig. 14-13). Alternatively, secondary ports provide flexibility in manipulation of instruments.

GASTRIC FOREIGN BODIES

Ratites are predisposed to gastrointestinal foreign bodies because their foraging selections include undigestible plastic and metal objects. These foreign objects are usually found in the proventriculus and ventriculus, which lie slightly to the left of the midline at the caudal border of the sternum. Although there are no reports of laparoscopically assisted proventricular foreign body removal, such techniques should be considered as a way to reduce morbidity with this condition. In smaller species, a laparoscopically assisted approach to the proventriculus may be possible as an alternative to an open procedure.

CLOSURE

Close the skin incision with one or two simple interrupted sutures of size 4/0 absorbable material on a small cutting needle. In small birds, suturing the incision sites may be omitted. Instead, close the skin edges with cyanoacrylate.

OTHER EXAMINATIONS USING RIGID ENDOSCOPY

Use a rigid telescope to examine the otic canals, oropharynx, esophagus, ingluvies (crop), and trachea. The choanal slit, which connects the sinuses to the glottis, is in the palate. Its size, form, and width vary with the species. Examine the oropharyngeal musculature, salivary glands, and laryngeal mound. The prominence and location of the salivary glands vary. The laryngeal mound is proximal to the glottis. Passing through the glottis, enter the trachea at the larynx. Tracheal rings are complete, circular, and usually prominent. The emu's tracheal rings are interrupted on the ventral surface by a cleft approximately 6 to 8 cm long, cranial to the thoracic inlet. In the emu chick, a thin membrane covers the cleft. As the bird matures, an expandable pouch forms cranial to the cleft. The cleft and pouch function to produce a booming vocalization.

Tracheobronchoscopy is easily accomplished in all birds except ratites and the smallest species. In applicable species, one can see the syrinx at the tracheal bifurcation in medium-sized to large birds by using a 180-mm, 2.7- to 4-mm telescope.[7] Smaller species may require a 1.7-mm scope. The syringeal membrane is frequently the site of infections by opportunistic bacteria and fungi.

Examine the esophagus by introducing a flexible endoscope or rigid telescope through the pharynx and past the laryngeal mound. Insufflating the esophagus provides a better view and makes it easier to pass the scope. Esophageal folds vary according to the bird's dietary restrictions. Carnivorous birds generally have a larger number of and more prominent folds than do seed-eating species. Members of the orders Galliformes, Psittaciformes, Columbiformes, and some members of Passeriformes have a true crop. In other species, the crop is less pronounced or absent. The crop can be examined more easily if it is insufflated. Use a sleeve with an insufflation channel or a small, flexible tube passed parallel to the telescope to introduce air cautiously with a syringe.[7] Fast the bird for several hours before examining the crop. Before performing ingluvioscopy, palpate the crop to detect the presence of ingesta. Flexible endoscopes are preferred for endoscopic examination of the proventriculus and ventriculus.

RECOVERY

Recovery from isoflurane inhalation anesthesia is usually rapid. Place the bird in a warm, darkened area for the few minutes until arousal, or hold the bird until it is awake.

Long-legged birds, such as storks and cranes, may severely injure themselves if they are left unassisted during the ataxic period of arousal. Hold these birds and assist in their recovery until they can stand in normal posture.

Mammals

The class Mammalia comprises 20 orders that vary in size from the smallest shrew to the megavertebrates such as elephants and whales. It is easiest to perform minimally invasive surgery on animals that are approximately the size of humans, because the instrumentation was developed for human procedures. The 1.7- and 2.4-mm laparoscopes make it possible to perform procedures on the smallest species, while custom-made larger telescopes allow procedures to be performed on the megavertebrates.

ANESTHESIA
Manual restraint is used in noninvasive procedures if the animal's size and demeanor permit. Such examinations usually involve the otic canals, nares, or oropharyngeal cavity. Specialized methods of immobilization and general anesthesia have been developed for many nondomestic mammals. If anesthesia is required, consult a knowledgeable zoologic veterinarian or an appropriate text to determine how best to approach the animal.

SURGICAL TECHNIQUE
Although it is difficult to make sweeping generalizations, mammals other than hoofed animals and megavertebrates are usually positioned in dorsal recumbency. Placing a ruminant in dorsal recumbency may increase the risk of regurgitation as gravity causes reflux of fluids through the relaxed esophageal sphincter. The megavertebrates are susceptible to myopathy and sciatic neuropathy if not properly padded while in dorsal recumbency.

Mammals have a complete diaphragm and maintain negative pressure in the pleural space. The one exception is elephants, in whom fibrous connective tissue adjoins the lung parenchyma to the chest wall to facilitate expansion of the immense lungs. For this reason, thoracoscopic procedures should not be attempted in elephants. In other species, thoracoscopic procedures are similar to those of domestic animals. After the procedure, one must reestablish negative pressure in the pleural space.

As in domestic species, the animal's size and the location of the organs of interest determine port location. Animals are usually positioned in dorsal recumbency, and the primary port is inserted at or near the umbilicus. In hoofed mammals and megavertebrates, the rumen or other specialized digestive tract variations may preclude entrance or visibility in some regions of the abdomen.

For maximum safety, use an open approach for primary trocar placement. Make a small incision through the skin, subcutaneous tissue, fascia, muscle, and peritoneum. Place the trocar cannula through this incision and secure it with sutures to the fascia. Maintain the optical cavity by insufflation of CO_2 with an automatic insufflator. Place additional ports as necessary. Tilt the surgical table so the region being examined is elevated. To examine the pelvis, elevate the foot of the table. To examine the cranial part of the abdomen, elevate the head of the table.

Techniques for minimally invasive procedures in nondomestic mammals are similar to those of related domestic animals or humans. For example, one would use techniques similar to human procedures to evaluate gorillas or baboons. Minimally invasive surgery of a tiger would have many similarities to a procedure on a domestic dog or cat. For details, refer to specific surgical procedures in domestic animals in this text.

RECOVERY
After the procedure has been completed, remove the ports and suture the incisions. Make every effort to secure and protect the surgical sites from trauma and self-mutilation. Use a subcuticular suture pattern in nonhuman primates, which may decrease picking at the incision with their digits. Felids and canids traumatize the incisions with their tongues. Cyanoacrylate applied over a sutured area with a top dressing of a noxious liquid, such as bitter apple, may discourage licking. When animals must be returned to warm outdoor enclosures, an insect repellent should be applied over the surgical site to prevent myiasis.

Recovery of nondomestic mammals is similar to that of domestic mammals except that on arousal, the animal can no longer be handled. The clinician must be prepared to move away from the waking animal and ensure that it is in a secure environment that is safe for both the caretakers and the animal.

OTHER APPLICATIONS OF RIGID ENDOSCOPY
A rigid telescope without a sheath can be used to examine the otic canals, nasal passages, oropharynx, esophagus, and trachea. Using either manual or anesthetic restraint, pass the telescope past the glottis and through the larynx to enter the trachea. Continue to pass the telescope distally to examine the tracheal bifurcation and bronchi. To examine the esophagus, introduce the telescope through the pharynx.

The respiratory tract of whales and dolphins in the vicinity of the nasal opening, or blowhole, can be examined with or without sedation. Although the rigid scope can be used, flexible endoscopic methods are usually preferred. Whales and dolphins have evolved unique respiratory adaptations for breathing oxygen in an aquatic environment. The blowhole opens on the dorsal surface of the head, usually on the midline. The opening proceeds ventrally where the larynx projects into, but is not attached to, its terminus. The animal controls the opening of this orifice, and one must wait for a breath before introducing the telescope.

REPRODUCTIVE STUDIES

Historically, minimally invasive surgery was first used in nondomestic animals to study or control reproduction. These applications continue to account for the greatest use of rigid endoscopy in nondomestic animals. The technique has been used to examine the ovaries of a woodchuck *(Marmota monax)*,[9] water buffalo *(Bubalus bubalis)*,[10] llamas *(Lama glama)* and alpacas *(Lama pacos)*,[11] red deer (elk) *(Cervus elaphus)*,[12] cheetahs *(Acinonyx jubatus)*,[13,14] cyclic jaguar *(Panthera onca)*,[13] Bengal tigers *(Panthera tigris)*,[13] and fallow deer *(Dama dama)*.[15] Oocyte aspiration in pumas *(Felis concolor)*[16] and gorillas *(Gorilla gorilla)*,[17] and embryo collection and transfer in suni *(Neotragus moschatus zuluensis)*,[18] have been performed laparoscopically. Intrauterine insemination of elds deer *(Cervus eldi thamin)*,[19] pumas *(Felis concolor coryi)*,[20,21] cheetah,[21,22] clouded leopard *(Neofelis nebulosa)*,[21,23] ocelots *(Felis pardalis)*,[24] and leopard cats have been performed with this technique. Laparoscopy was used to assist in the diagnosis of endometriosis in rhesus monkeys *(Macaca mulatta)*[25] and in reproductive organ evaluation of gorillas[26] and gelada baboons.[27]

Vasectomies in llamas *(Lama glama)* and alpacas *(Lama pacos)*,[28] crab-eating foxes *(Cerdocyon thous)*,[13] African lions *(Panthera leo)*,[13] Siberian and Bengal tigers,[13] and Rocky Mountain goats *(Oreamno americanus)*[29] have been performed laparoscopically. This surgical approach has been used to perform tubal ligations of African lions[30] and Rocky Mountain goats.[31]

Minimally Invasive Surgery Now and in the Future

Advances in optics and instrumentation allow a broad range of diagnostic and therapeutic procedures to be performed in nondomestic animals. In addition to exploratory laparoscopy and thoracoscopy and biopsy of selected tissues, with training and experience, advanced procedures are now feasible. Minimally invasive hysterectomy, cystotomy, nephrotomy, nephrectomy, intestinal resection and anastomosis, inguinal herniorrhaphy, splenectomy, adhesiolysis, cholecystectomy, and pulmonary resection can be performed. Arthroscopy may be used to diagnose and treat joint disease. For nondomestic animals, the application of this technology is in its infancy. Surgeons must have courage, imagination, and a willing-

ness to learn and apply these new techniques for nondomestic animals to realize the benefits of minimally invasive surgery.

REFERENCES

1. Stetter MD et al: Isoflurane anesthesia in amphibians: comparison of five application methods. *Ann Proc Am Assoc Zoo Vet* 255-257, Puerto Vallarta, Mexico, Nov. 3-8, 1996.
2. Hoogesteyn AL, Stetter ML, Cook RA: Oral Paste: a new bandage for the treatment of skin lesions in amphibians. *Bull Assoc Reptile Amphibian Veterinarians* 6:4-5, 1996.
3. King AS, McLelland J: Coelomic cavities. In Birds: their structure and function, Philadelphia, 1984, Balliere Tindall.
4. King AS, McLelland J: Respiratory system. In Birds: their structure and function, Philadelphia, 1984, Balliere Tindall.
5. Sauer FG, Sauer EM: The ratites. In Grzimek HC, editor: Grzimek's animal life encyclopedia, vol 7, Birds I, New York, 1972, Van Nostrand Reinhold.
6. Bush M: Laparoscopy in birds and reptiles. In Harrison R, Wildt DE, editors: Animal laparoscopy, Baltimore, 1980, Williams & Wilkins.
7. Taylor M: Endoscopic examination and biopsy techniques. In Ritchie BW, Harrison GJ, Harrison LR, editors: Avian medicine: principles and application, Lake Worth, Fla., 1994, Wingers Publishing.
8. Lumeij JT: Endoscopy: a contribution to clinical investigative methods for birds with special reference to the racing pigeon *(Colembia livia domestica)*. Utrech, PhD thesis, 1987.
9. Woolf A, Curl JL: A technique for laparoscopic examination of woodchuck ovaries. *Lab Anim Sci* 37:664-665, 1987.
10. Jainudeen MR, Bongso TA, Ahmad FB: A laparoscopic technique for in vivo observation of ovaries in the water buffalo *(Bubalus bubalis)*. *Vet Rec* 111:32-34, 1982.
11. Steptoe PC: Laparoscopy in gynaecology. Edinburgh, 1967, Livingstone.
12. Asher GW et al: Relationship between the onset of oestrus, the preovulatory surge in luteinizing hormone and ovulation following oestrous synchronization of farmed red deer *(Cervus elaphus)*. *J Reprod Fertil* 96:261-273, 1992.
13. Bush M, Seager SWJ, Wildt DE: Laparoscopy in zoo mammals. In Harrison R, Wildt DE, editors: Animal laparoscopy, Baltimore, 1980, Williams & Wilkins.
14. Wildt DE et al: Induction of ovarian activity in the cheetah *(Acinonyx jubatus)*. *Biol Reprod* 24:217-222, 1981.
15. Asher GW, Smith JF: Induction of oestrus and ovulation in farmed fallow deer *(Dama dama)* by using progesterone and PMSG treatment. *J Reprod Fertil* 81:113-118, 1987.
16. Miller AM et al: Oocyte recovery, maturation, and fertilization *in vitro* in the puma *(Felis concolor)*. *J Reprod Fertil* 88:249-258, 1990.
17. Loskutoff NM et al: Stimulation of ovarian activity for oocyte recovery in nonreproductive gorillas *(Gorilla gorilla)*. *J Zoo Wildl Med* 22:32-41, 1991.
18. Raphael BL et al: Embryo transfer and artificial insemination in suni *(Neotragus moschatus zuluensis)*. *Theriogenology* 31(1):244, 1989.
19. Monfort SL et al: Successful intrauterine insemination of Eld's deer *(Cervus eldi thamin)* with frozen-thawed spermatozoa. *J Reprod Fertil* 99:459-465, 1993.
20. Barone MA et al: Gonadotrophin dose and timing of anaesthesia for laparoscopic artificial insemination in the puma *(Felis concolor)*. *J Reprod Fertil* 101:103-108, 1994.

21. Howard JG et al: Ovulation induction sensitivity and laparo-scopic intrauterine insemination in the cheetah, puma and clouded leopard. *Proc Am Soc Androl J Androl* 14(suppl):55, 1993 (abstract 129).

22. Howard JG et al: Successful induction of ovarian activity and laparoscopic intrauterine artificial insemination in the cheetah *(Acinonyx jubatus). J Zoo Wildl Med* 23:288-300, 1992.

23. Seager SWJ et al: Laparoscopic sterilization in the female mountain goat. *Ann Proc Am Assoc Zoo Vet,* Louisville, Ky, 1984.

24. Swanson WF et al: Responsiveness of ovaries to exogenous gonadotrophins and laparoscopic artificial insemination with frozen-thawed spermatozoa in ocelots *(Felis pardalis). J Reprod Fertil* 106:87-94, 1996.

25. Stetter MD et al: Isoflurane anesthesia in amphibians: comparison of five application methods. *Ann Proc Am Assoc Zoo Vet,* Puerto Vallarta, Mexico, 1996.

26. Wildt DE et al: Laparoscopic evaluation of the reproductive organs and abdominal cavity content of the lowland gorilla. *Am J Primatol* 2:29-42, 1982.

27. Cornillie FJ et al: Morphological characteristics of spontaneous endometriosis in the baboon *(Papio anubis and Papio cynocephalus). Gynecol Obstet Invest* 34:225-228, 1992.

28. Bravo PW, Sumar J: Evaluation of intra-abdominal vasectomy in llamas and alpacas. *J Am Vet Med Assoc* 199:1164-1166, 1991.

29. Wildt DE et al: Induction of ovarian activity in the cheetah *(Acinonyx jubatus). Biol Reprod* 24:217-222, 1981.

30. Seager SWJ: Reproductive laparoscopy. In Jones BD, editor: *Vet Clin North Am Small Anim Pract* 20:1369-1374, 1990.

31. Seager SWJ et al: Laparoscopic sterilization in the female mountain goat. *Ann Proc Am Assoc Zoo Vet,* Louisville, Ky, 1984.

SUGGESTED READINGS
General Zoo Medicine
Fowler ME, editor: Zoo and wild animal medicine, Philadelphia, 1978, WB Saunders.

Fowler ME, editor: Zoo and wild animal medicine, ed 2, Philadelphia, 1986, WB Saunders.

Fowler ME, editor: Zoo and wild animal medicine, current therapy, ed 3, Philadelphia, 1993, WB Saunders.

Fowler ME, editor: Restraint and handling of wild and domestic animals, ed 2, Ames, Iowa, 1995, Iowa State University Press.

Harrison RM, Wildt DE, editors: Animal laparoscopy, Baltimore, 1980, Williams & Wilkins.

McKenzie AA, editor: The capture and care manual. Pretoria, Wildlife Decision Support Services CC, 1993.

Amphibians and Reptiles
Frye FL: Biomedical and surgical aspects of captive reptile husbandry, ed 2, 2 vols, Malabar, Fla., 1991, Krieger Publishing.

Hoff GL, Frye FL, Jacobson EL, editors: Diseases of amphibians and reptiles, New York, 1984, Plenum Press.

Mader DR, editor: Reptile medicine and surgery, Philadelphia, 1996, WB Saunders.

Birds
King AS, McLelland J: Birds: their structure and function, ed 2, Philadelphia, 1983, WB Saunders.

Smith SA, Smith BJ: Atlas of avian radiographic anatomy, Philadelphia, 1992, WB Saunders.

Redig PT et al, editors: Raptor biomedicine, Minneapolis, 1993, University of Minnesota Press.

Ritchie BW, Harrison GJ, Harrison LR, editors: Avian medicine: principles and application, Lake Worth, Fla., 1994, Wingers Publishing.

Mammals
Dierauf LA, editor: Handbook of marine mammal medicine: health, disease, and rehabilitation, Boca Raton, Fla., 1990, CRC Press.

Fowler ME: Medicine and surgery of South American camelids: llama, alpacas, vicana, guanaco. Ames, Iowa, 1989, Iowa State University Press.

Hartman GC, Straus WL, editors: The anatomy of the rhesus monkey, Baltimore, 1933, Williams & Wilkins.

Hillyer EV, Quesenberry KE: Ferrets, rabbits and rodents, Philadelphia, 1997, WB Saunders.

Raven HC: The anatomy of the gorilla, New York, 1950, Columbia University Press.

Mariappa D, editor: Anatomy and histology of the Indian elephant, Oak Park, Mich., 1986, Indira Publishing.

Nowak RM: Walker's mammals of the world, ed 5, 2 vols; Baltimore, 1991, Johns Hopkins University Press.

COMPANY	ADDRESS	TELEPHONE NO.	FAX NO.	INTERNET ADDRESS	SPECIAL INSTRUMENTS
Advanced Sterilization Products	33 Technology Drive Irvine, Calif. 92718	(800) 755-5900 (714) 581-5799	(714) 453-6353	www.sterrad.com http://www.jnj.com	Sterrad system for sterilization
Apple Medical	580 Main St. Bolton, Mass. 01740-1306	(800) 255-2926 (508) 779-2926	(800) 382-0349	http://www.applemed.com	Trocars, scissors
Aslan Medical Technologies	4110 S. 9th St. Kalamazoo, Mich. 49009	(800) 551-4561	(616) 372-9639	http://www. aslanmedical.com	General laparoscopy Minilaparoscopy instruments
Circon Corp.	6500 Hollister Ave. Santa Barbara, Calif. 93117	(805) 685-5100 (888) 5-CIRCON	(805) 968-1645	http://www. circoncorp.com	Videoendoscopic systems, trocars, laparoscopic equipment, monopolar and bipolar devices
Conmed Corp.	310 Broad St. Utica, N.Y. 13501	(800) 448-6506 (315) 797-8375	(315) 797-0321	http://www.conmed.com	Videoendoscopic equipment, trocars, laparoscopic equipment, electrosurgical generators, argon beam coagulators
Cook Urological, Inc.	1100 W. Morgan St. Spencer, Ind. 47460-9426	(800) 457-4448 (812) 829-4891	(812) 829-2022	http://www. cookgroup.com	Entrapment sac, needle holders, tissue morcellator, trocars
Core Dynamics, Inc.	11222 St. Johns Industrial Parkway Jacksonville, Fla. 32246	(800) 905-2673 (904) 641-6611	(904) 641-6467	http://www. coredynamics.com	Disposable trocars, forceps
Dexide	7509 Flagstone Drive Forth Worth, Texas 76118-6953	(800) 645-3378 (817) 589-1454	(817) 595-3300	http://www.dexide.com	FRED, trocars, clip appliers, specimen bags
Elmed	60 West Fay Ave. Addison, Ill. 60101-5198	(630) 543-2792	(630) 543-2102	http://www.elmed.com	Electrosurgical generators, trocars, laparoscopes
ERBE USA, Inc.	2225 NW Parkway, Suite 105, Marietta, Ga. 30067	(800) 778-3723 (770) 955-4400	(770) 955-4400	http://www.erbe-med.com	Electrosurgical generators
Ethicon Endo-Surgery, Inc.	4545 Creek Road Cincinnati, Ohio 45242-2839	(800) USE-ENDO (513) 786-7000	(513) 483-8113	http://www.ethicon-endo.com	Disposable trocars, laparoscopic equipment, monopolar and bipolar devices, scissors, staplers, harmonic scalpel
Ethicon, Inc.	U.S. Route 22 Somerville, N.J. 08876	(800) 4ETHICON (908) 218-0707	(908) 218-2813	http://ethicon.com	Endoscopic suture, mesh
Everest Medical Corp.	13755 First Ave. N Minneapolis, Minn. 55441-5454	(800) 852-9361 (612) 473-6262	(612) 473-6465	http://www. everestmedical.com	Bipolar graspers, scissors, dissecting/grasping forceps
General Surgical Innovations, Inc.	3172-A Porter Drive Palo Alto, Calif. 94304	(800) 980-0300 (415) 812-9730	(415) 812-9731	http://www.gsii.com	Balloon dissector/trocar
Gore & Associates, Inc., W.L.	555 Papermill Road Newark, Del. 19711-7513	(800) 368-4673 (302) 738-4880	(302) 731-9098	http://wlgore.com	Prosthetic materials, suture passer
Imagyn Medical Technologies, Inc.	8850 M-89 Richland, Mich. 49083-0351	(800) 253-7900 (616) 629-5811	(616) 629-4017	http://www.corp. Imagyn.com	Trocars, endoscopes, clip appliers, staplers
Innerdyne Medical	1244 Reamwood Ave. Sunnyvale, Calif. 94089	(800) 378-4733 (408) 745-6010	(408) 745-6570		Radially expanding trocars
Jarit Instruments	9 Skyline Drive Hawthorne, N.Y. 10532-2119	(800) 431-1123 (914) 592-9050	(914) 592-8056	http://www.jarit.com	Laparoscopes, trocars, laparoscopic equipment, monopolar and bipolar devices, 3.5-mm instruments
Johnson & Johnson Medical, Inc.	2500 Arbrook Blvd. Arlington, Texas 76014	(800) 433-5170 (817) 465-3141	(817) 784-5459	http://www.jnj.com	Cidex, Sterrad system for sterilization

Continued

MANUFACTURERS OF ENDOSCOPIC INSTRUMENTS

COMPANY	ADDRESS	TELEPHONE NO.	FAX NO.	INTERNET ADDRESS	SPECIAL INSTRUMENTS
Linvatec/Hall Surgical	11311 Concept Blvd. Largo, Fla. 34643-4908	(800) 237-0169 (813) 392-6464	(813) 399-5256	http://www. lindi.linvatec.com	Electrosurgical units, laparoscopic and arthroscopic equipment
Marlow Surgical Technologies, Inc.	1810 Joseph Lloyd Parkway Willoughby, Ohio 44094-8030	(800) 992-5581 (216) 946-2453	(216) 946-1997	http://www. coopersurgical.com	Videoendoscopic equipment, instruments, needle holders, specimen bags, trocars, suture ligator
Medical Dynamics, Inc.	99 Iverness Drive East Englewood, Colo. 80112-5115	(800) 525-1294 (303) 790-2990	(303) 799-1378	http://medy.com	Videolaparoscopic equipment
MIST, Inc.	3310 U.S. 70 West Smithfield, N.C. 27577	(800) 952-1660 (919) 989-6478	(919) 989-9092		Minilaparoscopy equipment, scopes and instruments
Olympus America, Inc.	2 Corporate Center Drive Melville, N.Y. 11747	(800) 645-8160 (516) 844-5000	(516) 844-5930	http://www. olympusamerica.com	Videolaparoscopic equipment, reusable trocars, instruments
Origin Medsystems, Inc.	135 Constitution Drive Menlo Park, Calif. 94025	(800) 457-8145 (415) 617-5000	(415) 617-5100	http://www.guidant.com	Gasless laparoscopy systems, instruments, trocars, videoendoscopic systems, Laparolift mechanical retractor
Ranfac Corp.	Avon Industrial Park 30 Doherty Ave. Avon, Mass. 02322-0635	(888) 821-0098 (508) 588-4400	(888) 821-0099	http://www.ranfac.thomas register.com	2-mm ports
Shor-Line Shroer Manufacturing Co.	2221 Campbell St. Kansas City, Mo. 64108	(816) 471-0488			Veterinary surgery tables
Snowden-Pencer	2058 Kilman Drive Tucker, Ga. 30084-3053	(800) 367-7874 (770) 496-0952	(770) 934-4922	http://www. genie.genzyme.com	Reusable instruments, needle holders
Steris Corp.	5960 Heisley Road Menton, Ohio 44060	(800) 548-4873 (216) 354-2600	(216) 639-4459		Steris system for sterilization
Storz Veterinary Endoscopy-America, Inc., Karl	175 Cremona Drive Goleta, Calif. 93117	(800) 955-7832 (805) 968-7776	(805) 685-2588	http://www.karlstorz.com	Veterinary endoscopes, trocars, instrumentation
Stryker Endoscopy	2950 Walsh Road Santa Clara, Calif. 95051	(800) 624-4422 (404) 435-0220	(408) 943-9260	http://www.endo. strykercorp	Videoendoscopic equipment
Tahoe Surgical Instruments	Miramar Plaza Center, Suite 304 San Juan, Puerto Rico 00907	(800) 824-6311 (787) 722-7075	(787) 722-4250	http://www. tahoesurgical.com	Ligature device
Unimar, Inc.	475 Danbury Road Wilton, Conn. 06897-2126	(800) 243-6608 (203) 762-9550	(203) 834-1762	http://www. coopersurgical.com	J-needle for wound closure
United States Surgical Corp.	150 Glover Ave. Norwalk, Conn. 06856	(800) 722-USSC (203) 845-1000	(203) 847-0635	http://www.ussurg.com	Disposable instruments, staplers, clip appliers
Valleylab, Inc.	5920 Longbow Drive Boulder, Colo. 80301-3202	(800) 255-8522 (303) 530-2300	(303) 530-6292	http://www.valleylab. com	Electrosurgical generator suction/irrigation devices, argon beam coagulator, laparoscopic handsets and electrodes
Wolf Medical Instruments Corp., Richard	353 Corporate Woods Parkway Vernon Hills, Ill. 60061-3110	(800) 232-WOLF (708) 913-1113	(708) 913-1488		Videoendoscopic equipment, reusable instruments

INDEX

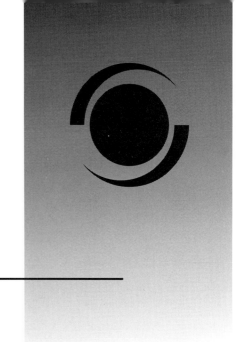